Advanced
Sports Nutrition

Dan Benardot, PhD, RD, FACSM

**HUMAN
KINETICS**

Library of Congress Cataloging-in-Publication Data

Benardot, Dan, 1949-
 Advanced sports nutrition / Dan Benardot.
  p. cm.
 "This book is a revised edition of 'Nutrition for serious athletes,' published in 2000 by Human Kinetics."
 Includes bibliographical references and index.
 ISBN 0-7360-5941-5 (soft cover)
 1. Athletes--Nutrition. I. Benardot, Dan, 1949- Nutrition for serious athletes. II. Title.
 TX361.A8B45 2006
 613.2'024'796--dc22

                                                      2005022895

ISBN-10: 0-7360-5941-5
ISBN-13: 978-0-7360-5941-1

This book is a revised edition of *Nutrition for Serious Athletes*, published in 2000 by Human Kinetics.

The Web addresses cited in this text were current as of October 2005, unless otherwise noted.

Acquisitions Editor: Jana Hunter; **Developmental Editor:** Kase Johnstun; **Assistant Editor:** Cory Weber; **Copyeditor:** Patricia MacDonald; **Proofreader:** John Wentworth; **Indexer:** Marie Rizzo; **Permission Manager:** Carly Breeding; **Graphic Designer:** Nancy Rasmus; **Graphic Artists:** Sandra Meier and Kathleen Boudreau-Fuoss; **Photo Manager:** Dan Wendt; **Cover Designer:** Keith Blomberg; **Photographer (cover):** All photos © Human Kinetics; **Art Manager and Illustrator:** Kareema McLendon-Foster; **Printer:** United Graphics

Human Kinetics books are available at special discounts for bulk purchase. Special editions or book excerpts can also be created to specification. For details, contact the Special Sales Manager at Human Kinetics.

Printed in the United States of America   10   9   8

The paper in this book is certified under a sustainable forestry program.

Human Kinetics
Web site: www.HumanKinetics.com

United States: Human Kinetics
P.O. Box 5076
Champaign, IL 61825-5076
800-747-4457
e-mail: humank@hkusa.com

Canada: Human Kinetics
475 Devonshire Road, Unit 100
Windsor, ON N8Y 2L5
800-465-7301 (in Canada only)
e-mail: info@hkcanada.com

Europe: Human Kinetics
107 Bradford Road
Stanningley
Leeds LS28 6AT, United Kingdom
+44 (0)113 255 5665
e-mail: hk@hkeurope.com

Australia: Human Kinetics
57A Price Avenue
Lower Mitcham, South Australia 5062
08 8372 0999
e-mail: info@hkaustralia.com

New Zealand: Human Kinetics
Division of Sports Distributors NZ Ltd.
P.O. Box 300 226 Albany
North Shore City, Auckland
0064 9 448 1207
e-mail: info@humankinetics.co.nz

The positive energy that my wife, Robin, infuses into my being
is limitless and makes every day joyful and meaningful.

My children, Jacob and Leah, maintain a zest for life
that infects me and everyone around them.

Alex, Lexie, and Ethan constitute the perfect extended family,
all dramatically unique people who fuse together wonderfully.

No matter how hard the work or how long the hours
these people make everything I do possible.

This book is for you.

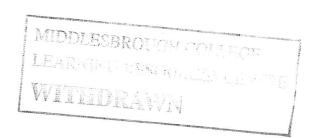

Contents

Foreword

Timing is everything in sporting endeavors, from split-second coordination in disciplines such as gymnastics and figure skating to budgeting of energy reserves in a daylong Ironman competition. Timing is everything from a nutritional perspective as well: Athletes must ensure that their metabolic needs are managed in such a way that performance is optimized. And the timing of the appearance of *Advanced Sports Nutrition* by Professor Dan Benardot of Georgia State University couldn't be better, either. In 2000 Professor Benardot wrote *Nutrition for Serious Athletes*, which quickly became a benchmark text for everyone leading a healthy athletic lifestyle. Timing was everything in that text as well. Benardot pioneered the concept that it isn't simply what you eat that is so critical; it's also the dynamic relationship between the timing of ingestion and exercise. In that first book Benardot put the fruits of his original research into practicality for the layperson and educated scientist as well.

Recently some thought was given to producing a second edition. So much has occurred in terms of advances in sports nutrition research during these past five years, however, that a rehash of the old stuff just did not pass muster with Benardot's thinking. After all, in addition to being a professional nutritionist (and a mighty good chef!), Benardot is also a fellow of the American College of Sports Medicine, given in respect to the quality and quantity of his own cutting-edge nutrition research. In keeping with his academic bent, *Advanced Sports Nutrition* is a total rewrite, a fresh new book filled with useful references summarizing the literature emphasizing the 2000 to 2005 period. The timing couldn't be better, because there is a great deal of excitement in the field of sports nutrition that needs visibility. It's a delightful read, with a ton of practical wisdom added to the research-based theory, thanks to Benardot's ongoing working relationships with top-level athletes in disciplines as varied as track and field, figure skating, and gymnastics. This new book is truly filled with food for thought!

David E. Martin, PhD, FACSM
Emeritus regents professor of health sciences
Department of cardiopulmonary care sciences
Georgia State University

Preface

This book is a comprehensive guide to nutrition for athletes and coaches and the health professionals who work with them. Ultimately, the information in this book should help athletes become healthier and help them understand what it takes to compete at the highest levels. Achieving a healthy state *and* competing at a top level are considered by many to be impossible. I have found, however, that athletes who have learned how to stay healthy while competing at a top level are nearly always able to have longer athletic careers, consistently improve in their sport, and reduce risks for chronic diseases. Doing the right things nutritionally can make the difference for staying healthy while pushing the body as hard as it can go.

With the expansion of professional sports franchises and the growing number of Olympic sports, the amount of elite athletes competing today is on the rise. Competitive athletes can now be found in most any age group. The Hawaii Ironman Triathlon has athletes in their 60s and 70s who are serious competitors in that age group. The rapidity with which this phenomenon has occurred has created a need for information on sports nutrition that is specialized for these diverse populations. Recognizing the changing demographics in athletics, this book includes chapters addressing the specific factors that affect nutritional needs, such as gender, age, body composition, and weight. High-altitude training also has a particular affect on nutritional needs and another chapter is devoted to this topic. And while superendurance competitions have become commonplace, there continues to be widespread misunderstanding about the nutritional stressors associated with this type of event. To clarify the nutritional aspects for optimal performance, there are chapters on oxygen efficiency, timing of energy intake, digestion and absorption, and fuel inhibitors.

A substantial amount of misinformation exists on the strategies for achieving peak athletic performance and health. Even a casual observer doesn't have to look too far to find "nutritional" products that are marketed with the idea that consuming them enhances performance. These products typically lack the research to back their claims, and the sports medicine literature is filled with cases of athletes who have used some of these products with disastrous, or even fatal, results. Investigations into commonly marketed ergogenic aids have discovered that these products frequently include banned substances that can put both the health and eligibility of athletes at risk. Compounding the potential for problems is the tendency for many beginning athletes to try to improve their athletic capabilities too quickly with training programs and dietary supplements that are intended to emulate the regimens of highly trained professionals. This is a formula for disaster that can result in overtraining injuries, malnutrition, and psychological stress—all of which have the potential to take talented young athletes out of a sport.

Given the realities of athletic competition and the enormous rewards that are available to athletes who have reached the pinnacle of their sport, it may be difficult for athletes to be wholly rational about the proper nutritional strategies that will help them best achieve their desired goals. Advertisers for nutritional products know that athletes are susceptible targets. While many products are backed by sound science and research, others are not. How is an athlete to know the difference? Is the health store staff a reliable source of information? There is an incredible attachment in our culture to beliefs about nutrition that long ago were proven false. The connection between high-protein diets and optimal athletic performance has been shown to be incorrect, yet athletes, coaches, and many others persist in advancing this myth. The truth is that most of the money spent on protein and amino acid pills is making someone richer but isn't making athletes any better.

The sports nutrition field is expanding rapidly. More researchers are concentrating on this area now, and an ever-increasing number of articles in scientific journals focus on the relationship between nutrition and athletic performance. As a result of this expanding knowledge base, old paradigms are clarified and new paradigms are created. To some extent, everyone involved in sports must keep their minds open enough to question old beliefs and allow new ones to settle in. Position papers dealing with sports nutrition from the American Dietetic Association and the American College of Sports Medicine are much more specific than they once were about the nutritional factors that enhance performance. Concerns about the short- and long-term effects that athletes face based on their nutrition habits are now emphasized in these position papers. A recent study on hydration emphasizes the importance of precise statements, because a misinterpretation can be lethal. The study suggested that high water consumption in poorly conditioned people competing in the Boston Marathon increases the risk of hyponatremia. However, not all consumed fluids are water, not all events take four hours to complete, and well-conditioned athletes have different sweat rates (both quantitatively and qualitatively) than poorly conditioned athletes. Nevertheless, newspapers translated this finding to suggest that you shouldn't drink much fluid because of the risk of hyponatremia, and they further suggested that the risk of dehydration is not all that serious. Of course, this is not what the study found. Because of the potential these results have for misinterpretation, athletes could be increasing their risk for dehydration and heatstroke.

If athletes follow a sound training and nutritional program, they are likely to be successful and healthy, but mistakes could result in career-ending injuries. Exercise and involvement in a sport can, should, and usually does lead to wonderful things. The underlying philosophy of this book is that involvement in sports should lead to a lifetime enhancement of health rather than a lifetime of problems, and good nutritional habits help make this happen. Doing the right things nutritionally will have a positive effect on an athlete's capacity to train well and compete successfully.

Acknowledgments

Working on this book as a member of an academic community has had a profound effect on how I view the world: I have friends and colleagues I knew were there, but also have many I didn't realize existed. These are selfless people who have their own careers to look after and are so busy it is hard to see how they manage to get their work done. Yet, there hasn't been a single instance where a request from me hasn't been responded to quickly, fully, and accurately. These are exceptional people who are full of good ideas, understand the science, and know the critical pieces of information that people can use to make their lives better. To put it simply, they are amazing folks who I acknowledge here as making a positive difference to this book and to the lives of athletes and coaches who will access the information contained in these pages.

Dr. David Martin, with whom I codirect the Laboratory for Elite Athlete Performance, has an encyclopedic understanding of the marathon. His knowledge of how environmental conditions and course elevations affect human running performance is without rival, and a major factor in the success of the USA marathoners at the 2004 Athens Olympic Games. His pre-event training camps for marathon competitors who represent the USA at world championships and Olympic games have become legendary and are must-attend events for these talented athletes and their coaches. Over the past years, Dave and I have traveled the world together, and he has *always* found a way to cleverly clarify complex issues in our discussions. One of my favorites, "The solution to pollution is dilution," cleverly answers many questions related to the confusing results derived from the assessment of dehydrated athletes. Dr. Dave, as he is lovingly called by those who know him, is a rare combination of ionospheric brilliance and plain old-fashioned fun. I owe him much.

Dr. Walter Thompson is an exercise physiologist with extraordinary talent and energy. He is deeply invested, both personally and professionally, in the well-being of inner-city youth, while carrying a full spectrum of committee assignments, research grants, and university teaching. Despite a schedule that would make most people wither, he still manages, with his wife Deon, to bottle some of the best merlot I have ever tasted. Walt has been a close colleague for many years (he was the best man at my wedding), and we have coauthored a number of papers and book chapters. It may seem an overstatement to say that I rely heavily on his council, but I do. He is one of the first people I bounce ideas off, and he *always* manages to instill clarity to my thoughts.

Dr. Mildred (Missy) Cody is a food scientist with a knowledge base that would make most people explode. But Missy maintains a quiet, pleasant, competent demeanor that often belies the powerhouse that she is. Missy is "cutting edge" in almost everything she does. She is the person people go to for a better grasp of new electronic media functionality, and she constantly tweaks course content and delivery to enhance the possibility that students will be exposed to more information in a better way. For me, besides being a friend and colleague, Missy is a fountain of creative ideas. You just never know what you might learn over lunch with her, which makes her a sheer joy to be around.

The people at Human Kinetics I have worked with on this book—particularly Jana Hunter and Kase Johnstun—are good and bright people who take the edge out of all the details associated with writing a book. Human Kinetics is lucky to have them, and I feel lucky that they were assigned to this project.

I work with athletes. They are too numerous to mention in the context of this acknowledgment, but you know who you are, and this paragraph is directed to you. Without you I would have nothing of use to anyone, so I owe you more than you could ever imagine. You are the best of the best, and you stimulate me to be better than I am. Thank you.

The ideas in this book represent an amalgam from all those mentioned above and many, many others, including my wife, Robin, who provides me with a constant and reliable sounding board. Ideas come from many places: an informal conversation with a coach, a speaker at a conference, lunch with a colleague, dinner with a group of athletes, observation of athletes competing—the soup from where I pulled the information has many ingredients and flavors. I know that every one of my words has someone else's influence on it, and I am thankful.

Part I

Nutritional Sources for Athletes

1 Energy Nutrients

The need for energy nutrients is high in athletes, and a great deal of science focuses on optimal distribution of the energy substrates to support exercise of different intensities and durations. Studies have demonstrated clearly that dependence on carbohydrate increases with greater exercise intensity, and many studies provide valuable guidelines on how best to deliver carbohydrate to optimize glycogen stores, how best to deliver carbohydrate during training and competition, and how energy substrates contribute to muscle recovery. The contribution of protein to muscle function and recovery is much better understood now than in the recent past, and there is some new science on the relationship between mental and muscle function that is mediated by carbohydrate, protein, and fat. The recent popularity of higher-protein, higher-fat, and lower-carbohydrate diets has serious implications for athletic performance. It is critical that athletes and coaches understand how to assess the appropriate energy intake and energy substrate distribution to optimize both mental and muscle function. This chapter presents the essential elements of carbohydrate, protein, and fat metabolism in exercise, along with a critical scientific view on how these substrates contribute to optimal athletic performance (see table 1.1).

Table 1.1   Basic Functions of the Energy Substrates

Carbohydrate (4 kcal/g)	Energy and muscular fuel (from starch, sugars, and glycogen) Cholesterol and fat control (from dietary fiber) Digestion assistance (from dietary fiber) Nutrient and water absorption (from sugars)
Protein (4 kcal/g)	Energy source (if carbohydrates are depleted) Delivery of essential amino acids (amino acids the body needs but can't make) Essential for developing new tissue (important during growth and injury repair) Essential for maintaining existing tissue (helps control normal wear and tear) Basic substance in the manufacture of enzymes, antibodies, and hormones Fluid balance (helps control water level inside and outside cells) Carrier of substances in the blood (transports vitamins, minerals, and fat to and from cells)
Fat (9 kcal/g)	Delivery of fat-soluble vitamins (vitamins A, D, E, and K) Delivery of essential fatty acids (fatty acids the body needs but can't make) Energy and muscular fuel (for low-intensity activity) Satiety control (helps make you feel satisfied from eating) Substance in many hormones

Carbohydrates

There are different types of carbohydrate, and each type is treated differently by our bodies. For instance, glucose and bran are both carbohydrates, but they are on different ends of the energy spectrum. Glucose enters the bloodstream quickly and initiates a fast and high insulin response, while the energy in bran never makes it into the bloodstream because of its indigestibility and tends to mediate the insulin response by slowing the rate at which other energy sources enter the bloodstream. These within-carbohydrate differences mandate that athletes should carefully consider the type of carbohydrate that might be best under different circumstances. Glucose is the main source of fuel for muscular activity, and the higher the exercise intensity, the greater the reliance on glucose as a fuel. When glucose runs out, the athlete stops performing. Therefore, understanding how to keep glucose from becoming depleted should become a major focus of an athlete's nutrition practices. Sustaining carbohydrate sufficiency is problematic because, unlike either protein or fat, humans have a limited storage capacity for carbohydrate. Carbohydrate adequacy becomes even more critical at higher levels of exercise intensity because there is a greater reliance on carbohydrate as a source of muscular fuel. Despite years of research confirming the importance of maintaining carbohydrate availability for sustaining muscular endurance and mental function, many athletes still believe protein is the critical substrate for achieving athletic success. Although all substrates are important, delivering the right amounts of carbohydrate at the right time optimizes the limited carbohydrate stores, ensures better carbohydrate delivery to the brain, and improves endurance performance. By comparison, the common focus on excess protein consumption does little to enhance performance or a sense of well-being.

Carbohydrate Types

Not all carbohydrates have the same form, function, and health impact. The basic unit of all carbohydrates is the monosaccharide, or single-molecule carbohydrate. The common monosaccharides all have six carbons, and while they vary only slightly in hydrogen–oxygen configuration, these subtle variations account for important metabolic differences. The basic metabolic unit for human cells is the monosaccharide glucose, and the other monosaccharides have biochemical pathways that enable them to be converted to glucose. The number of monosaccharides bonded together provides the main basis for classifying carbohydrates (see table 1.2).

Each of the three main monosaccharides (glucose, fructose, and galactose) has different characteristics of solubility, sweetness, and reactivity with the food environment in which it is found. With the exception of fructose, which is present in an increasingly wide variety of processed foods as high-fructose (corn) sweetener, most monosaccharides are delivered in the food supply as breakdown products of disaccharides, which are two-molecule carbohydrates (i.e., composed of two connected monosaccharides.)

There are three main disaccharides—sucrose, maltose, and lactose—each containing a different combination of monosaccharides (see table 1.3). Together, the monosaccharides and disaccharides are referred to as simple carbohydrates, or sugars, while the polysaccharides are commonly referred to as complex carbohydrates. The *indigestible* carbohydrates are also complex carbohydrates, but they are commonly

Table 1.2   Carbohydrate Classification

Simple carbohydrates	Sugars	Monosaccharides (single-molecule carbohydrates)	Glucose (also called dextrose) Fructose (also called levulose, or fruit sugar) Galactose	Some sugars, or simple carbohydrates, may cause a fast rise in blood sugar, thereby stimulating excess insulin production, which causes a fast drop in blood sugar. Glucose and maltose have the highest glycemic effect.
		Disaccharides (2-molecule carbohydrates)	Sucrose Lactose Maltose	

Table 1.2 *(continued)*

Complex carbohydrates	**Partially digestible polysaccharides**	Oligosaccharides (3- to 20-molecule carbohydrates)	Maltodextrins Fructo-oligosaccharides Raffinose Stachyose Verbascose	Partially digestible polysaccharides are commonly found in legumes and, while they may cause gas and bloating, are considered healthy carbohydrates.
	Polysaccharides	Digestible polysaccharides (20-plus-molecule starch carbohydrates)	Amylose Amylopectin Glucose polymers	These complex carbohydrates should provide the main source of carbohydrate energy. Glucose polymers are made from starch and are often used in sports drinks and athlete gels.
		Indigestible polysaccharides (20-plus-molecule nonstarch carbohydrates)	Cellulose Hemicellulose Pectins Gums Mucilages Algal polysaccharides Beta-glucans Fructans	These complex carbohydrates provide fiber, which is important for GI tract health and disease resistance.
	Other	Other carbohydrates	Mannitol Sorbitol Xylitol Glycogen Ribose (a 5-carbon sugar)	Mannitol, sorbitol, and xylitol (sugar alcohols) are nutritive sweeteners that do not produce tooth decay. They are commonly used in products because of their moisture retention and food-stabilizing characteristics, but they are digested slowly and are known to cause GI distress if consumed in high amounts. Glycogen is the main carbohydrate storage form in animals, while ribose is part of the genetic code (deoxyribonucleic acid, or DNA).

Table 1.3 **Relationship Between Monosaccharides and Disaccharides**

Disaccharide	Contains these monosaccharides
Sucrose (cane sugar)	Glucose Fructose
Lactose (milk sugar)	Glucose Galactose
Maltose (malt sugar)	Glucose Glucose

referred to as *dietary fiber*. The sugars (the mono- and disaccharides) have different sweetness characteristics, with fructose tasting the most sweet, followed by sucrose, glucose, and lactose (the least sweet). However, the sugars also differ in mouth feel and solubility (e.g., fructose is less soluble than sucrose), all of which influence food manufacturers in their choice of sugars in food preparation. Athletes now have a wide array of sports beverages from which to choose, with each containing different proportions of the mono- and disaccharides, and each trying to achieve the best combination of flavor, gut tolerance, gastric emptying, electrolyte replacement, and energy delivery to working muscles.

Carbohydrate Metabolism

Humans can store approximately 350 grams (1,400 kilocalories) in the form of muscle glycogen, an additional 90 grams (360 kilocalories) in the liver, and a small amount of circulating glucose in the blood (~5 grams, or about 20 kilocalories). The larger the muscle mass, the greater the potential glycogen storage but also the greater the potential need.

We have systems for maintaining blood glucose within a relatively narrow range (70 to 110 milligrams per deciliter) by recruiting insulin and glucagon. Insulin and glucagon are pancreatic hormones that work synergistically to control blood glucose (see figure 1.1). Excess production of insulin can result in hypoglycemia (low blood

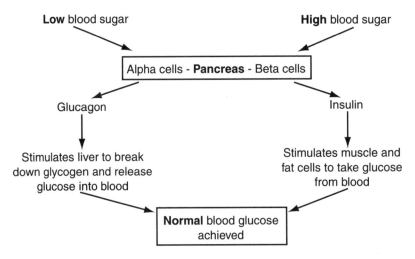

Figure 1.1 The impact of the pancreas on normalizing the blood glucose level.

sugar), with a resultant excess production of fat; inadequate insulin production results in hyperglycemia (high blood sugar) and diabetes.

Insulin is secreted by the beta cells of the pancreas, whereas glucagon is secreted by the alpha cells of the pancreas. The stimulus for insulin secretion is high blood glucose (the higher the glucose, the higher the insulin response), but a small amount of insulin is constantly being secreted by the pancreas even when blood glucose is in the normal range, causing a steady flow of glucose to the cells of the brain and muscles. Insulin lowers blood glucose by affecting the cell membranes of muscle and fat cells, thereby allowing glucose from the blood to enter the cell. This action causes a transfer from blood glucose to cell glucose and explains the blood-glucose-lowering effect of insulin; it also enables cells to receive a needed source of energy. (See figure 1.2 for an illustration of the possible pathways taken by blood glucose.)

With low blood glucose, as occurs between meals and during exercise, glucagon is secreted. Lower levels of blood glucose result in greater glucagon production. Glucagon causes catabolism of liver glycogen, which results in the release of some of its glucose molecules into the blood. Glucagon may also stimulate gluconeogenesis (the manufacture of glucose from nonglucose substances). The amino acid alanine, for instance, is derived from protein and is converted to glucose by the liver.

About 60 percent of the glucose released by the liver to sustain blood sugar is from liver glycogen stores, but the remainder is from glucose synthesized from lactate, pyruvate, glycerol, and amino acids.[1] The rate of liver glucose infused into the blood during exercise is a function of exercise intensity, with higher-intensity exercise causing a faster rate of liver glucose release.[2] The combination of lower blood insulin and higher epinephrine and glucagon during long-duration activity stimulates liver glucose release.[2]

Besides insulin and glucagon, two other hormones also influence blood glucose. Epinephrine (adrenaline) is a stress hormone that initiates an extremely rapid breakdown of liver glycogen to quickly increase blood glucose levels. Cortisol,

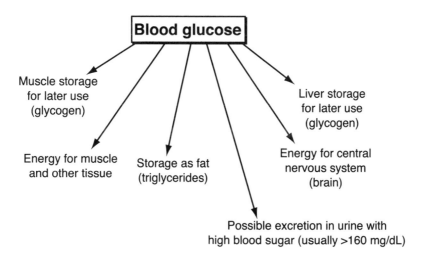

Figure 1.2   Possible pathways taken by blood glucose.

which is secreted from the adrenal gland, is also a stress hormone that promotes protein catabolism. This protein breakdown makes certain glucogenic amino acids available for gluconeogenesis, ultimately resulting in an increase in blood glucose. Both epinephrine and cortisol are released as a result of exercise-related stress, and both can be mediated through maintenance of blood glucose. Controlling epinephrine production helps preserve liver glycogen, and controlling cortisol helps preserve muscle protein. This is a strong argument for consuming carbohydrate during exercise.

The glucose circulating in the blood is derived mainly from dietary carbohydrate, with starch constituting the major source. Complex carbohydrates (starches) are digested into monosaccharides (glucose, fructose, and galactose) for absorption into the blood. In some cases, individuals have inadequate lactase to break milk sugar (lactose) into its component monosaccharides (glucose and galactose), causing the lactose to go indigested in the gut. Referred to as *lactose intolerance*, this leads to bloating, abdominal pain, diarrhea, and dehydration.

Excess glucose in the liver and muscle is stored as glycogen, but only up to the glycogen saturation point. The liver has a maximum glycogen storage capacity of approximately 87 to 100 grams (348 to 400 kilocalories), while the muscles can store approximately 350 grams (1,400 kilocalories), or more in larger individuals. Providing additional glucose to cells when glycogen stores are saturated leads to the excess being stored as fat (in both muscle and fat cells). The liver glycogen is primarily responsible for stabilizing blood glucose, while the muscle glycogen is mainly responsible for providing an energy source to working muscles that can be used both aerobically and anaerobically. Blood sugar is not easily maintained when liver glycogen is depleted, even when muscle glycogen stores are full.

Blood glucose is the primary fuel source for the central nervous system. Low blood sugar results in depressed central nervous system activity, coupled with increased irritability and a lower capacity to concentrate. For athletes, low blood sugar may be related to mental fatigue, which is related to muscle fatigue. Because liver glycogen and blood glucose stores are easily depleted during even short-duration activities, the intake of carbohydrate during activity is a critical factor in maintaining mental function and, ultimately, muscle function.

Glycolysis

ATP (adenosine triphosphate) is the high-energy compound for cells. We have a limited storage of immediately available ATP, so it must be generated quickly during exercise. The higher the exercise intensity, the faster the ATP must be regenerated. In steady-state, low-intensity activity, ATP can be adequately produced aerobically from the oxidation of carbohydrate and fat. However, as exercise intensity increases, athletes need a level of ATP production that cannot be fully supplied aerobically.[3, 4] (See table 1.4 for a summary of the energy metabolic systems.)

Glycolysis is the process through which a high volume of ATP can be produced through the breakdown of glycogen to glucose; it can occur in the presence of

Table 1.4   **Energy Metabolic Systems**

System	Characteristics	Duration
Phosphocreatine system (PCr)	Anaerobic production of ATP from stored phosphocreatine	Used for maximum-intensity activities
Anaerobic glycolysis (lactic acid system)	Anaerobic production of ATP from the breakdown of glycogen; the by-product of this system is the production of lactic acid	Used for extremely high-intensity activities that exceed the athlete's capacity to bring in sufficient oxygen; can continue producing ATP with this system no more than 2 min
Aerobic glycolysis	Aerobic production of large amounts of ATP from the breakdown of glycogen	Used for high-intensity activities that require a large volume of ATP but that are within the athlete's capacity to bring sufficient oxygen into the system
Oxygen system (aerobic metabolism)	Aerobic production of ATP from the breakdown of carbohydrate and fat	Used for lower-intensity activities of long duration that can produce a substantial volume of ATP but without the production of system-limiting by-products

oxygen (aerobic glycolysis) or without oxygen (anaerobic glycolysis). Aerobic glycolysis has the capacity to produce more ATP than anaerobic glycolysis and, unlike anaerobic glycolysis, can do so without producing lactic acid. For this reason, anaerobic glycolysis is also referred to as the *lactic acid system*. In activities where the intensity exceeds the capacity to bring sufficient oxygen into the system to meet energy demands, anaerobic glycolysis becomes the major pathway for ATP production. However, extremely high-intensity anaerobic activities are self-limiting because the lactic acid buildup permits activity to continue for a maximum of only 1.5 to 2 minutes. It is typical for high-intensity sports to have opportunities for recovery. For instance, the artistic gymnastics floor routine is 1.5 minutes long, after which the gymnast can rest and recover to prepare for the next high-intensity event; and hockey players are substituted frequently (a hockey player almost never skates continuously for more than 2 minutes) to allow for muscle recovery.

The lactic acid produced in anaerobic glycolysis can best be considered a form of stored energy, just waiting for sufficient oxygen to reenter the system. When exercise intensity is reduced and the athlete has enough oxygen in the system for aerobic metabolic processes, the lactic acid is converted to pyruvic acid and used to produce ATP aerobically.

Gluconeogenesis

Gluconeogenesis refers to the process of making glucose from noncarbohydrate substances. Blood glucose is critical for central nervous system function, aids in the metabolism of fat, and supplies fuel to working cells. However, because of its limited storage capacity, a minimum level of glucose is always available through the manufacture of glucose from noncarbohydrate substances. There are three systems for gluconeogenesis:

1. Triglycerides are the predominant storage form of fat in the human body and consist of three fatty acids attached to a glycerol molecule. The breakdown of triglycerides results in free glycerol molecules (a three-carbon substance), and the combination of two glycerol molecules in the liver results in the production of one glucose molecule (a six-carbon substance).

2. Catabolized muscle protein results in an array of free amino acids that constituted the building blocks of the muscle. One of these amino acids, alanine, can be converted by the liver to form glucose.

3. In anaerobic glycolysis, lactic acid is produced. This lactic acid, or *lactate*, can be converted back to pyruvic acid for the aerobic production of ATP, or two lactic acid molecules can combine in the liver to form glucose. The conversion of lactate to glucose is referred to as the Cori cycle (lactate removed from the muscle and glucose returned to the muscle). If blood glucose is low, pyruvic acid can be converted to lactate, and glucose can be produced via the Cori cycle.

Carbohydrate Utilization During Exercise

Low carbohydrate levels result in exercise fatigue. Since carbohydrate stores (or, *glycogen stores*) are limited (~350 kilocalories of glycogen in the liver; ~1,400 kilocalories of glycogen in muscles), athletes should consider how to initiate exercise with glycogen stores full and should establish a routine that keeps glycogen stores from running low. Even if muscle glycogen stores are adequate, low liver glycogen stores will result in hypoglycemia and mental fatigue, and mental fatigue leads to muscle fatigue.

The higher the exercise intensity, the greater the reliance athletes have on carbohydrate as an energy substrate. However, even low-intensity (i.e., mainly aerobic) exercise that derives most of its fuel from fat still requires some level of carbohydrate for the complete combustion of fat and to maintain blood glucose. Therefore, all modes of physical activity have some degree of carbohydrate dependence.

Several factors influence the proportionate contribution of carbohydrate to total fuel requirements during exercise. Factors that increase the reliance on carbohydrate include the following:

- High-intensity activity
- Long-duration activity
- Exercise in hot and cold temperature extremes

- Exercise at high altitude
- Age (higher in young boys than in men)

Factors that decrease the relative energy expenditure from carbohydrate include the following:

- Endurance training
- Good conditioning
- Temperature adaptation
- Gender

There is a common misconception that low-intensity activity (up to ~65 percent $\dot{V}O_2max$) is the most efficient means of fat loss. In fact, many popular exercise programs have been organized around the idea that a greater amount of fat is most efficiently "burned" with low-intensity aerobic exercise. However, the proportion of fat burned should not be confused with the volume of fat burned. While you're sitting there reading this sentence, you are very likely deriving the vast majority of your energy requirements from fat. However, the total volume of fat being burned is extremely low. (If this were not so, sitting in front of a TV would be a terrific means of initiating a fat-loss program.) When exercise intensity is increased, the proportion of energy derived from fat is decreased, and the proportion of energy derived from carbohydrate is increased, but some level of fat is always being burned. The total caloric requirement per unit of time is much greater in high-intensity activity than in low-intensity activity, and the volume of fat burned is greater in high-intensity activity (despite a lower proportion of fat meeting total energy requirements.) Therefore, athletes should work as intensely as possible within a given time frame to increase fat loss and optimize body composition (see chapter 12).

Carbohydrate is a critical fuel for athletes because we can more efficiently create energy per unit of oxygen from carbohydrate than from any other fuel. One liter of oxygen can yield approximately 5 calories from carbohydrate but only 4.7 calories from fat. In addition, aerobic glycolysis can produce ATP for muscular work in a larger quantity and

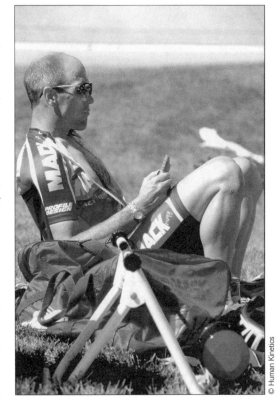

© Human Kinetics

As the intensity of exercise increases so does the need for carbohydrate intake, making the prerace high-carbohydrate meal a necessity.

at a faster rate than the oxidation of fat can produce it. The increased energy efficiency of carbohydrate helps explain the muscular fatigue that quickly occurs during high-intensity activities when muscle glycogen is nearly depleted. We simply cannot supply sufficient ATP to working muscles to maintain the workload.

Central Fatigue Theories

The conversion rate of adenosine diphosphate (ADP) to ATP is a critical step in the supply of energy to working muscles. Inadequate carbohydrate availability lowers the rate of ADP to ATP conversion, making it impossible for muscles to continue exercise at a high-intensity level. In addition, the failure to convert ADP to ATP causes a buildup of ADP that also contributes to muscle fatigue.[5]

A number of other factors involving the central nervous system are also involved in muscle fatigue.[6] As a group, these factors are referred to as *Central Fatigue Theory*. All of these theories involve mechanisms that cause more than the usual amount of the amino acid *tryptophan* to pass the blood–brain barrier, which stimulates an increase in the amount of serotonin (5-HT) that is produced. 5-HT is a neurotransmitter that causes people to feel relaxed and, if enough is produced, to feel sleepy. For the athlete, this could translate into muscular fatigue. Put simply, mental fatigue leads to muscle fatigue.

Theory 1   Low blood sugar and low muscle glycogen stores stimulate the muscle breakdown for gluconeogenesis. This results in an increased catabolism of branched-chain amino acids[7] (BCAAs), which causes a reduction in circulating blood BCAAs. BCAAs and tryptophan compete for the same receptor carriers that enable their passage through the blood–brain barrier. When BCAAs are high, the tryptophan passage to the brain is controlled. However, when the BCAA blood level is low (as happens when they are catabolized for energy), tryptophan can sequester more of the receptor carrier, and more tryptophan enters the brain. Tryptophan stimulates the formation of 5-HT. To prevent this from happening, blood and muscle glucose levels must be maintained to avoid gluconeogenesis.

Theory 2   Consumption of foods high in tryptophan (such as turkey) can increase the volume of tryptophan passing the blood–brain barrier, causing an increase in 5-HT production. The increase in 5-HT leads to premature fatigue.[8]

Theory 3   Fats compete for the same protein carrier in the blood as tryptophan. High fat intakes preferentially compete for this protein carrier, leaving a higher proportion of free tryptophan that can cross the blood–brain barrier. This causes an increase in 5-HT production, which may lead to premature fatigue.[8]

While it may be logical that the intake of both BCAAs and carbohydrate reduces 5-HT and, therefore, inhibits both mental and physical fatigue, studies have not been conclusive because of the difficulty in distinguishing between brain and muscle effects.[9] In addition, there may be interference from compounds such as caffeine, the ingestion of which has been shown to delay fatigue by temporarily stimulating the central nervous system.[10]

Carbohydrate Requirements

The Institute of Medicine recommends 130 grams (520 kilocalories) of carbohydrate per day, which is the average minimal usage of glucose by the brain.[11] The desirable range of carbohydrate intake is 45 to 65 percent of total caloric intake (also referred to as the Acceptable Macronutrient Distribution Range, or AMDR), and the Daily Value (DV) for carbohydrate on food labels is based on a recommended intake of 60 percent of total caloric consumption. These recommendations also generally advise that no more than 25 percent of carbohydrate intake be derived from sugars (mono- and disaccharides).[11, 12]

Dietary fiber consumption (from indigestible and partially digestible polysaccharides) should be at the level of 38 grams per day for adult men and 25 grams per day for adult women. Adequate fiber consumption aids in the maintenance of normal blood sugar, reduces heart disease risk, and lowers constipation risk. The difference between genders in recommended fiber consumption is based on the lower total food mass and calories typically consumed by women.

It has been suggested that our only true requirement for carbohydrate is for vitamin C, a six-carbon, glucose-like substance that most animals can derive through an enzyme conversion of glucose. There is some historical evidence that our human ancestors consumed very little carbohydrate and survived. However, when considering athletes and the mountain of research demonstrating that carbohydrate is the limiting substrate in athletic performance, it becomes clear that human survival and human performance are entirely different issues. Athletes need carbohydrate.

Athlete requirements for carbohydrate are based on several factors. Athletes must consume enough carbohydrate to

- provide energy to satisfy the majority of caloric needs;
- optimize glycogen stores;
- allow for muscle recovery after physical activity;
- provide a well-tolerated source of energy during practice and competition; and
- provide a quick and easy source of energy between meals to maintain blood sugar.

The traditional guideline for determining caloric intake has been to consider the amount of carbohydrate to be consumed as a proportion of total caloric intake. The recommendation for the general population is that carbohydrate should supply 50 to 55 percent of total calories,[13] and the Dietary Reference Intake (DRI) is 130 grams per day (520 calories per day) for male and female adults. However, the amount typically recommended for athletes is between 55 and 65 percent of total calories, assuming an adequate total caloric intake. Another, and clearly better, way of determining carbohydrate requirement is by taking into consideration the amount of carbohydrate to be consumed (in grams) per kilogram of body mass. The carbohydrate intake recommendations for endurance-trained athletes range from between

7 and 8 grams of carbohydrate per kilogram of body weight per day.[14, 15] Studies of carbohydrate consumption of different athlete groups have found differences in carbohydrate intakes. (See table 1.5 for a summary of carbohydrate intakes—often inadequate—of athletes involved in different sports.)

These data suggest that an athlete should consume between 5 and 10 grams of carbohydrate per kilogram of body mass, or between 20 and 40 kilocalories of carbohydrate, per kilogram of body mass. A hypothetical 155-pound (70 kilogram) athlete would take in between 1,400 and 2,800 calories from carbohydrate, which represents a far greater carbohydrate consumption than the DRI of 520 calories. Assuming this represents approximately 60 percent of total calories from carbohydrate, this athlete would consume a total of 2,300 to 4,700 kilocalories per day. Following the same logic, a 300-pound (136 kilogram) lineman on a football team would require 2,700 to 5,400 kilocalories just from carbohydrate each day, an amount that would be difficult to consume because carbohydrate has a relatively low energy density (i.e., only 4 kilocalories per gram). The generally recommended carbohydrate intake is based on the intensity and duration of exercise, with a higher requirement for greater duration and greater intensity. (See table 1.6 for examples of how much carbohydrate athletes should consume to optimize performance and recovery.)

Most carbohydrates are derived from cereals, legumes, fruits, and vegetables. There is no discernable amount of carbohydrate in meats, and only a small amount of carbohydrate in milk and cheese. A number of dairy products have sugars added (yogurt, ice cream) to make them more widely acceptable.

The glycemic index is a measure of how quickly consumed carbohydrates manifest themselves as blood glucose. Foods are compared with the ingestion of glucose, which enters the blood quickly because it requires no digestion and is readily absorbed. Glucose has a glycemic index score of 100, which is the basis of comparison for other foods. Foods are compared on an isocaloric basis (i.e., all providing the same number of calories), which is logical but is also the cause of some of the confusion associated

Table 1.5 **Carbohydrate Intakes of Different Athlete Groups***

Study reference	Sport	Moderate intake (g/kg)	High intake (g/kg)
Costill et al. 1988	Swimming	5.3	8.2
Lamb et al. 1990	Swimming	6.5	12.1
Kirwan et al. 1988	Running	3.9	8.0
Sherman et al. 1993	Running	5.0	10.0
Simonsen et al. 1991	Rowing	5.0	10.0
Sherman et al. 1993	Cycling	5.0	10.0

*Based on grams of carbohydrate per kilogram of body mass.

Adapted, by permission, from L.M. Burke, 2000, Dietary carbohydrates. In *Nutrition in Sport*, edited by R.J. Maughan (London, England: Blackwell Science), 82.

Table 1.6   Carbohydrate Requirement for Athletes

Activity or timing	Recommended intake	Example
Immediate recovery (0 to 4 hr) after exercise	1 g of carbohydrate per kg of body weight per hour (consumed at frequent intervals)	A 155 lb (70 kg) athlete would consume 70 g of carbohydrate (280 kcal) immediately after exercise, followed by an additional 70 g each hour for 4 hr.
Daily recovery from a moderate-duration, low-intensity training program	5 to 7 g of carbohydrate per kg of body weight per day	A 155 lb (70 kg) athlete would consume 350 to 490 g of carbohydrate (1,400 to 1,960 kcal) over the course of an entire day. (This amount includes the amount consumed for recovery immediately after exercise.)
Daily recovery from a moderate to heavy endurance training program	7 to 12 g of carbohydrate per kg of body weight per day	A 155 lb (70 kg) athlete would consume 490 to 840 g of carbohydrate (1,960 to 3,360 kcal) over the course of an entire day. (This amount includes the amount consumed for recovery immediately after exercise.)
Daily recovery from an extreme exercise program that includes 4+ hr per day	10 to 12 g of carbohydrate (or more) per kg of body weight per day	A 155 lb (70 kg) athlete would consume 700 to 840 g of carbohydrate (2,800 to 3,360 kcal) over the course of an entire day. (This amount includes the amount consumed for recovery immediately after exercise.)

Modified from L. Burke and E. Coyle, 2004, "Nutrition for athletes," *Journal of Sports Sciences* 22(1): 39-55.

with the glycemic index. For instance, carrots have a high glycemic index (>85) but the amount of carrots typically consumed is so low that the total calories of glucose from carrots entering the blood would be small.

Some foods have a surprisingly high glycemic index, while others are surprisingly low. Corn Flakes cereal, for instance, has a much higher glycemic index (84) than table sugar (65). When you assess the carbohydrate makeup of these two foods, however, it makes sense. The cereal grain in Corn Flakes is mainly composed of the disaccharide maltose, which is made of two glucose molecules. Table sugar, on the other hand, is made of sucrose (glucose plus fructose). The fructose must be converted by the liver to glucose, and this extra conversion slows the speed with which it manifests itself as blood glucose.

Because the volume of glucose and the speed at which it enters the blood can influence the amount of insulin produced, it is generally desirable for people (including athletes) to consume carbohydrates that have a medium to low glycemic index. However, there are times, such as during and immediately after exercise, when high-glycemic foods might be better for athletes. (See table 1.7 for examples of carbohydrate foods and their glycemic index.)

Generally speaking, carbohydrate foods higher in fiber have a lower glycemic index, so they are good choices for athletes. However, dietary fiber may be a source of gas and distention, making them poor choices for consumption just before or during competition. Soluble fiber foods may create less of a problem, but athletes should experiment to determine which foods are most easily tolerated. (See table 1.8 for a

Table 1.7   Examples of the Glycemic Index of Foods High in Carbohydrates

Classification	Food	Glycemic index
High (>70)	Glucose	100
	Baked potato	85
	Corn Flakes	84
	Instant mashed potatoes	83
	Honey	73
	White bread	70
Moderate (55-70)	Whole wheat bread	69
	Soft drink	68
	1-minute oatmeal cereal	66
	Sucrose (table sugar)	65
	Brown or white rice	59
	Orange juice	57
Low (<55)	Ripe banana	52
	Chocolate	49
	Orange	43
	All-Bran	42
	Pasta	41
	Baked beans	40
	Apple	36
	Kidney beans	27
	Fructose	20

Reprinted, by permission, from K. Foster-Powell and J.B. Miller, 1995, "International table of glycemic index," *American Journal of Clinical Nutrition* 62: 871S-893S.

Table 1.8   Foods High in Soluble and Nonsoluble Fiber

Good sources of soluble fiber	Good sources of nonsoluble fiber
Bananas	Barley
Barley	Beets
Beans and legumes	Brussels sprouts
Carrots	Cabbage
Citrus fruits	Cauliflower
Oat bran	Fruits and vegetables with skin
Oatmeal	Rice (except for white rice)
Peas	Turnips
Rice bran	Wheat bran
Strawberries	Wheat cereal
Sweet potatoes	Whole wheat breads

list of foods high in soluble and nonsoluble fiber.) Athletes often find that starchy carbohydrates with low fiber concentrations, such as pasta, are the most easily tolerated and deliver the high volume of carbohydrates athletes require.

Carbohydrates and Physical Activity

Because physical activity dramatically increases the rate of energy expenditure, athletes must strategize in order to best supply the needed energy to achieve success. It is critical for athletes to obtain sufficient total energy intake to support total energy requirements, including those for normal tissue maintenance, growth (in children and adolescents), tissue repair, and the energy requirements of the activity itself. It is impossible to discuss the ideal distribution of energy substrates without first conceptualizing how to best meet total energy needs. Although this may seem a logical and simple act, virtually all surveys have found that athletes fail to consume sufficient energy to fully satisfy their needs. This is much like planning to take a Ferrari on a 100-mile trip, and you appropriately put high-octane gas in the fuel tank—but only enough of it to go 80 miles. The Ferrari just won't get there, and poorly fueled athletes will also have difficulties doing what's required to be optimally competitive. Once a strategy has been established for obtaining sufficient energy, then athletes can reasonably consider how to parse the energy into the optimal distribution of energy substrates: carbohydrate, protein, and fat. It is generally accepted that athletes should consume sufficient carbohydrate to meet the majority of their exercise-related energy needs, plus enough carbohydrate to restore muscle glycogen stores between exercise sessions.[16]

Ideally, athletes should consume complex carbohydrates when possible but should consume simple carbohydrates during and immediately after exercise. Other energy substrates (protein and fat) should also be consumed to fulfill total nutrient requirements, but carbohydrate should remain the predominant energy source. It is difficult for athletes to take in sufficient energy and carbohydrate unless there is a well-established plan to do so. Athletes would do well to remember that training alone, without a sound nutrition plan to support the training, will be self-limiting.

Fat (Lipids)

Despite some recent literature wrongly espousing the benefits of high fat intakes (i.e., intakes of 30 percent or more of total calories from fat), fat is a highly concentrated fuel that does nothing to improve athletic performance, body composition, or weight when taken in excess. The adult AMDR for total fat intake is 20 to 35 percent of total calories, and there is no scientific information suggesting that more than 25 percent of total calories from fat is generally better for athletes. However, for athletes who may have difficulty sustaining weight because of a massive energy expenditure (such as cross-country skiers) or who must sustain high weights (such as linemen on football teams), higher fat intakes (up to the AMDR limit of 35 percent) may be necessary. Few Americans consume less than 35 percent of total calories from fat, so consumption of less fat is not easy, and unless steps are taken to provide sufficient energy from other substrates (mainly from more complex carbohydrates) to replace the eliminated fat, athletes may place themselves in an energy-deficit state that is, in itself, a detriment to performance. Therefore, while a reduction in fat intake is generally useful, a conscious effort should be made to provide enough total energy when fat intake is reduced. Since fat is more than twice as concentrated in calories than either protein or carbohydrate (9 calories per gram versus 4 calories per gram), more than twice as much food must be consumed to make up the difference in reduced fat.

Cholesterol, oils, butter, and margarine are all fats, or lipids, but each has slightly different characteristics. The one common attribute shared by lipids is that they are soluble in organic solvents but not soluble in water. (Anyone who has tried to mix Italian dressing knows this to be true. The oil in the dressing eventually rises to the top, no matter how hard the bottle is shaken.) The term *fat* is usually applied to lipids that are solid at room temperature, and the term *oil* is applied to lipids that are liquid at room temperature. The most commonly consumed form of lipid is triglyceride, which consists of three fatty acids and one glycerol molecule (thus the name triglyceride). Despite the numerous forms of lipids, we can obtain them all from the food supply, and we are also capable of making many types of lipids by combining carbon units from other substances. Nearly every cell in the body has the capacity to make cholesterol, which is why a person can have a high blood cholesterol level even when on a low-cholesterol diet. We can also manufacture phospholipids, triglycerides, and oils. In fact, it is this ability to effectively manufacture different types of lipids that limits the necessity to consume large amounts of lipids.

Fat Functions

A certain amount of fat, between 20 and 35 percent of total consumed calories, is necessary to ensure a sufficient energy and nutrient intake. The fat-soluble vitamins—vitamins A, D, E, and K—must be delivered in a fat package. The essential fatty acids, which are needed for specific body functions but that we are incapable of synthesizing, must also be consumed. Some dietary fat is also needed to give us a feeling of satiety during the meal, creating the important physiological signal that it is time to stop eating. Dietary fats have a longer gastric emptying time than do carbohydrates, which contributes to the feeling of satiety. Of course, fat also makes foods taste good.

Lipid Structure

Lipids have different levels of saturation, a term that refers to the number of double bonds in the carbon chain. Fatty acids with no double bonds are saturated, those with one double bond are monounsaturated, and those with more than one double bond are polyunsaturated. Single bonds are stronger and less chemically reactive than double bonds, so the greater the number of double bonds, the greater the opportunity for the fatty acid to react with its chemical environment. It is this differential reactive capacity that makes the number of double bonds an important factor in human nutrition.

Saturated fatty acids are most prevalent in fats of animal origin, palm kernel oil, and coconut oil. Monounsaturated fats are highest in olive oil and canola oil but are also present in fats of animal origin. Polyunsaturated fats are highest in vegetable oils (with the exception of olive oil, which is more than 75 percent monounsaturated). In the context of a fat intake that does not exceed 35 percent of total calories, mono- and polyunsaturated fats should make up the majority of the fats consumed. Saturated fats are associated with higher cholesterol levels, so they should be minimized when possible. This is most easily achieved by reducing the consumption of animal fats, chocolate candies (often high in saturated tropical oils), fried foods, and high-fat dairy products.

Triglycerides

The majority of consumed lipids are triglycerides, which contain three fatty acids and a glycerol molecule (see figure 1.3). Fat is stored in the form of triglycerides, which we manufacture when excess energy is consumed. We store triglycerides in adipose tissues (groups of fat cells) and inside muscle cells (intramuscular triglyceride), both of which are available as an energy source when needed. When fat is burned as a source of energy, the stored triglycerides are taken out of storage, and each molecule is cleaved into its component fatty acids and glycerol molecule. Each fatty acid can then be broken apart (two carbon units at a time) and thrown into the cellular furnaces for the creation of ATP to form heat and provide the energy for muscular work. This process is referred to as the beta-oxidative metabolic pathway because burning fat, besides requiring some carbohydrate for its complete oxidation, also requires oxygen.

Glycerol is a unique lipid that is burned like a carbohydrate rather than a fat and is also an effective humectant (it holds water). Some long-endurance athletes find that adding glycerol to water helps them retain more water (i.e., to superhydrate) than

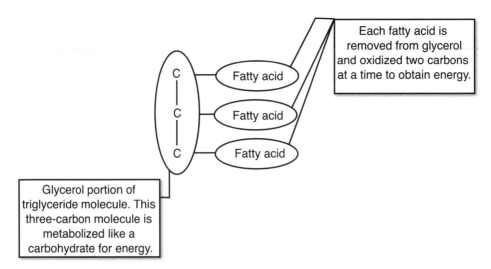

Figure 1.3   Triglyceride structure.

if they consumed water alone. (Refer to chapter 4 for more detailed information on glycerol as a superhydrating agent.) In an extremely hot and humid environment, water loss is likely to be higher than the athlete's fluid-replacement capacity, so beginning a competition in a superhydrated state may provide some advantages. In studies of tennis and Olympic distance triathlon, athletes consuming glycerol in water prior to competition experienced some protective hyperhydration benefits when exercising in high heat.[17, 18] However, being superhydrated is likely to impart a degree of discomfort that requires some adaptation. Athletes who consume fluids containing glycerol often describe the feeling of holding extra body water as making them feel "like a water bag," or "heavy," or "stiff." Still, they maintain that how they feel at the end of a race is more important than how they feel at the beginning, so adding glycerol to precompetition fluids has become a standard protocol for some athletes.

Essential Fatty Acids

Linoleic (omega-6) and linolenic (omega-3) fatty acids are the essential fatty acids; although they are needed for metabolic processes, we are incapable of synthesizing them. The "omega-6" classification means that these fatty acids, which are polyunsaturated, have the last double bond six carbons from the end of the carbon chain. The "omega-3" classification means that these fatty acids have the last double bond three carbons from the end of the carbon chain. Linoleic acid is an essential part of lipid membranes and is required for normal skin health. Linolenic acid is necessary for neural function and growth. The AMDR for omega-6 and omega-3 fatty acids is 5 to 10 and .6 to 1.2 grams per day, respectively.[11] Both fatty acids are easily obtained from vegetable oils (corn, safflower, canola, and so on) and the oils of cold-water fish.

Fish liver oils that are high in omega-3 acids have recently received much attention. These oils have been shown to reduce the ability of red blood cells to congregate, thereby decreasing the chance for an unwanted blood clot to form. This reduces the risk of a heart attack, which is most commonly caused by a clot formation in one of the major heart arteries. The oils from cold-water fish are the main source of the omega-3 fatty acids eicosapentanoic acid (EPA) and docosohexanoic acid (DHA). Even a once-weekly consumption of cold-water fish (salmon, albacore tuna, Atlantic herring) is sufficient to significantly reduce the risk of heart attack and stroke.[11] Despite these findings, excessive intake of these fish oils may cause problems, including an increase in cellular oxidative damage. The best rule of thumb is to make fish consumption a regular part of the weekly diet so that supplemental intake of omega-3 fatty acids is unnecessary.

Fat Requirements

From an exercise standpoint, there is little reason to believe that increasing fat consumption results in improving athletic performance, unless the increase in fat intake is the only reasonable means for the athlete to obtain sufficient energy. For the athlete who needs more than 4,000 calories each day to meet the combined demands of growth, exercise, and maintenance, moderate increases in dietary fat (preferably from plant and fish sources) may be needed. Since fat is a more concentrated form of energy than either carbohydrate or protein, more energy can be consumed in a smaller food package if the foods contain more fat. If an athlete tries to restrict fat completely, so much food needs to be consumed that it may be impossible to schedule enough meals or enough time during meals to consume the needed energy, leading to an inadequate energy consumption.

Lipids and Physical Activity

Even the leanest, healthiest athletes have a substantial energy pool of stored lipids. The average storage in adipose tissue ranges between 50,000 and 100,000 calories, or enough energy to walk or run 500 to 1,000 miles[19] (800 to 1,600 kilometers) without a refueling stop. In addition, athletes store approximately 2,000 to 3,000 calories of lipids inside the muscle tissue.[20] These lipids, which are stored in the form of triglycerides, are available as a fuel under the proper conditions of oxygen availability. Maximal fat oxidation occurs at 60 to 65 percent $\dot{V}O_2$max, but at higher levels of $\dot{V}O_2$max there is insufficient oxygen to derive the majority of energy used from fat catabolism.

Triglycerides stored in adipose tissue are cleaved into their component molecules of glycerol and fatty acids and transported to the blood plasma. The glycerol is available to all tissues for energy metabolism, and the free fatty acids are transported to working muscles where they are oxidized for energy. The triglycerides stored in working muscles are cleaved into glycerol and fatty acids, and the fatty acids can be oxidized for energy where they are resident. The glycerol can also be burned for energy in the working muscle or can be transported to the blood plasma as a source of energy for other tissues.

The lower the exercise intensity, the greater the proportion of fat burned to satisfy energy needs. As exercise intensity increases, the proportion of fat burned decreases and the proportion of carbohydrate burned increases. It is this basic reality that is behind why so many people do low-intensity activity to burn fat and lower body fat levels. However, the proportion of fat burned should not be confused by the total amount of fat burned at different intensities of physical activity. As exercise intensity increases, the total number of calories burned per unit of time also increases. Although there may be a decrease in the proportion of fat burned to satisfy total energy needs in higher-intensity activity, the total volume of fat burned is greater because the total energy requirement is higher (see figure 1.4). The take-away message from this metabolic reality is that athletes interested in lowering body fat should exercise at least as high as 65 percent of $\dot{V}O_2$max for the duration of their workouts to optimize the total mass of fat that is burned. Exercising at lower intensities burns a greater proportion of fat but less total fat than exercising at higher intensities.

Athlete Conditioning and Metabolizing Fat

Improving athletic endurance through a program of endurance training increases both the size and number of mitochondria (and related oxidative enzymes) inside cells, which increases the capacity of the athlete to use a greater amount of fat during physical activity. Since athletes store far more fat calories than carbohydrate calories, increasing the ability to use fat induces a proportionate reduction of carbohydrate

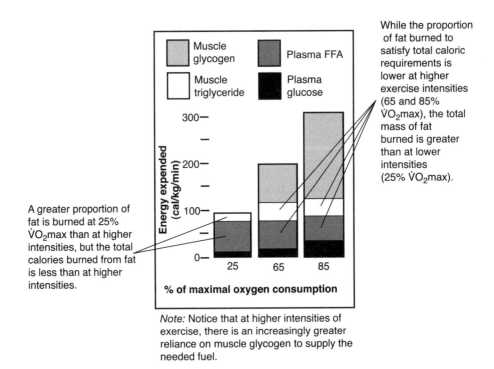

While the proportion of fat burned to satisfy total caloric requirements is lower at higher exercise intensities (65 and 85% $\dot{V}O_2$max), the total mass of fat burned is greater than at lower intensities (25% $\dot{V}O_2$max).

A greater proportion of fat is burned at 25% $\dot{V}O_2$max than at higher intensities, but the total calories burned from fat is less than at higher intensities.

Note: Notice that at higher intensities of exercise, there is an increasingly greater reliance on muscle glycogen to supply the needed fuel.

Figure 1.4   Energy substrate requirement at different levels of exercise intensity.

Reprinted, by permission, from J.A. Romijn, A.F. Coyle, J.F. Horowitz, L.S. Sideossis, A. Gastaldelli, E. Endert and R.P. Wolfe, 1993, "Regulation of endogenous fat and carbohydrate in relation to exercise intensity and duration," *Am J Physiol Endocrinol Metab* 265: E380-391.

reliance, thereby increasing endurance. Put simply, if you can burn more fat at higher exercise intensities, you can make your carbohydrate stores last longer so that your endurance is improved (see figure 1.5).

It is important to note, however, that fat oxidation cannot be improved to the point of eliminating the need for carbohydrate (muscle glycogen) during intense exercise. Also, a greater ability to metabolize fat for energy should not motivate an athlete to increase the proportionate intake of fat. Assuming an adequate caloric intake, athletes can manufacture and store the fat they need, and higher intakes of dietary fat are a clear risk factor in atherosclerotic heart disease. Even a short-term increase in fat intake with a concomitant decrease in carbohydrate intake for only 3 to 5 days leads to a reduction in endurance performance when compared with a high carbohydrate intake.[21]

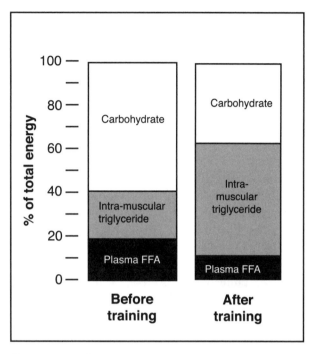

Figure 1.5   Change in fat reliance after endurance training.

Reprinted, by permission, from W.H. Martin, 3rd, G.P. Dalsky, B.F. Hurley, D.E. Matthews, D.M. Bier, J.M. Hagberg, M.A. Rogers, D.S. King and J.O. Holloszy,1993, "Effect of endurance training on plasma free fatty acid turnover and oxidation during exercise," *Am J Physiol Endocrinol Metab* 265: E708-714.

Medium-Chain Triglycerides (MCTs)

There is conflicting evidence that medium-chain triglyceride (MCT) oil (triglycerides with fatty acid chains that range from 6 to 12 carbon atoms) may have certain beneficial attributes for athletes. MCT oil is directly absorbed and rapidly catabolized into fatty acids and glycerol. It is easily and quickly oxidized for energy and appears to mimic the effects of carbohydrate metabolism rather than fat metabolism. There is also some evidence that it enhances the movement of fats from storage to be burned as energy, and it may also increase the rate at which energy is burned (i.e., a higher energy metabolism).[22-25] In a study assessing the relative impact of carbohydrate versus carbohydrate plus MCT oil on cycling time-trial performance, carbohydrate improved performance on the 100-kilometer distance, but the addition of MCT oil did not further improve performance.[26] Another study suggests that the timing of MCT oil consumption is an important factor in endurance performance. Consumption of 400 milliliters (13.5 ounces) of a 3.44 percent MCT oil solution before the time trial, plus a 10 percent glucose solution during the time trial, was associated with improved performance over the time-trial distance.[27] It was concluded that a reduced reliance on glycogen and an enhanced reliance on fat (MCT oil) was responsible for this observed performance enhancement. By contrast, a study of regular MCT oil consumption neither improved endurance nor altered energy metabolism in well-trained male runners.[28] In addition, there is some evidence that MCT oil supplementation may adversely alter the blood lipid concentrations, which should be seriously considered in athletes with family histories of heart disease.[29]

MCT oil consumption may offer an advantage for athletes having difficulty sustaining a desirable body composition. Healthy people who consume 5 to 10 grams (45 to 90 calories) of MCT oil experience a greater diet-induced thermogenesis than after the equivalent consumption of long-chain triglycerides (the most common form of fat found in foods), and this higher thermogenesis may stimulate weight loss.[30, 31]

Although it does not exist in concentrated amounts in any food, MCT oil is available in many stores, and because it is saturated, it is stable and has a long shelf life. For athletes who find it difficult to consume sufficient total energy, consumption of 2 to 3 tablespoons (30 to 45 milliliters) of MCT oil may prove to be beneficial. MCT oil is burned differently than other fats, so taking this small amount may be a good way to ensure that athletes who have difficulty taking in enough calories can meet their needs.

Please note that the maximum consumption of MCT oil for most athletes should not exceed 30 grams (270 calories). Exceeding this amount dramatically increases the risk of developing GI distress, including diarrhea.[32] MCT oil has, therefore, some inherent limitations in contributing to total energy intake.

Omega-3 Fatty Acids

Some attention has been given to the potential benefits of omega-3 fatty acids for athletic performance. According to Bucci,[33] these potential benefits include the following:

- Improved delivery of oxygen and nutrients to muscles and other tissues because of reduced blood viscosity
- Improved aerobic metabolism because of enhanced delivery of oxygen to cells
- Improved release of somatotropin (growth hormone) in response to normal stimuli, such as exercise, sleep, and hunger, which may have an anabolic effect or improve postexercise recovery time
- Reduction of inflammation caused by muscular fatigue and overexertion, which may improve postexercise recovery time
- Possible prevention of tissue inflammation

In general, studies evaluating the effectiveness of omega-3 fatty acids do not show consistent improvements in strength and endurance, nor is there consistent evidence that omega-3 fatty acids reduce muscle soreness.[34-36] The major impact of omega-3 fatty acid consumption appears to be a possible enhancement of aerobic metabolic processes, which is an important factor in both athletic performance and in an individual's ability to effectively burn fat as an energy substrate. This should not suggest that an increase in total fat consumption is either desirable or necessary to obtain these benefits. On the contrary, higher fat intakes are typically associated with reduced athletic performance. However, athletes might consider altering the types of fats consumed by including periodic but regular (once or twice weekly) 4- to 5-ounce (110 to 140 gram) servings of salmon, albacore tuna, Atlantic herring, and other cold-water fish in their diets to increase the proportion of omega-3 fatty acids available to them.

Protein

Many athletes consider protein to be the key to athletic success. It is difficult to find power athletes who can resist consuming some form of protein supplement, and most who do take supplements are convinced their successes are, at least partially, attributable to the extra protein. In fact, most athletes consume far too much protein and, in doing so, reduce the intake of other essential nutrients that are critical to achieving athletic success. Put simply, eating too much of one nutrient forces you into eating less of something else that may be equally important.

Athletes who typically need more protein (as a percentage of total energy consumption) very often have lower protein intakes. Endurance athletes, who appear thin and less muscular than power athletes, actually have a protein requirement nearly as high (per unit of body weight) as power athletes because they burn some level of protein as part of their normal endurance activities.[37, 38] By contrast, power athletes typically consume a great deal more protein than they need, and to make matters worse, many consume protein powders or amino acid supplements to increase their protein intake still further.[39] Considering that a single ounce of meat provides about 7,000 milligrams of amino acids and that a typical amino acid supplement provides between 500 and 1,000 milligrams, few of the protein intake strategies that many athletes follow are logical.

Protein Functions

Consumed proteins are digested into amino acids, and these amino acids join other amino acids produced by the body to constitute the amino acid pool. (See figure 1.6 for an illustration of amino acid structure.) The tissues take the amino acids from this pool to synthesize the specific proteins the body needs (muscle, hair, nails, hormones, enzymes, and so on). This amino acid pool is also available for use as energy (via a deamination process) to be burned if other fuels (carbohydrate and fat) cannot satisfy energy needs.

The major functions of protein include the following:

1. Protein provides a source of carbon for energy-yielding reactions. Certain amino acids can be converted to glucose and metabolized to provide ATP, while others can be stored as fat that can subsequently be catabolized to provide ATP.

2. Protein is a critical compound in controlling fluid volume and osmolarity in the blood and body tissues. This function is a major controlling factor in maintaining water balance.

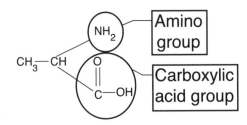

Example: Chemical structure of alanine (*Note:* Two alanine molecules can be combined with the nitrogen removed to make glucose in the liver via the glucose-alanine cycle. The process of making new glucose is referred to as *gluconeogenesis*).

Figure 1.6 Typical structure of amino acids.

3. Proteins are amphoteric,[40] with the capacity to buffer both acid and alkaline environments to maintain an optimal blood pH.

4. Antibodies are protein-based substances critical for maintaining health.

5. Proteins form enzymes that are involved in digestive and other cellular processes that create needed chemical end products.

6. Proteins are a critical component of body tissues, including the organs (heart, liver, pancreas, and so on), muscles, and bones.

7. Proteins are "smart" transporters of substances in the blood, moving substances to the correct receptor sites. For instance, transferrin is the protein transporter for iron.

8. Proteins are synthesized into specific hormones (such as insulin) and neurotransmitters (such as serotonin) that control body function.

See table 1.9 for a summary of amino acid and protein functions.

Protein Metabolism

Protein is composed of carbon, hydrogen, oxygen, nitrogen, and, in some cases, sulfur. Protein is the only nutrient that contains nitrogen, a fact that makes it both essential

Table 1.9   Amino Acid and Protein Functions

Working proteins (produce hemoglobin, enzymes, and hormones; maintain normal blood osmolarity; form antibodies; used as energy source)	Enzymes
	Antibodies
	Transport proteins
	Hormones
Structural proteins (constitute cell structure; help develop, repair, and maintain tissues)	Muscles, tendons, ligaments
	Skin
	Bone and teeth cores
	Hair and nails

and potentially toxic. Amino acid building blocks constitute the larger molecular structures of protein. Some of these amino acids can be synthesized from other amino acids (referred to as nonessential amino acids), while some must be obtained from the foods we eat (referred to as essential amino acids). There is widespread confusion about essential and nonessential amino acids because the word *nonessential* suggests that, although they are present, they are not really needed. This, however, could not be further from the truth. Both the essential and nonessential amino acids are equally important (and therefore equally essential) in human metabolic processes. (See table 1.10 for a list of the essential and nonessential amino acids.)

Amino acids combine together to make much larger proteins. The sequence of the amino acids and the secondary and tertiary structures of the protein determine its function. When dietary protein is consumed, it is digested into polypeptides (small protein molecules) and eventually into individual amino acids. The amino acids are absorbed into the blood and transported to different tissues, where they are manufactured into necessary proteins. Tissues manufacture the proteins that are needed through the amino acids available to them. To ensure that the tissues are capable of manufacturing needed proteins, the essential amino acids must be present for protein synthesis to take place. Some people believe that if you want healthy looking hair and nails, you should consume the primary protein that hair and nails are made of (gelatin). Gelatin is a low-quality protein with a poor distribution of the essential amino acids, so it would not encourage an optimal protein synthesis. Put simply, eating hair and nails does not encourage optimal synthesis of hair and nails. The best way to ensure an optimal synthesis of needed proteins is to make all the essential amino acids available to cells so they are capable of making whatever they need.

Several amino acids have specific effects on the central nervous system (see table 1.11). Because of these known effects, single amino acids have been sold with the purpose of imparting these known outcomes. Tryptophan, for instance, has been sold as an agent that causes relaxation or sleepiness. The dangers, however, of pushing high doses of single amino acids into the system are sufficiently large that this should not be done unless under the careful supervision of a physician. The best strategy is

Table 1.10 Nonessential and Essential Amino Acids

Nonessential amino acids (can be synthesized by humans from fragments of other amino acids)		Essential amino acids (cannot be synthesized by humans; must be obtained from consumed foods)	
Amino acid	Abbreviation	Amino acid	Abbreviation
Alanine	Ala	Histidine[a]	His
Arginine[CE]	Arg	Isoleucine[BC]	Ile
Asparagine	Asn	Leucine[BC]	Leu
Aspartic acid	Asp	Lysine	Lys
Cysteine[CE]	Cys	Methionine	Met
Glutamic acid	Glu	Phenylalanine	Phe
Glutamine[CE]	Gln	Threonine	Thr
Glycine[CE]	Gly	Tryptophan	Trp
Proline[CE]	Pro	Valine[BC]	Val
Serine	Ser		
Tyrosine[CE]	Tyr		

[BC]Branched-chain amino acids.

[CE]Conditionally essential amino acids (it may be necessary to consume these amino acids under certain metabolic conditions).

[a]Histidine, unlike the other eight essential amino acids, does not induce a protein-deficient state (i.e., negative nitrogen balance) when removed from the diet.

to supply the widest possible array of essential amino acids from food alone, which allows the individual tissues to synthesize the amino acids needed for optimal body function.

The liver is the central processing unit for protein synthesis, continually monitoring protein needs and synthesizing amino acids and proteins to satisfy a variety of needs. This protein synthesis is accomplished through transamination and deamination reactions. In transamination, the nitrogen from one amino acid is used for the manufacture of another amino acid; in deamination the amino group is removed from an amino acid and converted to ammonia (see figure 1.7). The remaining carbon structure is either reconstructed as fat and stored, converted to glucose (as happens with the amino acids alanine and glutamine), or burned for energy. Once all protein needs are met, the fate of all remaining amino acids is deamination. The ammonia created during deamination is toxic to the body, but enzymes in the liver convert the ammonia to urea. Urea is excreted from the body in the urine. Therefore, the

Table 1.11   Amino Acids With Neurotransmitter Products and Functions

Amino acid	Product	Function
Tryptophan	Serotonin Melatonin	Mood, pain, food intake, arousal
Tyrosine Phenylalanine	Dopamine Norepinephrine Epinephrine	Motor function, mood, arousal, attention, anxiety
Histidine	Histamine	Food intake, arousal, thermoregulation
Arginine	Nitric oxide	Arousal, anxiety, memory
Threonine	Glycine	Motor function

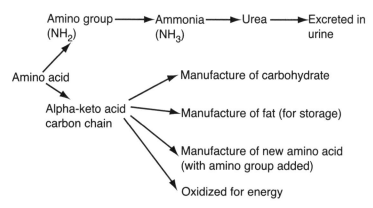

Figure 1.7   Deamination and the reconstruction of the remaining carbon structure.

greater the extra protein consumed, the greater the production of ammonia that must be removed from the system (as urea). The majority of the remaining deaminated carbon chains are typically stored as fat.

Protein Requirements

Protein yields approximately 4 calories per gram, which is the same energy concentration as carbohydrate. The recommended level of protein intake for the general population is 12 to 15 percent of total calories. Therefore, someone consuming 2,000 calories per day has an energy equivalent of 240 to 300 calories (60 to 75 grams) of protein per day. Most nonathletes do well with .8 grams of protein per kilogram of body weight. Using this guideline, a 165-pound (75 kilogram) nonathlete has a protein requirement of 60 grams per day. On a per kilogram basis, athletes have a higher protein requirement because of a greater lean mass, a greater need for tissue repair, and because a small amount of protein is burned during physical activity.

This increases the protein requirement for athletes to approximately double that of nonathletes (1.2 to 1.7 grams per kilogram). Therefore, a 165-pound (75 kilogram) athlete has a protein requirement of 120 grams (480 calories) per day. Although 120 grams of daily protein may seem high, it represents a relatively small proportion of total daily calories and is easily obtained by following the Dietary Guidelines for Americans (2005).[41] These guidelines focus on the premise that nutrient needs can and should be met mainly through food consumption. By comparison, the minimum recommended intake for carbohydrate is 30 calories per kilogram of body weight, so this 165-pound person has a requirement of 2,250 calories from carbohydrate alone. (See table 1.12 for the protein content of a 2,000-calorie meal plan).

Table 1.12   Protein Content of a 2,000-Calorie Meal Plan

Food	Calories	Protein (g)
Orange juice (1 cup)	112	1.74
Cracked wheat bread, toasted (2 slices)	132	4.37
Strawberry jam (1 tbsp)	55	0.12
Hard-boiled egg	88	6.29
Roast beef sandwich (1 sandwich, plain)	346	21.5
Low-fat (1%) milk (1 cup)	102	8.03
Apple, raw	87	0.26
Small tossed salad (3/4 cup)	27	1.3
Salad dressing (1 tbsp)	67	0.09
Chocolate chip cookies (5 small)	125	1.43
Gatorade (16 oz)	100	–
Chicken breast, broiled (1/2 breast)	152	26.67
Broccoli (1/2 stalk)	22	2.32
Baked potato	145	3.06
French bread (2 slices)	203	6.37
Vanilla ice cream (1/2 cup)	135	2.4
Total	1,898	85.95

Note: A 120-pound athlete requires approximately 1.5 grams of protein per kilogram of body weight. To convert pounds to kilograms, divide pounds by 2.2 (120/2.2 = 55 kg). Then multiply kilograms by 1.5 (55 × 1.5 = 82.5). The protein requirement for this 120-pound athlete is 82.5 grams (330 calories). The protein provided by this 2,000-calorie meal plan is more than 10 grams greater than the requirement.

Athletes require a higher protein intake than non-athletes for a number of reasons:

- Amino acids (from protein) contribute 5 to 15 percent of the fuel burned during exercise. The amount of protein used for energy rises as muscle glycogen decreases. It is generally thought that endurance exercise is more glycogen depleting than power exercise, so endurance activities are likely to cause a higher proportionate usage of protein.
- Exercise may cause muscle damage, which increases the protein requirement for tissue repair.
- Endurance exercise may cause a small amount of protein to be lost in the urine (where there is typically none or very little without exercise).

Despite the increased protein requirement for athletes, most athletes consume much more protein (from food alone) than they require. A look at the protein content of some commonly consumed foods demonstrates this point. Although most athletes have no difficulty consuming sufficient protein, the following groups of athletes should monitor protein intake carefully because it may be difficult for them to get enough:

- Young athletes who have the combined demands of muscular work and growth
- Athletes who are restricting food intake in an attempt to achieve a desirable weight or body profile
- Vegetarian athletes who do not eat meat, fish, eggs, or dairy foods
- Athletes who restrict food intake for religious or cultural reasons

As mentioned earlier, we can derive energy (calories) from protein. However, burning protein as a fuel is a bit like sprinkling your family diamonds on your breakfast cereal because you think it improves the texture. It's a complete waste of resources. Protein is so important for building and maintaining tissues and for making hormones and enzymes that burning it up as a fuel is wasteful. Besides, when protein is burned as a fuel, the nitrogen must be removed from the amino acid chains and excreted. When you increase the excretion of nitrogenous wastes, you also must increase the amount of water lost as urine. Thus, two undesirable things occur: You waste valuable protein by burning it up, and you increase the risk of dehydration because of the increased volume of water that is lost when nitrogenous wastes are excreted. In addition, high-protein diets are shown to increase the excretion of calcium in the urine (a clear problem for females who are at risk for bone disease later in life). Another potential problem is that high-protein diets tend to also be high in fat, which may increase the risk of cardiovascular disease. Therefore, the best way to make certain your protein needs are met is to consume a sufficient amount of food that focuses on carbohydrates but also contains small amounts of dairy products and meats (or plenty of legumes if you're a vegetarian). See table 1.13 for a list of plant sources of protein.

Table 1.13 Plant Sources of Protein

Source	Examples
Grains	Barley Bulgur Corn Rice Oats Pasta
Legumes	Dried beans Lentils Dried peas Soybeans
Seeds and nuts	Brazil nuts Cashews Peanuts Sesame seeds Walnuts
Vegetables (much poorer source of protein than other sources listed above)	Broccoli Carrots Potatoes Tomatoes

Meats and dairy products provide all the essential amino acids in a single food, but plant sources of protein do not. Therefore, vegetarians should be careful to combine foods in a way that optimizes essential amino acid availability. The general rule for ensuring a good distribution of all the essential amino acids is to combine cereals and legumes at the same meal. Both cereals and legumes are good sources of valine, threonine, phenylalanine, and leucine. Corn and other cereal grains are poor sources of isoleucine and lysine but are good sources of tryptophan and methionine. By contrast, legumes are good sources of isoleucine and lysine but poor sources of tryptophan and methionine. By combining cereal grains and legumes, the amino acid weakness of one food is complemented by the amino acid strength of the other food to provide a good quality protein.

Protein and Physical Activity

Protein utilization is, to a large degree, a function of total energy intake adequacy. An inadequate total energy intake forces athletes to burn protein for energy, making less protein available for other critical functions. Therefore, the protein requirement for athletes (i.e., 12 to 15 percent of total calories or 1.2 to 1.7 grams per kilogram) is based on the assumption that total energy intake is adequate.

A standard tenet in nutrition is that carbohydrate has a protein-sparing effect. This means that if you can supply sufficient carbohydrate to the system for fuel, then protein will be spared from being burned so it can be used for more important functions. Studies have generally found that the maximal rate of protein utilization for nonenergy uses is approximately 1.5 grams of protein per kilogram of body weight.[37-39] If this amount is exceeded, body tissues must make some decisions about what to do with the excess. The excess can be stored as fat, or some of the excess can be burned as energy. In either case, nitrogen must be removed from the amino acids, and this nitrogenous waste must be removed from the body. Virtually all studies that have looked at the total energy consumption of athletes indicate that athletes consume less total energy than they should to support the combined needs of activity, growth, and tissue maintenance. Since burning protein causes a lot of metabolic waste, it would be better to meet the energy requirement by providing a cleaner-burning fuel—carbohydrate.

A goal for most athletes is to remain in a nitrogen-balanced state in which as much nitrogen is coming into the system as is being excreted. A negative nitrogen balance suggests that more nitrogen is being excreted than is being consumed, a state that will inevitably lead to muscle loss. A positive nitrogen balance suggests that more nitrogen is being retained than is being excreted, a state that suggests that muscle is being gained. The amount of protein required to maintain a nitrogen-balanced state in nonathlete adults has been well studied and established at the level of .8 grams of protein per kilogram of body weight per day, while for athletes an intake of between 1.2 and 1.7 grams of protein per kilogram of body weight per day is needed. Both the athlete and nonathlete recommendations are based on the consumption of a total caloric intake that satisfies energy needs.

The higher protein recommendation for athletes is based on four factors:[37, 39, 42] (1) Athletes typically have a higher lean body mass that requires more protein to sustain; (2) athletes lose a small amount of protein in the urine, and nonathletes do not (the greater the intensity and duration, the greater the proteinuria); (3) athletes "burn" a small amount of protein (approximately 5 percent of total energy combustion) during physical activity; and (4) athletes require additional protein to recover from the muscle damage that occurs during training (see table 1.14).

The Institute of Medicine has stated that additional protein for healthy adults who exercise regularly is not needed because exercise increases protein retention. Nevertheless, both the American College of Sports Medicine and the American Dietetic Association recommend that protein intakes range between 1.2 and 1.7 grams per kilogram of body weight in physically active people. In reality, most athletes consume far more protein than they require, and typically more than the maximum recommended level of 1.7 grams per kilogram. Some strength and power athletes regularly consume 300 to 775 percent of the recommended level for protein

Table 1.14 Protein Requirements for Physically Active People

Athlete type	Total energy (calories/day)	Protein		
		g/kg/day	g/day	% of total calories/day
Endurance[a, b]	3,800	1.2-1.4	84-98	9-10
Strength[a, c]	3,200	1.6-1.7	112-119	14-15

[a]Assumes a resting energy expenditure of 40 calories per kg of body weight per day.

[b]Assumes a male runner who runs 10 miles/day (16 km/day) at a 6-minute/mile pace.

[c]Assumes an additional cost of 6 calories per kg of body weight per day for heavy resistance training.

Reprinted, with permission, from Dr. M.J. Gibala, 2002, "Dietary protein, amino acid supplements, and recovery from exercise," *GSSI Sports Science Exchange*, #87, 15(4).

(.8 grams per kilogram).[43, 44] Possible exceptions to high protein intakes may occur among vegetarian athletes and athletes in subjectively judged sports who strive to maintain low body weights (i.e., gymnasts, divers, figure skaters).

Protein oxidation during short-term, intense exercise is insignificant, but protein provides from 3 to 5 percent of total energy needs during endurance exercise.[45, 46] Protein utilization during exercise will rise to a level greater than 5 percent of total energy needs if glycogen levels are low, blood sugar is low, exercise intensity is high, or exercise duration is long.

There is a common misunderstanding that extra protein intake alone will support a larger muscle mass, and this theory is the main rationale for the large protein intakes seen in many athletes. In fact, additional total calories are required to support a larger muscle mass, and protein should constitute the same relative proportion of the extra calories consumed. For instance, if a 75-kilogram (165 pound) man wishes to increase his muscle mass by 3 kilograms (6.6 pounds), he would need to consume approximately 1.5 additional grams of protein for each kilogram of muscle mass desired. This amounts to only 4.5 grams of additional protein to support the larger muscle mass. By contrast, 30 grams per kilogram of additional carbohydrate, or 90 grams of additional carbohydrate in total, is required to support the larger muscle mass. Here is the total additional caloric requirement represented by the additional muscle:

- 4.5 grams protein × 4 calories per gram = 18 kilocalories from protein
- 90 grams carbohydrate × 4 calories per gram = 360 kilocalories from carbohydrate
- Total additional calories = 378 calories per day above current requirements to support a 3-kilogram increase in muscle mass

Of course, this athlete would also need to stimulate muscle enlargement by undertaking the appropriate strength-building exercises. Otherwise, the extra calories would manifest themselves as stored fat rather than additional muscle. It is likely that the large amount of protein consumed by so many athletes represents the extra calories they require to maintain or enlarge the muscle mass. Although it is certainly possible to use protein as a primary energy source, it is not the most desirable source because of the nitrogenous wastes produced with protein oxidation. In addition, protein can be an expensive source of calories when provided in supplement form. For instance, eggs (an extremely high-quality source of protein) cost approximately 13 cents per 8 grams of protein, while protein capsules cost approximately $1.20 per 8 grams of protein and may be of questionable quality.

High-protein foods have a long gastric emptying time so are not recommended immediately before or during exercise. In addition, there is no evidence that adding protein to a glucose- and sodium-containing sports beverage does anything useful for either endurance or power enhancement. In fact, protein added to a sports beverage that is consumed during competition increases the risk of gastrointestinal distress and may delay the delivery of fluids and carbohydrate to needy muscles. Protein added to a sports beverage reduces the content of what athletes really need: fluid,

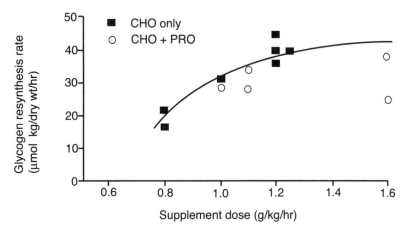

Figure 1.8   Postexercise carbohydrate and protein supplementation on glycogen resynthesis.

Reprinted, with permission, from Dr. M.J. Gibala, 2002, "Dietary protein, amino acid supplements, and recovery from exercise," *GSSI Sports Science Exchange*, #87, 15(4).

carbohydrate, and electrolytes. Therefore, the majority of energy in the preexercise meal and during exercise fluid replacement should be from carbohydrate.

An increasing body of evidence suggests that adding small amounts of protein to postexercise food and drink is useful for muscle recovery, although the benefit of protein is reduced if sufficient carbohydrate is ingested postexercise to replenish glycogen stores.[47] (See figure 1.8.)

Consuming a drink that contains approximately .1 gram of protein per kilogram (30 calories of protein for a 75-kilogram athlete) after heavy resistance training does appear to improve muscle protein balance.[48, 49] The general guideline is for endurance athletes to consume carbohydrate at the rate of a minimum of 1.2 grams per kilogram of body weight each hour during the first 3 to 5 hours after prolonged exercise. This strategy ensures muscle glycogen replenishment. The addition of some protein in this carbohydrate mix may be useful for muscle recovery, but the majority of postexercise substrate should clearly be from carbohydrate.

Vitamins and Minerals

Vitamins and minerals are essential for metabolizing energy substrates, for aiding in tissue building, for fluid balance in the intercellular and extracellular environments, and for carrying oxygen and other elements needed for metabolic work. In addition, vitamins and minerals play a role in reducing the exercise-induced oxidative stress experienced by athletes. Because of their higher rates of energy metabolism and higher muscular and skeletal stresses, athletes need more of many of the vitamins and minerals than do nonathletes. However, the amount of individual vitamins and minerals needed and the optimal delivery systems for ensuring adequate tissue levels are not well understood by most athletes, who often err on the side of providing an excessive vitamin and mineral load through high-dose supplementation. In addition, some companies now include selected vitamins in sports beverages without sufficient thought to their impact on increasing fluid osmolality and reducing the rate of fluid delivery to working muscles. The end result of this strategy is excess vitamin and mineral intake plus inferior fluid delivery.

This chapter discusses vitamin and mineral requirements for exercise, the functions of these nutrients, and the optimal delivery strategies to

Table 2.1   Dietary Reference Intakes Definitions

The Dietary Reference Intakes (DRIs) are quantitative estimates of nutrient intakes to be used for planning and assessing diets for healthy people. These values include both recommended intakes and tolerable upper intake levels. The DRIs are determined by the Institute of Medicine, a nonprofit group that provides health policy advice to the National Academy of Sciences. The DRIs are based on the scientific evaluation of the Recommended Dietary Allowance, the Adequate Intake, the Tolerable Upper Intake Level, and the Estimated Average Requirement.

- **Recommended Dietary Allowance (RDA):** the average daily dietary intake level that is sufficient to meet the nutrient requirement of nearly all (97 to 98 percent) healthy individuals in a particular life stage and gender group.
- **Adequate Intake (AI):** a recommended intake value based on observed or experimentally determined approximations or estimates of nutrient intake by a group (or groups) of healthy people that are assumed to be adequate—used when an RDA cannot be determined.
- **Tolerable Upper Intake Level (UL):** the highest level of daily nutrient intake that is likely to pose no risk of adverse health effects for almost all individuals in the general population. As intake increases above the UL, the potential risk of adverse effects increases.
- **Estimated Average Requirement (EAR):** a daily nutrient intake value that is estimated to meet the requirement of half of the healthy individuals in a life stage and gender group—used to assess dietary adequacy and as the basis for the RDA.

ensure athletes obtain what they need without adding to the cellular stress associated with excess or deficiency. Standards for nutrient intake adequacy have been established by the Institute of Medicine (see table 2.1). These standards, referred to as the Dietary Reference Intakes (DRIs), are based on the assessment of the Estimated Average Requirement (EAR), the Recommended Dietary Allowance (RDA), the Adequate Intake (AI), and the Tolerable Upper Intake Level (UL). Although the focus of the Recommended Dietary Allowance (the earlier standard for nutrient intake adequacy) was based on lowering the risk that someone would suffer from a nutrient-deficiency disease, the focus of the DRI is to lower the risk of developing chronic disease by ensuring a properly balanced nutrient intake.

Vitamins

Vitamins are substances needed by cells to encourage specific cellular chemical reactions. Some vitamins (particularly B vitamins) are involved in energy reactions that enable cells to derive energy from carbohydrate, protein, and fat. Since athletes burn more energy than do nonathletes, these vitamins are of particular interest in this book. Other vitamins are involved in maintaining mineral balance. Vitamin D, for instance, encourages greater absorption of dietary calcium and phosphorus. The synergism between vitamins and minerals is a critical factor in understanding their

---
Table 2.2   Maximizing Vitamin Intake

To maximize vitamin intake from your diet, try the following:

• Eat a wide variety of colorful fruits and vegetables.
• When possible eat fresh fruits and vegetables, especially those in season.
• Don't overcook vegetables—long cooking times reduce nutrient content.
• Steam or microwave your vegetables rather than boil them—nutrients seep out in
  boiling water only to be poured down the drain.

---

nutrient requirements. The fact that these nutrients have integrated functions should encourage athletes to present the widest possible spectrum of vitamins and minerals to their cells. Single vitamin or single mineral supplementation may corrupt nutrient balance and the delicate relationship between these nutrients. Table 2.2 gives some tips for maximizing vitamin intake.

Water-Soluble Vitamins

Vitamins are organized into fat-soluble and water-soluble categories. The fat-soluble vitamins require a fat-based environment in which to function, and the water-soluble vitamins require a water-based environment. To one degree or another, we have the capacity to store all vitamins. That is to say, if we ate a meal 2 days ago that contained a large amount of vitamin C but ingested no vitamin C in the foods we consumed yesterday, we wouldn't expect to suffer from symptoms of vitamin C deficiency today. Cells that require vitamin C are able to store more than they need, although there are no clear storage depots where large amounts of the vitamin can be stored. Fat-soluble vitamins, however, do have a large storage capacity. This difference in storage capacity is responsible for the commonly repeated recommendation that water-soluble vitamins should be consumed every day because they are *not* stored. It has also led to the myth that any excess in water-soluble vitamin intake is without problems because the excess is excreted in the urine. Although it is true that excess intake of fat-soluble vitamins, especially vitamins D and A, can produce severe toxicity, taking excess water-soluble vitamins may also lead to difficulties. A prime example of this is peripheral neuropathy (loss of feeling in the fingers), a neurological problem caused by excess intake of vitamin B_6 (500 milligrams per day over time is enough to create permanent damage). Another problem is that humans are adaptable to intake. Therefore, the more you take, the more you may need to get the same biological effect. A discussion of individual water-soluble vitamins follows. See tables 2.3 through 2.11 for a summary of the functions, sources, and possible problems associated with these vitamins.[1]

Vitamin B₁

Vitamin B_1 (thiamin) is present in a variety of food sources, including whole grains, nuts, legumes (beans and dried peas), and pork. It works in unison with other B vitamins to convert the energy in the foods we consume to muscular energy and heat. Thiamin contributes to this metabolic process by removing carbon dioxide in energy

Table 2.3   Vitamin B₁ Quick Guide

Alternate name	Thiamin
Dietary Reference Intake (DRI)	Adult males: 1.2 mg/day Adult females: 1.1 mg/day
Recommended intake for athletes	1.5 to 3.0 mg/day, depending on total calories consumed (high calories = more)
Functions	Carbohydrate metabolism, nervous system function
Good food sources	Whole grain cereals, beans, pork, enriched grains
Deficiency	Confusion, anorexia, weakness, calf pain, heart disease
Toxicity	None known (no safe upper limit established)

reactions with its active coenzyme thiamin pyrophosphate (TPP), an enzyme that is particularly important in carbohydrate energy metabolism.

Thiamin deficiency has not been reported in athletes, but deficiency disease does occur in alcoholics and populations consuming a low-quality diet of unenriched polished rice or other processed and unenriched grains. The DRI for thiamin (1.2 milligrams per day for males, 1.1 milligrams per day for females) may be inadequate for athletes. The actual requirement is based on approximately .5 milligrams of thiamin for each 1,000 calories consumed, and athletes often consume more than 3,000 calories (often 5,000 to 6,000 calories). It does appear that the upper limit for thiamin intake would be 3.0 milligrams per day, even for an athlete consuming more than 6,000 calories per day. It is reasonable, therefore, to recommend an intake of two times the DRI (~2.2 to 2.4 milligrams per day) for athletes consuming high levels of energy. Athletes commonly consume high-carbohydrate foods that are good sources of thiamin, making it likely that most well-nourished athletes already consume more than the recommended level of thiamin each day.

Vitamin B₂

Vitamin B₂ (riboflavin) is involved in energy production and normal cellular function through its coenzymes flavin adenine dinucleotide (FAD) and flavin mononucleotide (FMN). These coenzymes are mainly involved in obtaining energy from consumed carbohydrate, protein, and fat. Food sources of riboflavin include dairy products (e.g., milk, yogurt, cottage cheese), dark green leafy vegetables (e.g., spinach, chard, mustard greens, broccoli, green peppers), whole grain foods, and enriched grain foods.

No studies suggest that riboflavin-deficiency symptoms are common in athletes. Also, no apparent toxicity symptoms occur from consuming more than the DRI. Several studies have suggested that athletes may have higher requirements than the DRI, which is based on approximately .6 milligrams per 1,000 calories. In a series of studies performed on exercising women and women seeking to lose weight, the riboflavin requirement was found to range between .63 and 1.40 milligrams per 1,000 calories.[2-4]

Table 2.4   **Vitamin B$_2$ Quick Guide**

Alternate name	Riboflavin
Dietary Reference Intake (DRI)	Adult males: 1.3 mg/day Adult females: 1.1 mg/day
Recommended intake for athletes	1.1mg per 1,000 calories
Functions	Energy metabolism, protein metabolism, skin health, eye health
Good food sources	Fresh milk and other dairy products, eggs, dark green leafy vegetables, whole grain cereals, enriched grains
Deficiency	Inflamed tongue; cracked, dry skin at corners of mouth, nose, and eyes; bright light sensitivity; weakness; fatigue
Toxicity	None known (no safe upper limit established)

There is some evidence that physical activity increases the requirement to a level slightly higher than .5 milligrams per 1,000 calories, but not more than 1.6 milligrams per 1,000 calories.[5] However, even with this apparently higher requirement for athletes, no studies clearly demonstrate an improvement in athletic performance with intakes greater than the RDA. Since low-dose supplements of this vitamin induce no apparent toxicity symptoms, athletes could take a supplement delivering 1.6 to 3.0 milligrams of riboflavin as part of a B-complex supplement. This level of intake would serve as an adequate preventative measure to help the athlete avoid the symptoms—headache, nausea, weakness—associated with extremely high doses (more than 100 times the RDA).[6]

Niacin

Niacin is involved in energy production from carbohydrate, protein, and fat; glycogen synthesis; and normal cellular metabolism through its active coenzymes. These enzymes, nicotinamide adenine dinucleotide (NAD) and nicotinamide adenine dinucleotide phosphate (NADP), are essential for normal muscle function. Niacin deficiency is well documented in human populations suffering from famine or monotonous intakes of unenriched grain products, but there is no evidence of niacin deficiency in athletes.

Niacin is found in meat, whole or enriched grains, seeds, nuts, and legumes. Body cells have the capacity to synthesize niacin from tryptophan (60 milligrams of tryptophan yields 1 milligram of niacin), an amino acid found in all high-quality protein foods (e.g., meat, fish, poultry). Given the broad spectrum of foods that contain niacin, it is relatively easy for people to consume the DRI of 12 to 14 milligrams per day, or 6.6 niacin equivalents (NEs) per 1,000 calories. NEs are equal to 1 milligram of niacin or 60 milligrams of dietary tryptophan; you can obtain niacin directly from food or indirectly by consuming the amino acid tryptophan. The NE unit of measure takes both sources into account.

Table 2.5   Niacin Quick Guide

Alternate names	Niacinamide, nicotinic acid, nicotinamide
Dietary Reference Intake (DRI)	Adult males: 16 mg/day Adult females: 14 mg/day
Recommended intake for athletes	14 to 20 mg/day
Functions	Energy metabolism, glycolysis, fat synthesis
Good food sources	Foods high in tryptophan (an amino acid that can be converted to niacin): milk, eggs, turkey, chicken Foods high in niacin: whole grains, lean meat, fish, poultry, enriched grains
Deficiency	Anorexia, skin rash, dementia, weakness, lethargy Disease: pellagra
Toxicity	Tolerable upper limits: 10 to 15mg/day for young children (age 1-8) 20 to 35 mg/day for children and adults (age 9-70+) *Symptoms:* flushing, burning, and tingling sensations of extremities, hepatitis and gastric ulcers with chronic high intake

A deficiency of niacin results in muscular weakness, loss of appetite, indigestion, and skin rash. It is possible to produce toxicity symptoms from excess niacin intake; symptoms include gastrointestinal distress and feeling hot (becoming red faced or flushed). It may also result in a tingling feeling around the neck, face, and fingers. These symptoms are commonly reported in people taking large doses of niacin to lower blood lipids.

In studies evaluating the performance effects of niacin supplementation, endurance was reduced because the excess niacin caused a reduction in fat metabolism.[7-9] This resulted in a greater reliance on carbohydrate fuels (glucose and glycogen) to support physical activity. Because the storage of carbohydrate is limited, athletes taking niacin supplements had lower endurance. To date, there is no evidence that the requirement for niacin is increased with physical activity.

Vitamin B₆

Vitamin B_6 refers to several compounds (pyridoxine, pyridoxal, pyridoxamine, pyridoxine 5-phosphate, pyridoxal 5-phosphate, and pyridoxamine 5-phosphatepyridoxine) that all display the same metabolic activity. Vitamin B_6 is most concentrated in meats (especially liver) and is found also in wheat germ, fish, poultry, legumes, bananas, brown rice, whole grain cereals, and vegetables. Because the function of this vitamin is closely linked to protein and amino acid metabolism, the requirement is linked to protein intake (the higher the protein intake, the higher the vitamin B_6 requirement).

Table 2.6 Vitamin B₆ Quick Guide

Alternate names	Pyridoxine, pyridoxal, pyridoxamine
Dietary Reference Intake (DRI)	Adult males: 1.3 to 1.7 mg/day Adult females: 1.3 to 1.5 mg/day
Recommended intake for athletes	1.5 to 2.0 mg/day
Functions	Protein metabolism, protein synthesis, metabolism of fat and carbohydrate, neurotransmitter formation, glycolysis
Good food sources	High-protein foods (meats), whole grain cereals, enriched cereals, eggs
Deficiency	Nausea, mouth sores, muscle weakness, depression, convulsions, impaired immune system
Toxicity	Tolerable upper limits: 30 to 40 mg/day for young children (age 1-8) 60 to 100 mg/day for children and adults (age 9-70+) *Symptoms:* peripheral neuritis (loss of sensation in limbs), loss of balance and coordination

The adult requirement is based on .016 milligrams of B₆ per gram of protein consumed each day[1] and is satisfied in those consuming typical protein intakes. When you consider that high-protein foods are also typically high in vitamin B₆, those consuming protein from food (regardless of the amount) are most likely to have adequate B₆ levels as well. However, many athletes consume additional protein in purified supplemental forms (protein powders, amino acid powders), making it conceivable that athletes with high supplemental protein intakes may have an inadequate B₆ intake.

Vitamin B₆ functions in reactions related to protein synthesis by aiding in the creation of amino acids and proteins (transamination reactions) and is also involved in protein catabolism through involvement in reactions that break down amino acids and proteins (deamination reactions). It is involved, therefore, in manufacturing muscle, hemoglobin, and other proteins critical for athletic performance. The major enzyme of vitamin B₆, pyridoxal phosphate (PP), is also involved in the breakdown of muscle glycogen for energy through the enzyme glycogen phosphorylase.

A chronic deficiency of vitamin B₆ leads to symptoms of peripheral neuritis (loss of nerve function in the hands, feet, arms, and legs), ataxia (loss of balance), irritability, depression, and convulsions. An excess intake of vitamin B₆, primarily from consumption of supplements, does lead to toxicity symptoms that have been documented in humans. These symptoms are similar to those seen in B₆ deficiency and include ataxia and severe sensory neuropathy (loss of sensation in the fingers). Toxicity symptoms have been documented in women taking supplements that, on average, equal 119 milligrams per day to treat premenstrual syndrome and several types of mental disorders.[10, 11]

There is a theoretical basis for investigating vitamin B_6 and athletic performance. B_6 is involved in the breakdown of amino acids in muscle as a means of obtaining needed energy and in converting lactic acid to glucose in the liver.[12] Vitamin B_6 is also involved in the breakdown of muscle glycogen to derive energy. Other functions of vitamin B_6 that may be related to athletic performance include the formation of serotonin and the synthesis of carnitine from lysine. There is evidence that some athletes may be at risk of inadequate vitamin B_6 status.[13-15] Poor B_6 status reduces athletic performance.[16]

Because many athletes are always looking for that extra edge, there is an understandable attractiveness to natural substances that are legal. Vitamin B_6 is sometimes marketed as one of those natural and legal substances; besides its importance in energy metabolism, it is linked with the production of growth hormone, which can help increase muscle mass.[17] It appears as if the combined effect of exercise and vitamin B_6 on growth hormone production is greater than either of these factors individually.[18, 19]

Before athletes take vitamin B_6 supplements, the following factors should be considered:[20]

- Most athletes have adequate vitamin B_6 intakes and a healthy vitamin B_6 status.
- Those athletes with poor vitamin B_6 status are generally those with inadequate energy intakes.
- A greater proportion of female athletes and athletes participating in sports that emphasize low body weight (gymnastics, wrestling, figure skating) are likely to have inadequate energy and protein intakes and, therefore, inadequate vitamin B_6 intakes.
- High doses of vitamin B_6 have been shown to have toxic effects.
- While poor B_6 status is associated with reduced athletic performance, there is no good evidence that consuming more than the recommended intake has a beneficial effect on athletic performance.[21]
- Vitamin B_6 supplementation does not appear necessary to enhance athletic performance if a balanced diet with adequate energy is consumed.[22]

All things considered, these factors should encourage athletes to consume an adequate intake of energy substrates rather than resort to supplements of vitamin B_6.

Vitamin B_{12}

Vitamin B_{12} is the most chemically complex of all the vitamins. It contains the mineral cobalt (thus the name "cobalamin") and, while essential for all cell function, has a major involvement in red blood cell formation, folic acid metabolism, DNA synthesis, and nerve development.

Dietary sources of this vitamin are mainly foods of animal origin (meats, eggs, dairy products); it is essentially absent from plant foods. A small amount of absorbable vitamin B_{12} may also be produced by gut bacteria.[23] Vegetarian athletes who avoid all

Table 2.7   Vitamin B$_{12}$ Quick Guide

Alternate name	Cobalamin
Dietary Reference Intake (DRI)	Adult males: 2.4 mcg/day Adult females: 2.4 mcg/day
Recommended intake for athletes	2.4 to 2.5 mcg/day
Functions	Protein metabolism, protein synthesis, metabolism of fat and carbohydrate, neurotransmitter formation, glycolysis
Good food sources	Foods of animal origin (meat, fish, poultry, eggs, milk, cheese) and fortified cereals
Deficiency	Pernicious anemia (more likely caused by malabsorption of the vitamin than by dietary inadequacy, although vegans are at risk) *Symptoms:* weakness, easy fatigue, neurological disorders
Toxicity	Tolerable upper limits not established, although the DV is 6 mcg/day

foods of animal origin (i.e., they do not eat meat, nor do they consume eggs or dairy products) would therefore be at risk for vitamin B$_{12}$ deficiency.

B$_{12}$ deficiency results in pernicious anemia, a form of anemia that most commonly occurs in the elderly with compromised stomach function. The stomach normally produces intrinsic factor, which is required for vitamin B$_{12}$ absorption. Without intrinsic factor, even a normal dietary intake of vitamin B$_{12}$ will result in deficiency disease because of malabsorption. Symptoms of deficiency include fatigue, poor muscular coordination (possibly leading to paralysis), and dementia.

Athletes have abused vitamin B$_{12}$ for years. It was (and continues to be) common for many athletes to be injected with large amounts of vitamin B$_{12}$ (often 1-gram injections) before competitions.[24, 25] Despite the commonality of this strategy, there is no evidence that vitamin B$_{12}$ does anything whatsoever to improve performance when taken in excess.[26-28]

It certainly makes sense that athletes consume foods that will help them avoid deficiencies of any kind, including B$_{12}$ deficiency. The resulting anemia would clearly affect performance by reducing oxygen-carrying capacity, leading to reduced endurance. Potentially, muscular coordination could also be impaired. Unless someone has a genetic predisposition for B$_{12}$ malabsorption (typically because of an inadequate production of intrinsic factor), there is no basis for taking supplements if a balanced mixed-food diet is consumed. Vegan athletes, on the other hand, have good reason to be concerned about vitamin B$_{12}$ status. A supplement providing, on average, the DRI of 1.8 to 2.4 micrograms per day for vegan athletes makes good sense, as does the consumption of foods that are fortified with vitamin B$_{12}$ (such as some soy milk products).

Folic Acid

Folic acid is widespread in the food supply, with the highest concentrations in liver, yeast, leafy vegetables, fruits, and legumes. It is now also fortified in grain products (breads, cereals, spaghetti) within the United States, where fortified foods deliver approximately 140 micrograms of folate per 100 grams of food. It is easily destroyed through common household food preparation techniques and long storage times, so it is often most highly concentrated in fresh foods. Folate functions in amino acid metabolism and nucleic acid synthesis (RNA and DNA), and a deficiency leads to alterations in protein synthesis.[1] Tissues with a rapid turnover are particularly sensitive to folic acid, including red and white blood cells as well as tissues of the gastrointestinal tract and the uterus. Adequate folate intake immediately before and during pregnancy is associated with the elimination of fetal neural tube defects (most notably spina bifida).[29, 30]

Folic acid is measured in dietary folate equivalents (DFE), where 1 DFE equals

- 1 microgram of food folate;
- .6 micrograms of folate from fortified food or as a supplement consumed with food; or
- .5 micrograms of a folate supplement consumed on an empty stomach.

Because folate functions with vitamin B_{12} in forming healthy new red blood cells, a deficiency leads to megaloblastic anemia. Other deficiency problems include gastrointestinal distress (diarrhea, malabsorption, pain) and a swollen, red tongue. Folate toxicity from excess intake has not been reported in humans, and no studies have reported on the relationship between folic acid and athletic performance. However, since athletes have an above-normal tissue turnover because of the pounding the body takes in various sports, and with the evidence that red blood cell turnover is faster in athletes than in nonathletes[31, 32] there is good reason for athletes to be

Table 2.8   Folic Acid Quick Guide

Alternate name	Folate
Dietary Reference Intake (DRI)	Adult males: 400 mcg/day Adult females: 400 mcg/day
Recommended intake for athletes	400 mcg/day
Functions	Methionine (essential amino acid) metabolism, formation of DNA, formation of red blood cells, normal fetal development
Good food sources	Green leafy vegetables, beans, whole grain cereals, oranges, bananas
Deficiency	Megaloblastic anemia, neural tube defects (as a result of low intake during pregnancy) *Symptoms:* weakness, easy fatigue, neurological disorders
Toxicity	Tolerable upper limits: 300 to 400 mcg/day for young children (age 1-8) 600 to 1,000 mcg/day for children and adults (age 9-70+) *Symptoms:* none established

certain that adequate folic acid intake is satisfied. The best approach is through the regular consumption of fresh fruits and vegetables. If this is not possible, a daily supplement at the level of the DRI (400 micrograms per day) is an effective means of maintaining folate status.

Biotin

Biotin works with magnesium and adenosine triphosphate (ATP) to play a role in carbon dioxide metabolism; new glucose production (gluconeogenesis); carbohydrate metabolism; and synthesis of glycogen, fatty acids, and amino acids.[1] Good food sources of biotin include egg yolks, soy flour, liver, sardines, walnuts, pecans, peanuts, and yeast. Fruits and meats are poor dietary sources of the vitamin. Biotin is also synthesized by bacteria in the intestines. Because of this intestinal synthesis, a deficiency of this vitamin is rare but can be induced through the intake of large amounts of raw egg whites, which contain avidin, a protein that binds to biotin (20 raw egg whites would be needed to disturb biotin metabolism). When a deficiency does occur, symptoms include loss of appetite, vomiting, depression, and dermatitis. There is no evidence that athletes are at risk for biotin deficiency and no information exists on the relationship between biotin and athletic performance. Therefore, no recommendation on biotin intake for athletes above the suggested DRI can be made.

Table 2.9   Biotin Quick Guide

Alternate name	None
Dietary Reference Intake (DRI)	Adult males: 30 mcg/day Adult females: 30 mcg/day
Recommended intake for athletes	30 mcg/day
Functions	Glucose and fatty acid synthesis, gluconeogenesis, gene expression
Good food sources	Egg yolks, legumes, dark green leafy vegetables (also produced by intestinal bacteria)
Deficiency	Rare; if it occurs, due to high egg white intake *Symptoms:* anorexia, depression, muscle pain, dermatitis
Toxicity	Tolerable upper limits not established

Pantothenic Acid

Pantothenic acid is a structural component of coenzyme A (CoA), a compound of central importance in energy metabolic processes. It is involved, through CoA, in carbohydrate, protein, and fat metabolism. Pantothenic acid is widely distributed in the food supply, making it unlikely that an athlete would suffer from a deficiency, particularly with adequate total energy intake. If a rare deficiency does occur, symptoms include easy fatigue, weakness, and insomnia. The highest concentrations of pantothenic acid are found in meat, whole grain foods, beans, and peas. Supplemental doses of the vitamin are typically 10 milligrams per day (double the DRI of 5 milligrams per day) and, at this level, have not resulted in toxicity. However, few data are available on the potential for pantothenic acid toxicity, so athletes should be cautious about high-dose supplementation with this vitamin.

A possible relationship exists between pantothenic acid supplementation and exercise performance, but more information is needed before a sound recommendation can be made on pantothenate intake for athletes. In studies that have experimented with pantothenic acid supplements to determine a requirement level, the typical dosage has been 10 milligrams per day. At this level of intake, 5 to 7 milligrams per day are excreted in the urine.[1] Therefore, it appears that taking supplements at the level of 10 milligrams per day is excessive.

Table 2.10 Pantothenic Acid Quick Guide

Alternate name	Pantothenate
Dietary Reference Intake (DRI)	Adult males: 5 mg/day Adult females: 5 mg/day
Recommended intake for athletes	4 to 5 mg/day
Functions	Energy metabolism as part of coenzyme A, gluconeogenesis, synthesis of acetylcholine
Good food sources	Present in all *but* processed and refined foods
Deficiency	Unknown in humans
Toxicity	Tolerable upper limits not established, although DV is 10 mg *Symptoms:* unknown

Vitamin C

Vitamin C functions as an antioxidant and is also involved in reactions that form the connective-tissue protein *collagen*. Fresh fruits and vegetables are the best sources of vitamin C. Meats and dairy products are low in vitamin C, and cereal grains contain none (unless fortified). Vitamin C is easily destroyed by cooking (heat) and exposure to air (oxygen). It is also highly water soluble, making it easily removed from foods cooked in water. The deficiency disease scurvy is almost nonexistent today. Toxicity from high, regular supplemental intakes of the vitamin is rare, but may include a predisposition to developing kidney stones and a reduction in tissue sensitivity to the vitamin. Doses of 100 to 200 milligrams per day will saturate the body with vitamin C,[33] yet many people take supplemental doses of 1,000 to 2,000 milligrams per day, well above the 75 to 90 milligrams per day of the DRI.

Table 2.11   **Vitamin C Quick Guide**

Alternate names	Ascorbic acid, ascorbate, dehydroascorbate, L-ascorbate
Dietary Reference Intake (DRI)	Adult males: 90 mg/day Adult females: 75 mg/day
Recommended intake for athletes	200 mg/day
Functions	Collagen formation, iron absorption, epinephrine formation
Good food sources	Fresh fruits (particularly citrus and cherries) and vegetables
Deficiency	Rare; if it occurs, results in scurvy Symptoms: bleeding gums, deterioration of muscles and tendons, sudden death
Toxicity	Tolerable upper limits: 400 to 650 mg/day for young children (age 1-8) 1.2 to 2.0 g/day for children and adults (age 9-70+) Increased risk of kidney stone formation with chronic intake of 1g/day or more

A number of studies have evaluated the relationship between vitamin C intake and athletic performance, although the results are inconsistent. Part of the problem with many of these studies is poor standardization between subjects and a general lack of comparative controls. Nevertheless, according to a review of studies that used controls and provided vitamin C supplements at or below 500 milligrams per day (remember that the DRI is 75 milligrams for adult women and 90 milligrams for adult men), there was no measurable benefit to athletic performance.[34] One study noted that when a 500-milligram dose of vitamin C was provided shortly (4 hours) before testing, there was a significant improvement in strength and a significant reduction in maximal oxygen consumption, but no impact on muscular endurance.[35] When subjects were provided with the same amount for 7 days, the result was an improvement in strength but a decrease in endurance. When these same subjects were provided with 2,000 milligrams each day for 7 days, the athletes' $\dot{V}O_2$max was lowered, but no change was evident in endurance performance.

Athletes involved in concussive sports—where muscle soreness occurs or an injury requires more collagen formation—may benefit from a slightly higher level of vitamin C. Studies on animals suggest that vitamin C improves the healing process, and inadequate vitamin C inhibits healing.[36] It has also been suggested that muscle soreness may be more rapidly relieved when consuming moderate supplemental doses of vitamin C and other antioxidants.[37]

It is difficult to make a rational recommendation on vitamin C and performance, but athletes should keep the safe upper limit (2,000 milligrams per day) of this vitamin in mind before investing in supplements. Because some studies demonstrate that high doses may cause endurance problems, the intake level should be kept below the point of causing performance deficits. Vitamin C is known to enhance iron absorption. In 1993, there were three reported deaths due to iron overload, and the people who died were taking large daily doses of vitamin C.[38] Also consider that many athletes already consume more than 250 milligrams of vitamin C each day from food alone because of their high intake of fresh fruits and vegetables. A reasonable recommendation is to eat an abundant amount of fresh fruits and vegetables (wonderful sources of carbohydrate and many other nutrients besides vitamin C). If that's not possible, a reasonable strategy is to take a moderate daily supplement containing the DRI (between 75 and 90 milligrams per day). Except for athletes chronically consuming diets that are inadequate in energy, athletes meet the DRI and consume more vitamin C than the general nonathlete population.[39] Even someone consuming a low but regular intake of fruits and vegetables is likely to meet the DRI for vitamin C, but a low-level supplement may provide an appropriate safety buffer.

Fat-Soluble Vitamins

Fat-soluble vitamins are carried in a fat solute and represent an important reason why athletes should not consume a diet excessively low (i.e., below 20 percent of calories) in fat. There are four fat-soluble vitamins—A, D, E, and K—and each is effectively stored to be used as needed. See tables 2.12 through 2.15 for a summary of the functions, sources, and possible problems associated with these vitamins.[33, 40, 41] There are limits to the storage capacity of fat-soluble vitamins, so chronically high intakes may lead to serious disease states. To emphasize this point, the two most potentially toxic substances in human nutrition are vitamins A and D. Achieving toxic-level doses of these vitamins is difficult if consuming the usual foods, but toxic doses may be easily obtained from a regular supplemental intake of these vitamins. Generally speaking, however, our storage capacity for these vitamins eliminates the need for supplemental intake.

Vitamin A

The active form of vitamin A is retinol, which we obtain from foods of animal origin, including liver, egg yolks, fortified dairy products (e.g., vitamin A and D milk), margarine, and fish oil. The DRI ranges between 700 retinol activity equivalents (RAE) for women and 900 RAE for men. One RAE equals

- 1 microgram of retinol,
- 12 micrograms of beta-carotene,
- 24 micrograms of alpha-carotene, or
- 24 micrograms of beta-cryptoxanthin.

Vitamin A has a well-established relationship with normal vision; helps keep bones, skin, and red blood cells healthy; and is also needed for the immune system to function normally. There is no evidence that taking extra vitamin A aids athletic performance. Since the vitamin has clearly toxic effects when taken in excess (the

Table 2.12 Vitamin A Quick Guide

Alternate name	Retinol (precursor: beta-carotene)
Dietary Reference Intake (DRI)	Adult males: 900 mcg/day Adult females: 700 mcg/day
Recommended intake for athletes	700 to 900 mcg/day
Functions	Maintaining healthy epithelial (surface) cells, eye health, immune system health
Good food sources	Retinol: liver, butter, cheese, egg yolks, fish liver oils Beta-carotene: dark green and brightly pigmented fruits and vegetables
Deficiency	Dry skin, headache, irritability, vomiting, bone pain, night blindness, increased risk of infection, blindness
Toxicity (high toxicity potential)	Tolerable upper limits: 600 to 900 mcg/day for young children (age 1-8) 1.7 to 3.0 mg/day for children and adults (age 9-70+) *Symptoms:* liver damage, bone malformations, death

maximum upper limit that poses the risk of adverse effects is 3,000 RAE for women and men), athletes should be cautioned against taking supplemental doses. Toxicity of vitamin A manifests itself in several ways, including dry skin, headache, irritability, vomiting, bone pain, and vision problems. Excess vitamin A intake during pregnancy is associated with an increase in birth defects.

A precursor to vitamin A is beta-carotene. (A precursor is a substance that, under the proper conditions, is converted to the active form of the vitamin.) Therefore, consuming foods with beta-carotene is an indirect way of obtaining vitamin A. Beta-carotene is found in all red, orange, yellow, and dark green fruits and vegetables (carrots, sweet potatoes, spinach, apricots, cantaloupes, tomatoes, and so on). It is a powerful antioxidant, protecting cells from oxidative damage that could lead to cancer, and it can be converted to vitamin A as we need it. Unlike preformed vitamin A (retinol), beta-carotene does not exhibit the same clear toxic effects if excess doses are consumed. However, a consistently high intake of carrots, sweet potatoes, and other foods high in beta-carotene may cause a person to develop a yellowish skin tone as the beta-carotene accumulates in subcutaneous fat.

It is conceivable that beta-carotene may, as an antioxidant, prove to be effective in reducing postexercise muscle soreness and may aid in postexercise recovery. However, this is a theoretical connection only; no study makes a direct link between beta-carotene intake and reduced soreness and improved recovery. Nevertheless, given its relatively low toxicity potential and its potential benefits, the U.S. Olympic Committee has recognized beta-carotene's potential as an antioxidant.[42]

Vitamin D

Vitamin D is the most potentially toxic vitamin in human nutrition, with an upper limit (UL) of 50 micrograms per day. We can obtain the vitamin in an inactive form from food and sunlight exposure. Ultraviolet radiation (sunlight) exposure of the skin transforms a cholesterol derivative (7-dehydrocholesterol) into an inactive form of vitamin D called cholecalciferol. To be functional, this inactive form of vitamin D must be activated by the kidneys. Therefore, kidney disease may be the cause of vitamin D-related disorders. Dietary sources of vitamin D include eggs, fortified milk, liver, butter, and margarine. Cod liver oil, which was once given commonly as a supplement, is a concentrated source of the vitamin. The adult DRI for vitamin D is 5 micrograms per day of cholecalciferol or 200 international units (IU) of vitamin D (1 microgram of calciferol equals 40 IU of vitamin D).

Vitamin D promotes growth and mineralizes bones and teeth by increasing the absorption of calcium and phosphorus. A diet with an adequate intake of calcium and phosphorus but without adequate vitamin D leads to calcium and phosphorus deficiency. The childhood deficiency disease rickets and the adult deficiency disease osteomalacia are diseases of calcium deficiency that are caused either by inadequate levels of vitamin D or the inability to convert vitamin D to the active (functional) form. However, because of vitamin D's potential toxicity, caution must be taken not to consume too much. Excess vitamin D intake may lead to vomiting, diarrhea, weight loss, kidney damage, high blood calcium levels, and death.

No existing studies suggest that high levels of vitamin D intake, either through foods or supplementation, aid athletic performance. There is also no theoretical basis for performance enhancement to occur. It is possible, however, that vitamin D may

Table 2.13   Vitamin D Quick Guide

Alternate names	Cholecalciferol, calcitriol, calciferol
Dietary Reference Intake (DRI)	Adult males: 5 mcg/day Adult females: 5 mcg/day
Recommended intake for athletes	5 to 15 mcg/day
Functions	Absorption of calcium and phosphorus, healthy skin
Good food sources	Ultraviolet light exposure, fish liver oil; lesser amounts in eggs and canned fish; fortified milk and margarine
Deficiency	Rickets (children), osteomalacia (adults), increased risk of stress fractures, increased risk of osteoporosis
Toxicity (high toxicity potential)	Tolerable upper limits: 50 mcg/day for all age groups *Symptoms:* nausea, diarrhea, loss of muscle function, organ damage, skeletal damage

play an indirect role in injury resistance. Athletes in some sports may have dramatically lower sunlight exposure because all training sessions take place inside a building. This lower UV exposure may reduce vitamin D synthesis to a point where both growth and bone density are negatively affected. Lower bone densities are known to place athletes at higher risk for developing stress fractures, an injury that can end an athletic career.[43-45] In a survey of U.S. national team gymnasts, the factor most closely related to bone density was sunlight exposure. Those with higher densities had the greatest exposure.[46] Also, sunlight exposure was more important as a predictor of bone density in this group than vitamin D or calcium intake from food.

Vitamin E

Vitamin E is a generic term for several of the tocopherols that have similar activity, and the unit of measure is based on the level of tocopherol with an activity equivalent to that of alpha-tocopherol. Beta-tocopherol[47] has a lower level of activity than alpha-tocopherol[48] so more of it would be necessary for the same effect. The adult DRI for vitamin E is 15 milligrams per day, a level easily obtained by consuming green leafy vegetables, vegetable oils, seeds, nuts, liver, and corn. However, a failure to consume sufficient vegetables, nuts, or vegetable oil may place adults at risk of an inadequate intake. It is difficult to induce a vitamin E deficiency in humans, and it also appears to be a relatively nontoxic vitamin (there is no evidence of toxicity from consuming the vitamins from food). The Institute of Medicine indicates that adverse effects from vitamin E supplementation may include hemorrhagic toxicity.

Vitamin E is a potent antioxidant that protects membranes from destruction by peroxides. Peroxides are formed when fats (especially polyunsaturated fats) become oxidized (rancid). These peroxides are called free radicals because they bounce around unpredictably inside cells, altering or destroying them. Since vitamin E is

Table 2.14 Vitamin E Quick Guide

Alternate names	Tocopherol, alpha-tocopherol, gamma-tocopherol
Dietary Reference Intake (DRI)	Adult males: 15 mg/day Adult females: 15 mg/day
Recommended intake for athletes	15 mg/day
Functions	Antioxidant protection of cell membranes
Good food sources	Polyunsaturated and monounsaturated vegetable and cereal oils and margarines (corn, soy, safflower, olive); lesser amounts in fortified cereals and eggs
Deficiency	Rare; if it occurs, possible increased risk of cancer and heart disease
Toxicity	Tolerable upper limits: 200 to 300 mg/day for young children (age 1-8) 600 to 1,000 mg/day for children and adults (age 9-70+)

an antioxidant, it helps capture oxygen, thereby limiting the oxidation of fats to protect cells.

Several studies on vitamin E and physical performance have been conducted, but none has found an improvement in either strength or endurance with vitamin E supplementation.[49-52] Studies evaluating whether vitamin E supplementation reduces exercise-induced peroxide damage have mixed results. Some suggest that a clear reduction in peroxidative damage occurs,[53, 54] but others have found that vitamin E has no benefit.[55] It seems clear that more information on vitamin E is needed before a definitive exercise-related benefit can be claimed. However, the theoretical basis related to a reduction in peroxidative damage through a slight increase in additional vitamin E consumption is sound. Vitamin E supplements may be sold in international units (IU). One milligram of alpha-tocopherol is equivalent to approximately 1.5 IU of vitamin E.

Vitamin K

Vitamin K is found in green leafy vegetables and also, in small amounts, in cereals, fruits, and meats. Bacteria in the intestines also produce vitamin K, so the absolute dietary requirement is not known. This vitamin is needed for the formation of prothrombin, which is required for blood to clot. It is possible for people who regularly take antibiotics that destroy the bacteria in the intestines to be at increased risk for vitamin K deficiency. A deficiency would cause an increase in bleeding and hemorrhages. The DRI for vitamin K is 90 micrograms per day for adult women and 120 micrograms per day for adult men. There is no established UL for this vitamin. Vitamin K appears to be relatively nontoxic, but high intakes of synthetic forms may cause jaundice. Supplemental doses also interfere with anticoagulant drugs. People taking warfarin (a blood thinner) must be aware that vitamin K or foods containing vitamin K may reduce the effectiveness of their medication.

Table 2.15 Vitamin K Quick Guide

Alternate names	Phylloquinone, menoquinone, antihemorrhagic vitamin
Dietary Reference Intake (DRI)	Adult males: 120 mcg/day Adult females: 90 mcg/day
Recommended intake for athletes	700 to 900 mcg/day
Functions	Formation of blood clots, enhancement of osteocalcin function to aid in bone strengthening
Good food sources	Phylloquinone: a variety of vegetable oils and dark green leafy vegetables (cabbage, spinach) Menoquinone: formed by the bacteria that line the gastrointestinal tract
Deficiency	Rare; if it occurs, results in hemorrhage
Toxicity	Tolerable upper limits not established

Vitamin K has also been linked to bone density. People with low levels of vitamin K have lower bone density, which can be improved with vitamin K supplementation.[56] In addition, women obtaining a minimum of 110 micrograms of vitamin K are at significantly lower hip fracture risk than women who have a lower intake.[57] The Framingham Heart Study also found a relationship between higher vitamin K intake and reduced hip fracture risk.[58] Vitamin K is found in so many foods, and with bacterial production in the gut, it would seem difficult to not get enough. Nevertheless, a survey has found that an important segment of Americans, particularly children and young adults, does not obtain sufficient vitamin K.[59]

No studies have examined the relationship between vitamin K and athletic performance. Further, it is difficult to think of a theoretical framework in which such a relationship might exist. It seems clear that, especially for athletes involved in contact sports, adequate vitamin K is necessary to avoid excessive bruising and bleeding. However, there is no documented evidence that athletes are at a particularly high risk for a deficiency.

Minerals

Minerals are unique in that, unlike other nutrients, they are inorganic. Nevertheless, they work in unison with other organic nutrients (vitamins and energy substrates). An obvious example of this inorganic–organic integration is the well-established relationship between the mineral calcium and vitamin D. Individually these nutrients are essentially useless, but when available together, they work in concert to sustain bone density. Minerals have numerous functions, including the following:

- Adding to the strength and structure of the skeleton, keeping it strong and resistant to fracture.

- Maintaining the relative acidity or alkalinity of the blood and tissue. For athletes, hard physical activity tends to lower the pH level (i.e., increase the relative acidity), so having a healthy system to control acid–base balance is critical for endurance performance.

- Serving as bridges for electrical impulses that stimulate muscular movement. Since all athletic endeavors rely on efficient and effective muscular movement and coordination, this function is critically important.

- Metabolizing cells. Physical activity increases the rate at which fuel is burned. Therefore, the effective control of this fuel burned at the cellular level is necessary for athletic endeavors.

All of these functions are important for athletes. Athletes with low-density bones are at increased risk for stress fractures; poor acid–base balance leads to poor endurance; poor nerve and muscle function results in poor coordination; and altered cell metabolism limits a cell's ability to obtain and store energy.

The established roles of minerals in the development of optimal physical performance include involvement in glycolysis (obtaining energy from stored glucose), lipolysis (obtaining energy from fat), proteolysis (obtaining energy from protein), and the phosphagen system (obtaining energy from phosphocreatine).[60] Inorganic mineral nutrients are required in the structural composition of hard and soft body tissues. Minerals also participate in the action of enzyme systems, muscle contractions, nerve reactions, and blood clotting. These mineral nutrients, all of which must be supplied in the diet, are of two classes: major elements (macrominerals) and trace elements (microminerals).[33, 40, 41]

Macrominerals

The total mineral content of the body is approximately 4 percent of body weight. Macrominerals are present in the body in relatively larger amounts than microminerals (thus the name) and include calcium, phosphorus, magnesium, sodium, chloride, and potassium. Calcium makes up approximately 1.75 percent of total body weight, phosphorus makes up approximately 1.10 percent of total body weight, and magnesium makes up approximately .04 percent of total body weight. See tables 2.16, 2.17, 2.18, 2.19, 2.22, and 2.23 for a summary of the functions, sources, and possible problems associated with macrominerals.

Calcium

Calcium is an important mineral for bone and tooth structure, blood clotting, and nerve transmission; it has a DRI of 1,000 milligrams per day for adult men and women. Deficiencies are associated with skeletal malformations (as in rickets), increased skeletal fragility (as in osteoporotic fracture and stress fractures), and blood pressure abnormalities. There are few reports of toxicity from taking high doses of calcium,

Table 2.16   Calcium Quick Guide

Symbol	Ca
Dietary Reference Intake (DRI)	Adult males: 1,000 mg/day Adult females: 1,000 mg/day
Recommended intake for athletes	1,300 to 1,500 mg/day
Functions	Bone structure and strength, acid–base balance, nerve function, muscle contraction, enzyme activation
Good food sources	Dairy products, dark green leafy vegetables, calcium-fortified orange juice and other calcium-fortified foods, soy milk, legumes
Deficiency	Osteoporosis, rickets, poor muscle function
Toxicity	Tolerable Upper Intake Level (UL): 2,500 mg/day for all age groups *Symptoms:* constipation, malabsorption of other bivalent minerals (iron, magnesium, and zinc), kidney stones, cardiac arrhythmia

but it is conceivable that a high and frequent intake of calcium supplements may alter the acidity of the stomach (making it more alkaline), thereby interfering with protein digestion. Since there is competitive absorption between bivalent minerals (calcium, zinc, iron, and magnesium) in the small intestine, it is also possible that a high amount of calcium may interfere with the absorption of other minerals if they are present in the gut at the same time. Therefore, taking high-dose calcium supplements with a meal that contains iron, for example, may result in the malabsorption of iron and eventually lead to iron-deficiency anemia.

Food sources of calcium include dairy products (milk, cheese, yogurt), dark green vegetables (collards, spinach, chard, mustard greens, broccoli, green peppers), and dried beans and peas (lentils, navy beans, soy beans, and split peas). Calcium and several other minerals (especially iron, magnesium, and zinc) are easily bound to the oxalic acid in dark green vegetables, making the minerals unavailable for absorption. Therefore, although dark green vegetables are potentially good sources of calcium and several other minerals, these foods don't make the minerals easily available to us unless they are properly prepared. Oxalate is water soluble, so by dipping the vegetables for a few seconds into boiling water (blanching), a good deal of the oxalate is removed but the minerals remain. The vegetables can then be prepared as needed. This technique dramatically improves the delivery of calcium from vegetables and has been used by cultures that have not traditionally consumed dairy products (especially in Asia) for thousands of years. As a side benefit, vegetables that are blanched may also be more acceptable to eat. Oxalic acid has a bitter taste. Therefore, removal of oxalate has the added benefit of making the vegetables more pleasant tasting.

Numerous studies have assessed the relationships among calcium intake, physical activity, and bone density. Athletes most often take calcium supplements to reduce the risk of fracture (i.e., by improving bone density), not for the purpose of improving physical performance. Physical activity is known to enhance bone density, just as physical inactivity is known to lower bone density. However, the development and mineralization of bone are complex processes involving several factors, including growth phase (childhood and adolescence are associated with faster bone development), hormonal status (especially estrogen for women), energy adequacy, vitamin D availability, and calcium intake.

Since the early 1990s, the increased availability of an accurate bone-density measuring device called DEXA (dual energy X-ray absorptiometry) has dramatically improved the ability to measure bone density and determine fracture risk. Studies that used DEXA indicate that children and adolescents who have a calcium intake at or slightly above the RDA (up to 1,500 milligrams) have higher bone densities. Adequate calcium intake in adults may not increase bone density, but it lays the groundwork for stabilizing the bone. It seems prudent, therefore, to make certain that calcium intake is maintained at the DRI level, that adequate physical activity is maintained (not a problem for most athletes), and that the intake of vitamin D is adequate. A survey of elite gymnasts indicates that sunlight exposure is more related to bone mineral density than is calcium intake. This points to the integrated relationship between calcium and vitamin D and how critical it is to have nutrients working together to ensure optimal health.[61]

Another concern of many female athletes is amenorrhea (cessation of menses), which is strongly associated with either poor bone development in young athletes or bone demineralization in older athletes. The causes of amenorrhea are complex and include inadequate energy intake, eating disorders, low body fat levels, poor iron status, psychological stress, high cortisol levels, and overtraining. Put simply, elite female athletes who train hard are at risk. Anything that might lower risk, such as maintaining a good iron status and consuming enough energy, is useful for lowering the risk of developing amenorrhea. Even if an amenorrheic athlete has sufficient calcium intake, that alone would not suffice to maintain or develop healthy bones because the lower level of circulating estrogen associated with amenorrhea would inhibit normal bone development or maintenance.

Phosphorus

Phosphorus is present in most foods and is especially plentiful in protein-rich foods (meat, poultry, fish, and dairy products) and cereal grains. It combines with calcium (about two parts calcium for every part phosphorus) to produce healthy bones and teeth. It also plays an important role in energy metabolism, affecting carbohydrate, fat, and protein. The energy derived for muscular work comes largely from phosphorus-containing compounds called adenosine triphosphate (ATP) and creatine phosphate (CP). As with calcium, the absorption of phosphorus is dependent on vitamin D, and the adult RDA is 700 milligrams per day.

Because phosphorus is so omnipresent in the food supply, phosphorus deficiencies are uncommon. If deficiencies occur, they are most likely to be seen in people on

Table 2.17   Phosphorus Quick Guide

Symbol	P
Dietary Reference Intake (DRI)	Adult males: 700 mg/day Adult females: 700 mg/day
Recommended intake for athletes	1,250 to 1,500 mg/day
Functions	Bone structure and strength, acid–base balance, B-vitamin function, component of ATP
Good food sources	All high-protein foods, whole grain products, carbonated beverages
Deficiency	Unlikely; if it occurs, results in low bone density and muscle weakness
Toxicity	Tolerable Upper Intake Level (UL): 3,000 mg for young children (age 1-8) and adults over 70 4,000 mg for children and adults (age 9-70) Toxicity is unlikely, but if it occurs, results in low bone density and GI distress

long-term antacids containing aluminum hydroxide.[62] This type of antacid binds with phosphorus, making it unavailable for absorption.[63] The adult UL for phosphorus is 4,000 milligrams per day, above which there may be interference with calcium absorption.

Phosphorus supplementation has been used for a long time to enhance physical activity. During World War I, Germany commonly provided its soldiers with high-phosphorus foods and supplements for the purpose of improving strength and endurance.[64] This large-population experience with phosphorus suggests that large doses of phosphorus are relatively well tolerated over time. However, there is no direct evidence that strength and endurance were actually improved with this high intake. The results of more recent studies on the effect of phosphorus supplementation yield mixed results. Runners, rowers, and swimmers taking 2 grams of sodium dihydrogen phosphate 1 hour before exercise all experienced performance improvements, while only half the unsupplemented athletes showed improvements.[65] Another study found that $\dot{V}O_2$max was improved on a treadmill test after short-term phosphorus supplementation.[66] However, a study evaluating the effect of phosphate supplementation on muscular power observed no apparent benefit from taking the phosphate.[67] The mixed results of these studies make it difficult to conclude that a preexercise supplement of phosphorus actually improves performance. Clearly, more well-designed studies are needed before an answer to this question can be attempted.

Magnesium

Magnesium, a mineral present in most foods, is essential for human metabolism and for maintaining the electrical potential in nerve and muscle cells. When associated with widespread malnutrition, especially in alcoholics, a magnesium deficiency results in tremors and convulsions. Magnesium is involved in more than 300 reactions in which food is synthesized to new products, and it is a critical component in the processes that create muscular energy from carbohydrate, protein, and fat.[68] The adult DRI for magnesium ranges between 310 and 320 milligrams per day for females and 400 and 420 milligrams per day for males. The safe upper limit for magnesium is similar to the DRI but represents the intake from supplement doses only and does not include the amount obtained from foods and water.

It is possible that athletes training in hot and humid environments could lose a relatively large amount of magnesium by sweating. Were this to occur, a magnesium deficiency could, given the importance of magnesium in muscle function processes, cause athletes to underachieve athletically. In one study where magnesium supplements were given to athletes, an improvement in physical performance was shown.[69] There is some limited evidence that taking magnesium supplements at the level of the DRI may positively affect endurance and strength performance in athletes with blood magnesium levels at the low end of the normal range.[70, 71] In a study assessing the effect of magnesium supplements (365 milligrams per day) on well-trained marathon runners, the supplements had no impact on performance, did not improve resistance to muscle breakdown, and did not enhance muscle recovery after the race.[72] With the exception of athletes who are known to reduce total energy intake to maintain or lower body weight (wrestlers, gymnasts, figure skaters), it appears that

Table 2.18 Magnesium Quick Guide

Symbol	Mg
Dietary Reference Intake (DRI)	Adult males: 420 mg/day Adult females: 320 mg/day
Recommended intake for athletes	400 to 450 mg/day if from food sources; 350 mg/day if from supplements
Functions	Protein synthesis, glucose metabolism, bone structure, muscle contraction
Good food sources	Milk and milk products, meat, nuts, whole grains, dark green leafy vegetables, fruits
Deficiency	Unlikely; if it occurs, results in muscle weakness, muscle cramps, and cardiac arrhythmia
Toxicity	Tolerable Upper Intake Level (UL): 350 mg if taken as supplements *Symptoms:* nausea, vomiting, diarrhea

most male athletes consume the DRI or more, and most female athletes consume at least 60 percent of the magnesium DRI.[73, 74] The limited number of studies assessing magnesium and performance suggest that this level of intake is sufficient to sustain athletic performance and that supplemental intake does little or nothing to enhance performance when magnesium tissue levels are at or near normal.

Sodium

Sodium is an essential mineral commonly referred to as salt. (Table salt is actually a combination of sodium and chloride.) It is involved in body water balance and acid–base balance and is the major extracellular (outside the cell, including blood and fluid) mineral. Sodium is present in small quantities in most natural foods and is found in high amounts in processed, canned, cooked, and fast foods. Although most people are capable of excreting excess sodium, some individuals are sodium sensitive because they lack this capacity. In these people, excess sodium retention causes edema (an excess accumulation of extracellular fluid) and contributes to high blood pressure. Sodium-sensitive individuals can limit intake by concentrating food choices on natural, whole foods and avoiding high-sodium (i.e., salty) commercially prepared foods. Food labels provide information about sodium content (see table 2.20). The 2004 Institute of Medicine's recommendation for sodium intake is 1.5 grams per day,[75] while the tolerable upper limit (UL) is 2.3 grams of sodium per day.

One of the key ingredients in sports beverages is sodium because it helps drive the desire to drink and because it helps maintain blood volume. Maintenance of blood volume is a key factor in athletic performance; it is related to the ability to deliver nutrients to cells, to the removal of metabolic by-products from cells, and to the maintenance of the sweat rate. Additional information on sodium is included in chapter 3.

Table 2.19 Sodium Quick Guide

Symbol	Na
Adequate Intake (AI)	Adult males: 1.5 g/day Adult females: 1.5 g/day
Recommended intake for athletes	>1.5 g/day; high sweat losses of sodium may increase requirement to >10 g/day
Functions	Water balance, nerve function, acid–base balance, muscle contraction
Good food sources	Processed and canned foods, pickles, potato chips, pretzels, soy sauce, cheese
Deficiency	Hyponatremia, with muscle cramping, nausea, vomiting, anorexia, seizures, and coma (potentially extremely dangerous)
Toxicity	Tolerable Upper Intake Level (UL): 2.3 g/day (about 5.8 g of table salt); athletes may have a requirement that far exceeds the UL Major symptom: hypertension

Table 2.20 Sodium on Food Labels: Understanding the Terms

Term	Definition
Sodium-free	Less than 5 mg of sodium per standard serving
Low sodium	• 140 mg of sodium or less per standard serving • If the serving weighs 30 g or less, 140 mg sodium or less per 50 g of food • If the serving is 2 tbsp or less, 140 mg sodium or less per 50 g of food
Very low sodium	• 35 mg of sodium or less per standard serving • If the serving weighs 30 g or less, 35 mg of sodium or less per 50 g of food • If the serving is 2 tbsp or less, 35 mg sodium or less per 50 g of food
Reduced or less sodium	A minimum of 25% lower sodium content than the food it is compared with

Because of sweat losses, athletes are likely to require more than the 1.5 grams of sodium recommended for the general public. On hot and humid days when sweat losses of sodium are high, athletes may require more than 10 grams of sodium per day, a level that dramatically exceeds the UL of 2.3 grams per day. Therefore, the Institute of Medicine's recommendation for sodium intake is not applicable to most athletes and should not be followed. On the contrary, athletes should regularly consume salty foods and beverages when exercising or competing in hot and humid conditions. The higher athlete requirement for salt is recognized in the recommendations of the Institute of Medicine, which state that the general recommendation is not applicable to those who sweat regularly.[76]

Chloride

Chloride is an extracellular mineral that is essential for the maintenance of fluid balance and, therefore, normal cell function. It is also an important component of gastric juices. Virtually all the chloride we consume is associated with table salt (sodium chloride), so sodium and chloride intakes parallel each other. Because chloride losses are closely linked to sodium losses, a deficiency of one is related to a deficiency of the other. Deficiencies typically occur with heavy sweating, frequent diarrhea, or frequent vomiting.[76] Sweat losses are likely to deplete chloride and sodium to a greater degree than other minerals, including potassium and magnesium.[77] Most people consume excessive amounts of salt (which is 60 percent chloride), so chloride intake is typically 6,000 milligrams (6 grams) or more, a level that is well above normal requirements.[76] The DRI-estimated chloride requirement is 2.3 grams per day for both adult men and women, while the safe upper limit for chloride is 3.6 grams per day. Excess chloride and sodium may both contribute to the development of hypertension.

Hyponatremia

A failure to consume sufficient sodium when fluid and sodium losses are high can lead to hyponatremia. The word *hyponatremia* literally means low (hypo) sodium (Na) in the blood (emia). This condition commonly results from the production of a large volume of sweat, which contains both sodium and water, and the consumption of a replacement fluid that has an inadequate concentration of sodium. The sodium dilution that results leads to a reduced blood volume, which is the cause of the symptoms of hyponatremia. The sodium concentration of sweat varies greatly between individual athletes but typically falls within the range of 2.25 to 3.4 grams of sodium per liter of sweat. Given the volume of sweat that can be lost during a race (may exceed well over 1 liter per hour), it is conceivable that an athlete could lose more than 40 grams of sodium over the course of an Ironman competition. If the fluid replacement the athlete chooses has no sodium or is too low in sodium, hyponatremia can result. (See table 2.21 for a summary of the different forms of hyponatremia.)

It has been suggested that commonly consumed NSAIDs (aspirin, ibuprofen) and any substances that induce a diuretic effect may alter kidney function in a way that exacerbates the risk of hyponatremia during long-duration events.[11] Hyponatremia can be caused by many medications, and athletes should check with their doctors regarding the medications they use. Given the very real risks associated with hyponatremia, all reasonable steps should be taken to avoid this condition.

(continued)

Table 2.21 Different Forms of Hyponatremia

Hypovolemic hyponatremia	Total body water (TBW) decreases; total body sodium (Na^+) decreases to a greater extent. The extracellular fluid (ECF) volume is decreased. This is likely to be the most common form seen in long-endurance events, and it occurs as sodium and body water are lost and replaced by inappropriately hypotonic fluids, such as tap water. Sodium may also be lost through renal or nonrenal routes. Nonrenal routes include GI losses, excessive sweating, and body water shifts from peritonitis, pancreatitis, and burns.
Euvolemic hyponatremia	TBW increases while total sodium remains normal. The ECF volume is increased minimally to moderately, but edema is not present. Euvolemic hyponatremia suggests that sodium stores are normal but that there is a total body excess of free water. This occurs in people who consume excess fluids.
Hypervolemic hyponatremia	Total body sodium increases, and TBW increases to a greater extent. The ECF is increased markedly, and edema is present. This occurs when sodium stores are excessive, usually a result of renal malfunction, such as acute or chronic renal failure, when kidneys are unable to excrete the excess ingested sodium.
Redistributive hyponatremia	Water shifts from the intracellular to the extracellular compartment, with a resultant dilution of sodium. The TBW and total body sodium are unchanged. This condition occurs with hyperglycemia.
Pseudo-hyponatremia	The blood volume is diluted by excessive proteins or lipids. The TBW and total body sodium are unchanged. This condition is seen with hypertriglyceridemia and multiple myeloma.

Used with permission from eMedicine.com, Inc., 2005. Craig S. Hyponatremia. *eMedicine Journal* [serial online]. 2005. Available at: http://www.emedicine.com/EMERG/topic275.htm. [January 20, 2005].

Hyponatremia becomes physiologically important when free water shifts from the blood to the intracellular space. Cellular edema, although well tolerated by many tissues, is not well tolerated by the brain. Therefore, the serious symptoms of hyponatremia are related mainly to cerebral edema. Hyponatremia symptoms include nausea, cramping, slurred speech, disorientation, and general confusion. If allowed to progress, athletes may experience coma and death. Put simply, hyponatremia is a potentially fatal condition that can be avoided if athletes consume only sodium-containing beverages and avoid plain water during a long-duration event.

Athletes experiencing any of the initial symptoms of hyponatremia, such as muscle cramping, may find that consumption of salty foods and sodium-containing sports beverages satisfactorily resolves the symptoms. However, slurred speech, disorientation, and confusion are serious symptoms that require immediate medical attention.[78]

Table 2.22   Chloride Quick Guide

Symbol	Cl
Dietary Reference Intake (DRI)	Adult males: 2.3 g/day Adult females: 2.3 g/day
Recommended intake for athletes	2.3 g/day or more to match the increase in sodium intake with high sweat losses
Functions	Water balance, nerve function, parietal cell (stomach) HCl production
Good food sources	Table salt (~60% chloride and 40% sodium)
Deficiency	Associated with frequent vomiting; although rare, may lead to convulsions
Toxicity	Tolerable Upper Intake Level (UL): 3,500 mg/day, or the equivalent of 5,800 mg of table salt Cl intake is associated with sodium intake, so an excess intake is typically associated with hypertension (from the sodium)

Potassium

Potassium is the main mineral found inside cells (an intracellular electrolyte) at a concentration that is 30 times greater than the concentration of potassium found outside cells. It is involved in water balance, nerve impulse transmission, and muscular contractions. Dietary deficiency is rare and typically occurs only with chronic diarrhea and vomiting or laxative abuse. Individuals taking medications for high blood pressure force the loss of sodium, and in this process potassium is also lost. These individuals are encouraged to replace this lost potassium through the intake of potassium supplements or foods high in potassium (fruits, vegetables, and meats). Typical intakes of potassium range from 1,000 to 11,000 milligrams per day (1 to 11 grams per day); people consuming large amounts of fresh fruits and vegetables have the highest intakes.

There is evidence that a potassium intake of about 3,500 milligrams per day is useful in controlling high blood pressure.[76] Adequate intakes of potassium help counteract the impact of excess sodium intake, thereby helping to control high blood pressure. It also reduces the risk of developing a lower bone density and lowers the risk of developing kidney stones.[76] The DRI for potassium is 4.7 grams per day for both adult men and women. Although there is no established safe upper limit, potassium toxicity appears to develop with an intake of approximately 18 grams and may lead to cardiac arrest.[76] People with chronic renal disease or diabetes appear to be at particular risk of death from hyperkalemia, most often resulting from high intake of salt substitutes or potassium supplements. Because of the risk of sudden cardiac arrest with an excess potassium intake, potassium supplementation is generally not recommended.

Table 2.23   **Potassium Quick Guide**

Symbol	K
Dietary Reference Intake (DRI)	Adult males: 4.7 g/day Adult females: 4.7 g/day
Recommended intake for athletes	4.7 g/day or more with high levels of sweat loss
Functions	Water balance, glucose delivery to cells
Good food sources	Citrus fruits, potatoes, vegetables, milk, meat, fish, bananas
Deficiency	Hypokalemia, which is associated with anorexia, arrythmias, and muscle cramping
Toxicity	Hyperkalemia, a condition that may lead to arrythmias and altered heart function (may lead to death) Potassium supplements are generally NOT recommended for this reason.

It is well established that potassium is critical for heart and skeletal muscle function. However, the relatively small amount of potassium lost in sweat does not seriously affect body stores, so it does not typically have an impact on athletic performance in well-nourished athletes.[79]

Microminerals

Microminerals (trace elements) are present in body tissues in extremely small amounts but have critically important roles to play in human nutrition. The required intake of each micromineral is less than 100 milligrams per day, and the total body content of these minerals is less than 5 grams. They include iron, zinc, iodine, selenium, copper, manganese, and chromium. See tables 2.24 and 2.27 through 2.32 for a summary of the functions, sources, and possible problems associated with microminerals.

Iron

Iron is needed to form the oxygen-transporting compounds hemoglobin (in blood) and myoglobin (in muscle) and is also found in a number of other compounds involved in normal tissue function. Iron absorption is limited because there is no effective mechanism for excreting the excess once it is absorbed. To a large degree, the amount absorbed is driven by the amount of iron in storage (in ferritin and hemosiderin). The lower the iron storage level, the higher the rate of iron absorption; however, overall absorption rates rarely go above 10 to 15 percent of the iron content of consumed food. This variable absorption mechanism is aimed at maintaining a relatively constant level of iron while avoiding an excess iron uptake. Despite this variable absorption rate, people with marginal iron intakes are at risk of developing iron deficiency and, eventually, iron-deficiency anemia.

Iron-deficiency anemia is characterized by poor oxygen-carrying capacity, a condition that causes endurance problems in athletes. Iron deficiency is also associated with poor immune function, short attention span, irritability, and poor learning ability. In the United States, children experiencing fast growth, women of menstrual age, vegetarians, and pregnant women are at increased risk for developing iron-deficiency anemia. Periods of growth and pregnancy are associated with a higher requirement of iron because of a fast expansion of the blood volume, and iron is an essential component of red blood cells. Women of childbearing age have higher requirements because of the regular blood (and iron) losses associated with the menstrual period. For this reason, women of childbearing age have a higher DRI for iron (18 milligrams) than do men of the same age (8 milligrams). Some people are at risk of developing iron toxicity because they are missing the mechanisms for limiting absorption. Young children in particular may be at risk for iron toxicity if they ingest supplements intended for adults. Although the iron DRI for children (~7 to 10 milligrams per day) is similar to that for male adults, many iron supplements intended for adults contain iron levels more than 300 percent of the DRI. Iron overload disease is potentially fatal.

Iron is available in a wide variety of foods, including meats, eggs, vegetables, and iron-fortified cereals. Milk and other dairy products are poor sources of iron. The most easily absorbed form of iron is "heme" iron, which comes from meats and other foods of animal origin. Nonheme iron, which is not as easily absorbed, is found in fruits, vegetables, and cereals. However, nonheme iron absorption may be enhanced by consuming foods high in vitamin C. On the other hand, nonheme iron absorption may be inhibited by phytic acid (a substance associated with bran in cereal grains), antacids, and calcium phosphate. In general, red meats are considered to provide the most abundant and easily absorbable source of iron. For this reason, vegetarians

Table 2.24   Iron Quick Guide

Symbol	Fe (Fe^{2+} = ferrous iron; Fe^{3+} = ferric iron)
Dietary Reference Intake (DRI)	Adult males: 8 mg/day Adult females: 18 mg/day
Recommended intake for athletes	15 to 18 mg/day
Functions	Oxygen delivery (as hemoglobin and myoglobin), part of numerous oxidative enzymes, essential for aerobic metabolism
Good food sources	Meat, fish, poultry, and shellfish; lesser amounts in legumes, dark green leafy vegetables, and dried fruit; cast-iron cookware increases iron content of cooked foods
Deficiency	Fatigue, lower infection resistance, low energy metabolism (with possible hypothermia)
Toxicity	Toxic levels of tissue iron (hemochromatosis) and liver damage

are considered to be at increased risk of iron-deficiency anemia. Nevertheless, with proper planning; consumption of vegetables, iron-fortified grain products, and fruits high in iron; and sound cooking techniques that aid iron absorption, vegetarians can obtain sufficient iron. Table 2.25 lists a few ways to improve iron absorption in a vegetarian diet.

Iron Status and Athletic Performance   Athletes have good reason to be concerned about iron status because oxygen-carrying capacity and oxidative enzyme function are critical factors in physical endurance. Iron deficiency is one of the most common nutrient deficiencies of the general public, and it appears that iron deficiency and iron-deficiency anemia have the same incidence level in athletes.[80] (See table 2.26 for common causes of iron deficiency in athletes.)

Dietary Intake   The dietary intake of athletes, particularly endurance athletes, typically focuses on carbohydrate foods and diminishes the intake of meats. This eating pattern is generally associated as ideal from the perspective of providing an optimal distribution of energy substrates, but it may marginalize the intake of iron. Meat clearly provides a higher concentration of iron than other foods, despite the fact that cereal grains are currently fortified with iron as a public health measure to lower iron-deficiency anemia prevalence. Vegetarian athletes, through their avoidance of foods that are highest in iron, are at greatest risk for deficiency.

Low Iron Absorption   Iron absorption is relatively low (rarely more than 10 percent of total dietary consumption), even in those with the greatest need. The absorption of iron is enhanced by the intake of meat and diminished by the intake of nonmeat foods. In addition, certain components of vegetables (oxalic acid) and cereals (phytic acid) bind iron and other divalent minerals and make them unavailable for absorption.

Table 2.25   Maximizing Iron Intake in a Vegetarian Diet

Food type	Normal absorption	Improving absorption rate
Vegetables (all varieties)	Contain iron in the nonheme form, which has a lower rate of absorption than iron in meats.	Add vitamin C to the vegetables by squeezing lemon or orange juice on them before eating.
Dark green vegetables	Contain iron, but also contain oxalic acid, which reduces availability of iron for absorption.	To remove the oxalic acid, blanch the vegetables by putting in a pot of boiling water for 5 to 10 seconds. Much of the oxalate is removed, but the iron remains.
High-fiber cereals (with a high bran content)	Contain large amounts of phytic acid, which binds with iron and reduces the availability for absorption.	To maximize absorption, replace bran-added cereals in the diet with whole grain cereals.

Table 2.26 Summary of Iron-Deficiency Causes in Athletes

Low dietary intake of iron	Athletes may consume foods containing an inadequate level of iron.
Consumption of foods with low iron absorption rates	Vegetable sources of iron have lower iron concentrations and lower iron absorption rates than meats.
Increased iron losses (hematuria)	Red blood cell breakdown may occur at a faster rate because of higher intravascular compression, resulting in hemolysis. This may result in small amounts of iron (as hemoglobin and myoglobin) being lost in the urine because of a rupturing of red blood cells.
Loss of iron in sweat	Iron losses in sweat are low but may contribute to iron deficiency in athletes with marginal iron intakes.
Loss of iron from bleeding	A loss of blood, through GI losses or through abnormal menstrual losses, increases iron-deficiency risk.
Dilutional pseudoanemia (also commonly referred to as sports anemia)	Physical training results in an expansion of the blood volume, which may result in a dilution, albeit temporarily, of red blood cells.

Iron is competitively absorbed with other divalent minerals (most notably calcium, magnesium, and zinc), so an excessive intake of one or more of these minerals may diminish the absorption rate of iron. Given the common supplementary intake of calcium in particular, reduced iron absorption may be likely.

Increased Red Blood Cell Breakdown   A number of studies have documented higher rates of intravascular hemolysis in athletes than in nonathletes.[81] Hemolysis occurs when exertional forces cause a ballistic and premature breakdown of red blood cells (RBCs). Athletes have RBCs with a life expectancy of approximately 80 days, while in nonathletes RBCs last approximately 120 days. Runners, because of frequent foot strike, and other athletes involved in concussive sports may be at increased risk of hemolysis, but hemolysis has also been documented in swimmers and dancers.[76] The importance of foot strike on hemolysis is evident—the phrase "foot-strike hemolysis" is commonly used to describe this condition. Typically, the harder the surface the runner works out on, the greater the potential for hemolysis.[81, 82]

Loss of Iron in Sweat   The concentration of iron in sweat is low (approximately .2 milligrams per liter of sweat), but the sweat loss in long-duration activities may be sufficiently high (possibly more than 2 liters of sweat per hour) that a significant amount of iron can be lost.[83] Although it appears that those athletes engaging in extremely long-duration training sessions are at risk of losing a substantial amount of iron through this route, other athletes are likely to have negligible iron losses through sweat.[84]

Loss of Iron From Blood Loss   Loss of blood is typically from menstrual losses or through the gastrointestinal tract. Of course, athletes who donate blood also lose a significant amount of iron. Blood loss through the GI tract appears to be significant and has been found in up to 85 percent of athletes engaged in intense endurance events.[85] It seems likely that nonsteroidal anti-inflammatory drugs (NSAIDs) such as aspirin and ibuprofen, frequently taken by athletes to control muscle pain, may result in a degree of GI tract irritation and blood loss.[81]

Dilutional Pseudoanemia (Sports Anemia)   Sports anemia is experienced by most athletes, typically at the beginning of an intensive training period. The initiation of intensive training is associated with an enlargement of the blood volume, which causes a dilution of the blood constituents. Because there is no reduction in blood constituents, as occurs with any form of blood loss, oxygen-carrying capacity remains at previous levels (thus the name pseudoanemia). After several weeks, the constituents of the blood (including red blood cells) have an opportunity to increase so as to normalize their concentrations. Exhaustive exercise typically results in a reduction in plasma volume, which experiences a positive recovery and expansion after rehydration in the postexercise period.[86] Harder training, particularly in endurance activities, is associated with the greatest plasma volume increase and will persist for up to 5 days after exercise cessation.[81] True iron-deficiency anemia is associated with a smaller red cell volume (i.e., lower mean cell volume, or MCV) and lower stored iron (i.e., lower ferritin), but athletic pseudoanemia is not associated with either of these biomarkers.

Iron Deficiency and Iron-Deficiency Anemia   Athletes should make every effort to avoid an iron-deficient state because oxygen-carrying capacity is of central importance for athletic endurance. Besides its obvious importance in oxygen transport, iron is also important in a large number of energy-transport enzymes and is also involved in normal nerve and behavioral function and in immune function.[87]

Iron deficiency is seen in approximately 20 percent of females of childbearing age and has a much smaller incidence (1 to 5 percent) in postmenopausal females and males.[88] Iron deficiency with anemia (i.e., low hemoglobin, low hematocrit, low MCV, low ferritin) has a lower prevalence (1 to 3 percent of the population). Athletes may have a higher prevalence of iron deficiency but not iron-deficiency anemia. Further, athletes might respond differently to the presence of frank anemia (reduction in the number and size of red blood cells) versus iron-deficiency anemia (low serum iron and low stored iron but normal red blood cells).[89] Those at highest risk for iron-deficiency anemia appear to be elite endurance runners, although the condition has been reported in virtually every athlete group that has been assessed.[90, 91]

Although iron-deficient athletes are known to experience a performance deficit, there appears to be no benefit in providing iron supplements to athletes who have a normal iron status.[92] Further, iron supplementation is often associated with nausea, constipation, and stomach irritation. However, in athletes with blood tests that demonstrate either an anemia or a marginal level of stored iron, iron supplementation is warranted. The usual iron replacement therapy is to provide oral ferrous sulfate, but in athletes with GI distress, ferrous gluconate can be used and appears to be better tolerated. Intermuscular injections of iron are generally not recommended because of their association with potentially serious side effects.[81]

The frequency of iron supplement intake remains a topic of ongoing debate. Some suggest that the best means of providing iron supplements to reduce the chance of potential negative side effects is to take 25 to 50 milligrams every third or fourth day instead of daily doses.[93] This approach may prevent GI distress and may impart the same benefits seen with daily supplementation. Of course, taking iron supplements in the absence of iron deficiency or iron-deficiency anemia should be avoided. Besides increasing the risk of hemochromatosis (iron overload disease), which may affect 1 percent of people of northern European descent, iron supplementation may mask celiac disease and colon cancer.[94] Excess iron stores may be observed among professional road cyclists who habitually consume excessive iron supplements.[95]

Zinc

Zinc helps form a large number of enzymes, many of which function in energy metabolism and in wound healing. Inadequate dietary intake of zinc causes a variety of health problems, including stunted growth, slow wound healing, and failure of the immune system.[96] Zinc also plays an important role in the removal of carbon dioxide from cells and is part of an important antioxidant enzyme called superoxide dismutase. Excessive intake can lead to anemia, vomiting, and immune system failure.

Table 2.27 Zinc Quick Guide

Symbol	Zn
Dietary Reference Intake (DRI)	Adult males: 11 mg/day Adult females: 8 mg/day
Recommended intake for athletes	11 to 15 mg/day
Functions	Part of numerous enzymes involved in energy metabolism, protein synthesis, immune function, sensory function, and sexual maturation
Good food sources	Meat, fish, poultry, shellfish, eggs, whole grain foods, vegetables, nuts
Deficiency	Impaired wound healing and immune function, anorexia, failure to thrive (in children), dry skin
Toxicity	Tolerable Upper Intake Level (UL): 40 mg/day *Symptoms:* impaired immune system, slow wound healing, hypogeusia, hyposmia, high LDL:HDL cholesterol ratio, nausea

Meat, liver, eggs, and seafood are good sources of zinc. The adult RDA for zinc is 12 to 15 milligrams per day.

Zinc levels at the lower end of the normal range, or lower, have been observed in male and female endurance runners. Athletes with lower serum zinc values had lower training mileage, probably from not being able to train as hard, than those who had higher values.[97-99] Therefore, there appear to be training deficits in the small number of athletes who have poor zinc status. The effect of zinc supplementation on performance has not been extensively studied, and the level of supplementation in these studies has been extremely high (around 135 milligrams per day). Also, the athletes tested were not assessed for zinc status before the initiation of the research protocol. Nevertheless, this intake level did lead to an improvement in both muscular strength and endurance.[100] A recent study of elite athletes found an important positive relationship between normal zinc status and the athletes' ability to respond to the antioxidant mechanisms associated with intense exercise.[101] Perhaps the greatest potential problem associated with inadequate zinc is in athletes who have inadequate diets and who also use sweat loss as a means of achieving desirable weight. Athletes, usually gymnasts and wrestlers, with inadequate diets and heavy sweat losses are reported to have impaired growth and zinc deficiency.[102]

Athletes should be cautioned that chronically high zinc intakes have never been tested over time and may well have negative side effects. Toxicity and malabsorption of other nutrients are both likely and possible with high supplemental intake.[103-105]

Iodine

Iodine is needed to synthesize a key hormone of the thyroid gland, thyroxine, which is involved in regulating metabolic rate, growth, and development. An iodine deficiency leads to goiter, a swelling of the thyroid gland in the front of the neck. Goiter

Table 2.28   Iodine Quick Guide

Symbol	I
Dietary Reference Intake (DRI)	Adult males: 150 mcg/day Adult females: 150 mcg/day
Recommended intake for athletes	120 to 150 mcg/day
Functions	Forms thyroid hormone thyroxine, which is involved in metabolism control
Good food sources	Iodized salt and seafood (depending on soil, some vegetables may also be good sources)
Deficiency	Goiter (enlarged thyroid gland with inadequate thyroxine production), with associated obesity
Toxicity	Inadequate thyroxine production

was once common in the United States, but the use of iodized salt has eliminated the condition in this country. An excessive intake of iodine depresses thyroid activity, so taking supplemental doses of iodine is not recommended.

Selenium

Selenium is an important mineral antioxidant in human nutrition. Since exercise (particularly endurance exercise) is associated with an increased production of potentially damaging oxidative by-products (peroxides and free radicals) in muscle fibers, it is possible that selenium may play a role in reducing muscular oxidative stress.[106] A selenium deficiency may result in muscle weakness and increased recovery time after exhaustive exercise.[107] There is little evidence, however, that increasing the intake of supplemental selenium increases exercise performance.[108] The adult male and female DRI for selenium is 55 micrograms per day. Nutritional supplements, including sodium selenite and high-selenium yeast, are effective sources of selenium, but excessive intake may be toxic, so proper care in taking appropriate supplement levels is important. The safe upper limit is set at 400 micrograms per day for adults, with brittle hair and nails a sign of toxicity.

Table 2.29   Selenium Quick Guide

Symbol	Se
Dietary Reference Intake (DRI)	Adult males: 55 mcg/day Adult females: 55 mcg/day
Recommended intake for athletes	50 to 55 mcg/day
Functions	Antioxidant (part of glutathione peroxidase)
Good food sources	Meat, fish, seafood, whole grain foods, nuts (depending on soil, some vegetables may also be good sources)
Deficiency	Unlikely; if it occurs, results in heart damage
Toxicity	Tolerable Upper Intake Level (UL): 400 mcg/day for adults (lower for children) Toxicity is rare; if it occurs, results in nausea, GI distress, and hair loss

Copper

Among the more important trace elements is copper, which is present in many enzymes and in copper-containing proteins found in the blood, brain, and liver. Copper is important for preventing oxidative damage to cells through the enzyme *superoxide dismutase*. Deficiency is associated with the failure to use iron in the formation of hemoglobin and myoglobin. The adult DRI for copper is 900 micrograms per day, and the safe upper limit for adults is set at 10,000 micrograms per day. Excess consumption may result in GI distress or liver damage. Good sources of copper include shellfish, soybean products, legumes, nuts, seeds, liver, and potatoes. As another good example of why nutritional balance is important, excessive consumption of calcium, phosphate, iron, zinc, and vitamin C all reduce copper absorption.

Very few studies have been performed on the relationship between copper and athletic performance. Studies of blood copper concentrations in athletes and non-athletes have not revealed any significant differences, but the athletes have a slightly higher (3 to 4 percent) concentration of serum copper than do nonathletes.[109] In a study evaluating the copper status of swimmers during a competitive season, there was no difference in pre- and postseason copper status. In this study, the majority of swimmers were consuming adequate levels of copper (more than 1 milligram per day) from food.[110]

Table 2.30 Copper Quick Guide

Symbol	Cu
Dietary Reference Intake (DRI)	Adult males: 900 mcg/day Adult females: 900 mcg/day
Recommended intake for athletes	900 mcg/day
Functions	Part of iron-transport protein ceruloplasmin, oxidation reactions
Good food sources	Meat, fish, poultry, shellfish, eggs, nuts, whole grain foods, bananas
Deficiency	Rare; if it occurs, results in anemia (inability to transport iron to red blood cells)
Toxicity	Tolerable Upper Intake Level (UL): 10 mg/day Toxicity is rare; if it occurs, leads to nausea and vomiting

Manganese

Manganese is a trace mineral involved in bone formation, immune function, antioxidant activity, and carbohydrate metabolism.[111] Although manganese deficiency is rare, deficiencies are associated with skeletal problems (undermineralized bone and increased risk of fracture) and poor wound healing. It appears that the greatest risk of deficiency is found in people on diets (inadequate intake) or where malabsorption occurs. Manganese is in competition with calcium, iron, and zinc for absorption, so an excess intake of these other minerals may decrease manganese absorption and lead to deficiency symptoms. Much like iron, manganese absorption is enhanced with vitamin C and meat intake. Food sources of manganese include coffee, tea, chocolate, whole grains, nuts, seeds, soybeans, dried beans (navy beans, lentils, split peas), liver, and

Table 2.31   **Manganese Quick Guide**

Symbol	Mn
Dietary Reference Intake (DRI)	Adult males: 2.3 mg/day Adult females: 1.8 mg/day
Recommended intake for athletes	2.0 to 2.5 mg/day
Functions	Energy metabolism, fat synthesis, bone structure
Good food sources	Whole grain foods, legumes, green leafy vegetables, bananas
Deficiency	Poor growth and development in children
Toxicity	Tolerable Upper Intake Level (UL): 11 mg/day *Symptoms:* neurological problems, confusion, easy fatigue

fruits. As with several other minerals, the intake of foods high in oxalic acid (present in dark green leafy vegetables) may inhibit manganese absorption. (See calcium section on pages 56-58 for ways of reducing the oxalic acid content of foods.) The adult DRI for manganese is 2.3 milligrams per day for men and 1.8 milligrams per day for women. The safe upper limit is set at 11 milligrams per day for both men and women, with an excess intake causing neurological symptoms. As with copper, excessive intakes of calcium, phosphorus, iron, zinc, fiber, and oxalic acid all decrease manganese absorption.

Chromium

Chromium is also known as glucose tolerance factor (GTF) because of its involvement in helping cells use glucose. Chromium deficiency is associated with poor blood glucose maintenance (either hypo- or hyperglycemia), an excessive production of insulin (hyperinsulinemia), excessive fatigue, and a craving for sweet foods. (Hypoglycemia is low blood sugar; hyperglycemia is high blood sugar). It is also associated with irritability (a common condition with poor blood glucose control), weight gain, adult-onset diabetes, and increased risk of cardiovascular disease.[112] There is some evidence that frequent intense exercise, which is common for serious athletes, may increase the risk of chromium deficiency. High consumption of simple sugars (sweets) may also place people at risk for deficiency. Dietary sources of chromium include whole grain breads and cereals, and meats. Nutritional supplements, commonly in the form of chromium picolinate, are taken as a means of reducing weight or body fat, but studies on this supplement have produced mixed results. Initial studies of chromium picolinate supplementation suggest that this supplement is effective for increasing muscle mass and decreasing body fat in bodybuilders and football players.[113] However, subsequent controlled studies have failed to reach the same conclusions.[114, 115] Other

Table 2.32   **Chromium Quick Guide**

Symbol	Cr
Dietary Reference Intake (DRI)	Adult males: 35 mcg/day Adult females: 25 mcg/day
Recommended intake for athletes	30 to 35 mcg/day
Functions	Glucose tolerance (glucose–insulin control)
Good food sources	Brewer's yeast, mushrooms, whole grain foods, nuts, legumes, cheese
Deficiency	Glucose intolerance
Toxicity	Unlikely

supplements for chromium include chromium polynicotinate, chromium chloride, and high-chromium yeast. The adult DRI for chromium is 25 micrograms per day for females and 35 micrograms per day for males. There is no established safe upper limit, although an excess intake may result in chronic renal failure.

Because chromium is not well absorbed, there is little evidence to suggest that an excessive intake of chromium will result in toxicity. However, the toxicity of chromium has not been directly tested, so athletes should be cautious about taking supplements. One study suggests that chromium picolinate has the potential to alter DNA and thus produce mutated, cancerous cells.[116] Taken together, studies of this trace mineral suggest that to maintain optimal chromium nutriture, athletes should consume foods low in sugar and a diet that contains whole grains and some meat (if not a vegetarian).

3 | Fluids and Electrolytes

Perhaps the single most important factor associated with sustaining a high level of athletic performance is maintenance of fluid balance during exercise. Despite this, most athletes experience deterioration in hydration state (with a resultant drop in blood volume) during training and competition. Studies demonstrate that, even in the presence of available fluids, athletes experience a degree of voluntary dehydration that has an inevitably negative impact on performance. Given the tremendous amount of heat that must be dissipated during exercise through sweat evaporation, athletes have no reasonable alternative for sustaining exercise performance other than to pursue strategies that can sustain the hydration state. A failure to do so will result in premature fatigue and may also lead to potentially life-threatening heatstroke. This chapter discusses the strategies related to achieving and sustaining an optimal hydration state and reviews studies that have assessed the optimal concentration of carbohydrate and electrolytes for the "ideal" sports beverage.

Water is the main component of blood, which delivers oxygen, nutrients, hormones, and a multitude of other substances to cells and removes metabolic by-products from cells. Water also has a protective function, cushioning the spinal cord and brain from sudden-impact injury, and is a critical component of our temperature regulation mechanism. Water and its electrolyte components are involved in the control of osmotic pressure, regulating the amount of fluid inside and outside cells. (See table 3.1 for a breakdown of the body's water composition.)

Well-hydrated athletes are referred to as being euhydrated or normohydrated; those with below-normal body water levels are referred to as hypohydrated or, if severe, dehydrated; and those with above-normal body water levels are referred to as hyperhydrated. We have systems for the normal control of body water levels, involving an increased retention of body water or an increased loss of body water, all mediated through a series of hormones stimulated by osmoreceptors that monitor blood osmolality and volume receptors that monitor the volume of extracellular water.

Excretion of fluids and metabolic by-products is a main function of the kidneys, which are stimulated by hormones and enzymes to adjust the volume of water and electrolytes excreted or retained. The concentration of sodium is a primary influence on the osmolality of extracellular fluid, which is maintained within a narrow range. Because sweat is hypotonic, prolonged exercise results in a higher plasma osmolality (more water is lost than sodium). As a means of preserving body water volume, urine production during and shortly after exercise is slightly decreased.[1, 2]

If the blood has a relatively high concentration of sodium, protein, or glucose per unit volume of fluid (i.e., is hypertonic), water is drawn from cells to normalize the concentration of electrolytes. Receptors in the hypothalamus detect the fact that the blood is hypertonic through its osmoreceptors, which leads to the release of antidiuretic hormone (ADH) from the pituitary gland. ADH forces the kidneys to reabsorb more water by producing a more concentrated urine.[3] For this reason, a common test for adequate hydration status is urine color, with dark urine indicating a greater degree of underhydration than light urine. The osmoreceptors can also induce the sensation of thirst, although this sensation rarely occurs before the loss of 1.5 to 2.0 liters of water (1 liter equals approximately 1 quart; see table 3.2). Since

Table 3.1   **Where's the Water?**

- 66% of a person's total body weight is from water.
- 65% of total body water is intracellular.
- 35% of total body water is extracellular.
- Well-hydrated muscles are about 75% water.
- Bones are about 32% water.
- Fat is essentially anhydrous, having only about 10% water content.
- Blood is about 93% water.
- Average males are about 60% water weight.
- Average females are about 50% water weight.
- Obese individuals are about 40% water weight.
- Athletes are about 70% water weight.

Note: The higher the musculature and the lower the body fat, the higher the contribution of body water to total body mass.

Table 3.2 Common Conversions

- To convert Fahrenheit to Celsius, subtract 32 degrees and divide by 1.8.
- To convert Celsius to Fahrenheit, multiply by 1.8 and add 32 degrees.

- To convert quarts to liters, multiply quarts by .946.
- To convert liters to quarts, multiply liters by 1.057.

---

it is nearly impossible for athletes to consume sufficient fluids during physical activity to maintain the body water level, waiting for the thirst sensation before drinking fluids guarantees that the athlete will be exercising in a progressively worsening state of underhydration.

In a state of hyperhydration, the concentrations of electrolytes, protein, and glucose are lower than normal in the blood. This condition shuts down the production of ADH so that diluted urine is produced. Fluid tends to migrate from blood to cells to adjust for this hypotonic state.

Blood volume is affected by the concentration of sodium, the main extracellular electrolyte. A high sodium concentration is associated with an eventual enlargement of the blood volume, which results from the body's attempt to normalize the concentration of sodium per unit of fluid volume. The reverse situation, a low sodium concentration, is typically associated with an eventual reduction of the blood volume. To adjust for the natural variations in sodium intake, the hormone aldosterone is produced to retain more sodium in a low-sodium environment, and aldosterone production ceases when sodium concentrations are high so as to cause the excretion of more sodium.

Under normal circumstances, the combination of volumetric controls, osmoreceptors, antidiuretic hormone, and aldosterone maintains a relatively steady blood volume even with variations in fluid and sodium consumption. Exercise leads to an increased production of ADH and aldosterone, both of which conserve

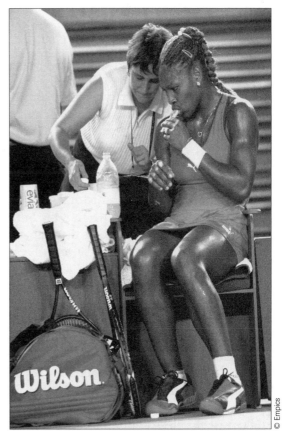

Athletes need to combat dehydration by consuming sufficient fluids before competition rather than waiting until the onset of thirst, as waiting almost guarantees underhydration.

body water and sodium. This system is sufficiently effective that fluid deficiencies leading to physiological problems are rare, even in athletes. However, exercise at high intensity or of long duration (or both), particularly in a hot and humid environment, places the athlete at hydration risk because fluid loss (through sweat) may exceed the athlete's capacity to consume and absorb fluids. This can lead to a progressive reduction in blood volume, a reduced sweat rate, and other problems that negatively affect performance and health; therefore, it is important for athletes to always maintain fluid balance. (See table 3.3 for the specific benefits of maintaining fluid balance.)

Table 3.3   Benefits of Maintaining Fluid Balance

Maintaining fluid balance during exercise helps sustain athletic performance through the following:

• Attenuation of increased heart rate
• Attenuation of increased core temperature
• Improvement in stroke volume
• Improvement in cardiac output
• Improvement in skin blood flow
• Attenuation of higher plasma sodium, osmolality, and adrenaline
• Reduction in net muscle glycogen usage

A Balance of Fluid Loss and Intake

Physical activity creates heat, and this heat must be dissipated for the athlete to continue performing the activity. Failure to dissipate heat will eventually lead to heatstroke and, potentially, death. One of the main mechanisms for dissipating heat is sweat production; sweat cools the body down when it evaporates off the skin. The inability to produce sufficient sweat will cause the body to overheat. Since athletes have a finite storage capacity for water, and a tremendous ability to produce sweat, fluids must be consumed during physical activity to maintain the sweat rate.

Athletes working intensely in the heat can lose 2.5 liters of sweat per hour. Sweat contains electrolytes (mainly sodium chloride but also potassium, calcium, and magnesium), with a sodium concentration that ranges from 20 to 80 millimoles per liter, depending on common sodium consumption in the diet, the sweat rate, acclimatization to the heat (better acclimatization results in lower sodium loss), and content and amount of rehydration beverages.[4] (See table 3.4 for concentrations of electrolytes in sweat, plasma, and intracellular water.)

Because the electrolyte concentration of sweat is different from that of plasma and intracellular water, there are concerns that an electrolyte imbalance will develop with intense physical activity. Of greatest concern is the potential sodium imbalance that could occur. The loss of a single liter of sweat containing 50 millimoles per liter of sodium translates into a loss of nearly 3 grams of sodium chloride. Athletes who lose

Table 3.4   Concentrations of Electrolytes in Sweat, Plasma, and Intracellular Water

	Sweat (mmol/L)	Plasma (mmol/L)	Intracellular water (mmol/L)
Sodium	20-80	130-155	10
Potassium	4-8	3.2-5.5	150
Calcium	0-1	2.1-2.9	0
Magnesium	<.2	.7-1.5	15
Chloride	20-60	96-110	8
Bicarbonate	0-35	23-28	10
Phosphate	.1-.2	.7-1.6	65
Sulphate	.1-2.0	.3-.9	10

Reprinted from R.J. Maughan, 1994, Fluid and electrolyte loss and replacement in exercise. In *Oxford textbook of sports medicine,* edited by M. Harries, et al., pp. 82-93, by permission of Oxford University Press.

2.5 liters of sweat per hour will lose almost 15 grams of sodium in 2 hours, a level that could easily exceed normal daily sodium intakes.[5]

Temperature regulation represents the balance between heat produced or received (heat-in) and heat removed (heat-out). When the body's temperature regulation system is working correctly, heat-in and heat-out are in perfect balance, and body temperature is maintained. Both internal and external factors can contribute to body heat. Radiant heat from the sun contributes to body temperature, as does the heat created from burning fuel (carbohydrate, protein, or fat). Somehow, athletes must find a way to dissipate from the body the same amount of heat that has been added to the body to maintain a constant body temperature.

The two primary systems for dissipating, or losing, heat involve (1) moving more blood to the skin to allow heat dissipation through radiation and (2) increasing the rate of sweat production. These two systems account for about 85 percent of heat removal when a person is at rest. Heat losses through conduction (the natural transmission of heat from a hotter body to the cooler air environment) and convection (heat transfer from tissue to the blood and through the skin) account for the remaining 15 percent of heat-out. During exercise, however, virtually all heat loss occurs via evaporation (sweat). (See figure 3.1.)

Both of these systems rely on maintenance of an adequate blood volume. A lower blood volume results in a reduced movement of blood to the skin, and sweat production is also reduced. Working muscles demand more blood flow to deliver nutrients and to remove the by-products of burned fuel. However, at the same time there is a need to shift blood away from the muscles and toward the skin to increase the sweat rate. With low blood volume, one or both of these systems fail, with a resultant decrease in athletic performance. In fact, the maintenance of blood volume is rightly

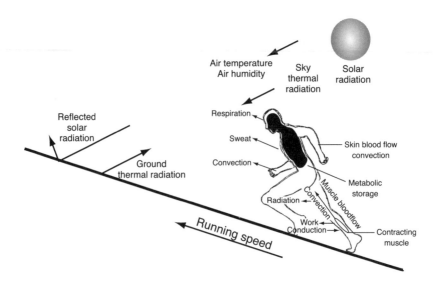

Figure 3.1   Systems for adding and removing heat in an exercising athlete.

Reprinted, by permission, from M.N. Sawka, W.A. Latzka and S.J. Montain, 2000, Effects of dehydration and rehydration on performance. In *Nutrition in sport*, edited by R.J. Maughan (London, England: Blackwell Science), 205.

considered by many to be the primary indicator of whether an athlete's performance can be maintained at a high rate.

Energy metabolism is only about 20 to 40 percent efficient, meaning that only 20 to 40 percent of food energy can be converted to the mechanical energy of muscular work. The remaining 60 to 80 percent of the food energy that is burned is lost as heat. However, when the rate of energy burn goes up, as happens during physical activity, the amount of heat added to the system is dramatically increased, so the heat-out systems must be "turned up." In fact, heavy exercise can produce 20 times the amount of heat produced at rest. Without an efficient means of heat removal, body temperature will rise quickly. The upper limit for human survival is about 110 degrees Fahrenheit (43.3 degrees Celsius), or only 11.4 degrees Fahrenheit (or 6.3 degrees Celsius) higher than normal body temperature. Body temperature has the potential to rise approximately 1 degree Fahrenheit every 5 minutes. It is conceivable, therefore, that an underhydrated athlete could be at risk for heatstroke and death less than 1 hour after the initiation of exercise.

Athletes doing very mild exercise that burns 300 kilocalories of energy during 30 minutes would use approximately 75 kilocalories for muscular work, and 225 kilocalories would be lost as heat.[6] This excess heat must be dissipated to maintain normal body temperature. Athletes working twice as intensely would create 450 kilocalories of excess heat that would need to be dissipated over the same 30 minutes to maintain body temperature. It is estimated that 1 milliliter of sweat can dissipate .5 kilocalories,[7] so over this 30-minute period the athlete would lose approximately 900 milliliters (almost 1 liter) of sweat. In 1 hour of high-intensity activity, approximately 1.8 liters of water would be lost. On sunny and hot days when the heat of the sun is added to the heat generated from muscular work, the athlete must produce more sweat to remove more heat. The fluid requirement is compounded when exercising intensely

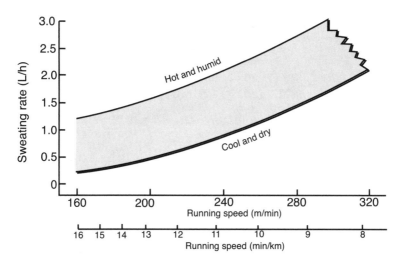

Figure 3.2 Seating rates in different climactic conditions and during different exercise intensities.

Reprinted, by permission, from M.N. Sawka, W.A. Latzka and S.J. Montain, 2000, Effects of dehydration and rehydration on performance. In *Nutrition in sport*, edited by R.J. Maughan (London, England: Blackwell Science), 217.

on a hot and humid day (see figure 3.2). Sweat doesn't evaporate off the skin as easily when it is humid, so even more sweat must be produced. In these conditions, a person can easily lose between 1 and 2 liters of fluid (via sweat) per hour.

Well-trained athletes exercising in a hot and humid environment may lose more than 3 liters of fluid per hour. To protect athletes from placing themselves at increased heat-stress risk, the heat index was developed (see table 3.5). This index simultaneously considers environmental temperature and relative humidity to establish exercise risk.

Factors Affecting Fluid Loss

Because sweat has a lower osmolality than does plasma (i.e., sweat is hypotonic), profuse sweating increases plasma osmolality. Whether or not this increased plasma osmolality affects body temperature or cooling capacity in an exercising individual is, as yet, unclear, but a sufficient change in osmolality and volume does stimulate the kidneys to excrete sodium and reduce urine output by producing more concentrated urine.

Several factors affect the rate at which an athlete can produce sweat. Higher ambient temperatures result in a greater potential for sweat production. Higher humidity is also responsible for higher sweat production, but because the vapor pressure gradient and skin is low, the cooling potential (i.e., the rate of evaporation off the skin) is lower in humid environments. The same problem also exists with clothing that traps sweat against the skin (i.e., does not breathe). This type of clothing results in a reduced cooling efficiency that forces a greater sweat rate. (Sweat-soaked clothing doesn't mean an athlete is effectively controlling body temperature, it just means he or she is losing water.) Some new materials designed for athletes actually wick sweat

Table 3.5 The Heat Index

Relative humidity	Environmental temperature °F (°C)										
	70 (21)	75 (24)	80 (27)	85 (29)	90 (32)	95 (35)	100 (38)	105 (41)	110 (43)	115 (46)	120 (49)
	Apparent temperature °F (°C)										
0%	64 (18)	69 (20)	73 (23)	78 (26)	83 (28)	87 (30)	91 (33)	95 (35)	99 (37)	103 (39)	107 (42)
10%	65 (18)	70 (21)	75 (24)	80 (27)	85 (29)	90 (32)	95 (35)	100 (38)	105 (41)	111 (44)	116 (47)
20%	66 (19)	72 (22)	77 (25)	82 (28)	87 (30)	93 (34)	99 (37)	105 (41)	112 (44)	120 (49)	130 (54)
30%	67 (19)	73 (23)	78 (26)	84 (29)	90 (32)	96 (36)	104 (40)	113 (45)	123 (51)	135 (57)	148 (64)
40%	68 (20)	74 (23)	79 (26)	86 (30)	93 (34)	101 (38)	110 (43)	123 (51)	137 (58)	151 (66)	
50%	69 (20)	75 (24)	81 (27)	88 (31)	96 (36)	107 (42)	120 (49)	135 (57)	150 (66)		
60%	70 (21)	76 (24)	82 (28)	90 (32)	100 (38)	114 (46)	132 (56)	149 (65)			
70%	70 (21)	77 (25)	85 (29)	93 (34)	106 (41)	124 (51)	144 (62)				
80%	71 (22)	78 (26)	86 (30)	97 (36)	113 (45)	136 (58)					
90%	71 (22)	79 (26)	88 (31)	102 (39)	122 (50)						
100%	72 (22)	80 (27)	91 (33)	108 (42)							

Apparent temperature	Heat-stress risk with physical activity or prolonged exposure.
90-104 °F (32-40 °C)	Heat cramps or heat exhaustion possible.
105-129 °F (41-53 °C)	Heat cramps or heat exhaustion likely. Heat stroke possible.
130 °F and up (54 °C and up)	Heat stroke very likely.

Caution: This chart provides guidelines for assessing the potential severity of heat stress. Individual reactions to heat will vary. Heat illnesses can occur at lower temperatures than indicated on this chart. Exposure to full sunshine can increase values up to 15 °F.

away from the skin to improve evaporative efficiency. Athletes with large body surface areas may also have an enhanced sweat production capacity and, therefore, an enhanced evaporative heat loss. But these athletes may also gain more heat from the environment through radiation and convection in hot weather.[8] The conditioning or training state of an athlete makes a difference. Well-conditioned athletes have a higher sweat volume potential that results in an enhanced cooling potential. However, this higher sweat rate requires a greater during-exercise fluid consumption to avoid higher heat-stress risk.

An athlete's state of fluid balance also plays a factor. The better the hydration state, the greater the sweat potential. As athletes become progressively dehydrated, the sweat rate is reduced, and body temperature rises. This is a problem because fluid consumption during activity is rarely greater than 2 cups (480 milliliters) per hour, or only 30 to 40 percent of the amount of fluid lost in sweat, an amount that will inevitably lead to the athlete's becoming dehydrated. Consider that marathoners competing in a cool temperature of 50 to 54 degrees Fahrenheit (10 to 12 degrees Celsius) lose between 1 and 5 percent of total body mass.[9] Marathoners competing in warm weather lose about 8 percent of total body mass, or between 12 and 15 percent of total body water.[10]

Factors Affecting Fluid Intake

The two main factors influencing fluid intake are thirst and taste. Thirst is a sensation of dryness in the mouth and throat related to the body's need for additional fluids. Taste is the response humans have (either good or bad) to substances in the mouth. Humans are more likely to consume more of what they like, or more of what tastes good to them. Most athletes induce "voluntary dehydration" because they don't drink enough despite having plenty of fluids readily available. Insufficient consumption of fluids by athletes is probably due to a lack of the thirst sensation.

The onset of thirst may be the result of habit, ritual, or the need for a warming (hot fluids) or cooling (cold fluids) effect.[11] A rise in plasma osmolality of between 2 and 3 percent is needed to produce the sensation of thirst, and sensitivity to a reduction in fluid volume is even less responsive, requiring nearly a 10 percent decrease in blood volume to stimulate thirst.[12, 13] The thirst sensation, often considered delayed in athletes because it doesn't appear until an athlete has already lost 1.5 to 2.0 liters of body water, is therefore a poor indicator of fluid needs in athletes.[14] There is no hope that an athlete can return to an adequately hydrated state during exercise if fluid consumption begins at the same time the thirst sensation occurs. This apparent delay in the thirst mechanism is a primary reason for athletes to train themselves to consume fluids on a schedule, whether they feel thirsty or not.

Color, taste, odor, temperature, and texture all play important roles in determining if the beverage will be considered desirable and whether it will be consumed. It appears that athletes prefer cool beverages with a slightly sweet flavor. Heavily sweetened beverages (around a 12 percent carbohydrate solution) are not as widely tolerated during exercise as beverages with a 6 or 7 percent carbohydrate solution.[15, 16] When not exercising, however, the reverse may be true, pointing to an interesting phenomenon of exercise: Food and drink taste differently while exercising than when not exercising. Therefore, athletes are wise to determine the fluids they find most desirable for exercise while they are exercising.

Gastric Emptying and Fluid Delivery to Working Muscles

Several factors influence the rate at which fluids leave the stomach. Gastric emptying describes the volume of food or drink that leaves the stomach per unit of time. Food or drinks with a slower gastric emptying take longer to completely leave the stomach. This means that these substances enter the small intestine more slowly, and some of the food or drink will remain in the stomach longer.

Carbohydrate Concentration of the Solution   Sports beverages and other beverages consumed by athletes commonly contain carbohydrate. When the concentration of carbohydrate in a fluid rises above 7 percent, gastric emptying time decreases. At concentrations below 7 percent carbohydrate, gastric emptying time is not significantly affected, showing gastric emptying characteristics similar to water.[17] For this reason, the recommended carbohydrate concentration in sports beverages is below 8 percent.[18] Having said that, some ultraendurance athletes "train" their guts to tolerate greater concentrations because they desperately need the additional carbohydrate.

Type of Carbohydrate in the Solution   Carbohydrates are not all the same, coming in different molecular sizes and in different molecular combinations. For instance, glucose[19] is a monosaccharide (a single-molecule carbohydrate), sucrose is a disaccharide (two monosaccharides held together with a bond), and starch is a polysaccharide (many molecules of monosaccharides held together with bonds). The smaller the length of a carbohydrate chain, the slower the gastric emptying time. Therefore, on an isocaloric basis, pure glucose (a monosaccharide) will take longer to leave the stomach than table sugar (a disaccharide), and table sugar will take longer to leave the stomach than a simple starch (a polysaccharide).[20]

Amount of Fluid Consumed   The amount of fluid consumed at one time has a major influence on gastric emptying time. When a large volume of fluid is consumed, gastric emptying time is initially faster, and when the volume of fluid in the stomach is reduced, gastric emptying time slows. To achieve a hydrated state before competition or practice, 14 to 22 ounces (420 to 660 milliliters) of fluid should be consumed, followed by frequent sipping on fluid to maintain fluid volume in the stomach and, therefore, a faster gastric emptying time.[21, 22]

Temperature of the Solution   Beverage temperature only slightly affects gastric emptying time. When people are at rest, fluids at body temperature leave the stomach more quickly than either very hot or very cold fluids.[23] During exercise, however, it appears as if cool fluids leave the stomach more quickly than room-temperature or body-temperature fluids.[24] An important consideration, although not affecting gastric emptying, is that athletes may consume more cool fluids.

Carbonation of the Solution   Athletes commonly believe that consuming a carbonated beverage causes gastric distress and delayed gastric emptying (the first "sports beverage" was probably a defizzed cola), but there is little scientific evidence that this occurs. However, studies evaluating the impact of fluid carbonation on gastric emptying time have typically relied on few subjects. In general, the studies suggest that, all other things being equal (carbohydrate concentration, volume, temperature, and so on), carbonation has little impact on gastric emptying.[25, 26] Nevertheless, carbonation does make athletes feel more full, thereby reducing the drive to drink. Nothing should take away the athletes' drive to drink because this can negatively affect hydration state.

Relative Hydration State of the Athlete   Progressive dehydration and higher body temperatures associated with high-intensity activity cause a slower gastric emptying rate.[27] This is an excellent rationale for athletes to maintain hydration state during activity. Dehydration will make it almost impossible for the athlete to return to an adequately hydrated state during exercise, and if this is attempted through consumption of a large volume of fluid, it will likely lead to a sense of discomfort rather than faster rehydration.

Degree of Mental Stress   The mental stress and anxiety associated with athletic competition is a major factor in gastric emptying. Higher levels of mental stress and anxiety are associated with a reduced gastric emptying that can have a serious impact on the ability to adequately rehydrate during competition.[28, 29] The mental training techniques that can be learned from a sports psychologist to reduce stress are important for reducing the physiological effects of sports-related stress and anxiety.

Type of Physical Activity   High-intensity activity is associated with a slower gastric emptying rate than lower-intensity activity, but the differences are minor. Additionally, the type of activity (running, swimming, cycling) does not appear to have a large influence on gastric emptying rate.[30]

Athlete Conditioning, Adaptation, and Age

The human body has wonderful adaptive mechanisms (see table 3.6), and the ability to adapt to higher or lower glucose concentrations and faster or slower rates of fluid ingestion is no exception. It seems clear that athletes can train to enhance their potential for achieving optimal hydration. Therefore, each athlete should start with general recommendations for fluid intake to maintain hydration state, then make modifications that are best suited to them.

Heat tolerance is highly influenced by physical fitness: Poor physical fitness dramatically increases the risk of heat illness similarly in both men and women. However, this improved heat tolerance is the result of an enhanced sweat rate. Since children have fewer sweat glands and each gland produces less sweat, child athletes have a lower potential for adaptation to heat and are generally considered to have a lower heat tolerance than well-conditioned adults.[31] Poorly conditioned athletes with higher

Table 3.6   Body Adjustments During Acclimatization

- Plasma volume expands to increase total blood volume.
- The heart is then able to pump more blood per beat.
- More blood flows to muscles and skin.
- Less muscle glycogen is used as an energy source during exercise.
- Sweat glands hypertrophy and produce 30% more sweat.
- Salt in sweat decreases by about 60% to conserve electrolytes.
- Sweating starts at a lower core temperature.
- Core temperature will not rise as high or as rapidly as in unacclimatized state.
- Psychological feeling of stress is reduced at a given exercise rate.

body fat levels also have lower heat tolerance. Put simply, fat deters heat loss. In summary, well-conditioned adult athletes with low body fat levels must develop strategies for constantly increasing fluid intakes as their conditioning improves because sweat rates increase with better conditioning. Children and adults with higher body fat are likely to have a lower heat tolerance, making maintenance of adequate hydration even more critical for these individuals.

Intestinal Absorption

As fluids leave the stomach and enter the small intestine, the water and carbohydrate that make up the solution must pass through the intestinal mucosa for take-up by blood. The main factor influencing the speed with which water and carbohydrate are absorbed is the concentration of carbohydrate in the solution that enters the intestines.[32] Slightly lower concentrations of carbohydrate and electrolytes, relative to the concentration of plasma, result in faster absorption of water than a solution that has either a much higher or much lower concentration.[33] A 6 to 7 percent carbohydrate solution appears to offer the best balance for speedy absorption. Consumption of highly concentrated carbohydrate solutions during exercise may cause a temporary shift of fluids away from muscle cells and into the intestines to dilute the solution before absorption. This would have a negative impact on both muscle function and sweat rates because it would cause, at least temporarily, a degree of plasma and tissue dehydration.

Fluid-Related Problems

Heat balance (see figure 3.3) can be described by the following equation:[34]

$$S = M \pm R \pm K \pm C - E \pm WK$$

Heat balance (S) = metabolic heat production (M), as corrected for the net heat exchange by radiation (R), conduction (K), convection (C), and evaporation (E), and as further corrected by the amount of work performed (WK).

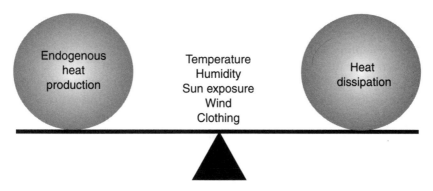

Figure 3.3   Heat balance.

Dehydration

Dehydration occurs when more fluids are lost than are consumed. By definition, dehydration means that the amount of body water is below optimal. As little as a 2 percent drop in body water results in a measurable reduction in athletic performance. Common risks for dehydration include the following:

- Vomiting
- Diarrhea
- Inadequate fluid replacement
- Induced high sweat rates (as in saunas)
- Laxatives
- Diuretics (and substances with a diuretic effect, such as high intakes of caffeine)
- Dieting
- Febrile illness

Ideally, dehydration avoidance is the best policy. The only way to avoid dehydration is to rightly assume there is a constant output of fluids that must be dealt with by having an equally constant input of fluids. It is important for athletes to recognize the signs of dehydration. Thirst is an obvious sign, but athletes should learn to monitor urine output for volume and color. Both low urine output and dark urine color are signs of dehydration that may precede the sensation of thirst.

Some athletes dehydrate themselves to try to look better or to make a competitive weight classification, or they fail to consume fluids even when they are readily available to them (referred to as voluntary dehydration); other athletes become dehydrated as a result of heavy training, particularly in hot and humid environments, when adequate fluid consumption is difficult (referred to as involuntary dehydration). Regardless of the cause, athletes can be certain that dehydration will result in negative performance outcomes and reduced mental function.[35, 36]

Heat Cramps

Heat cramps—painful spasms in the legs and abdomen—are typically the result of a fluid and electrolyte imbalance caused by severe dehydration. They are most likely to occur in people who sweat heavily and who lose a higher than normal amount of sodium and other electrolytes (including potassium, calcium, and magnesium) in the sweat (see table 3.7). For these individuals, drinking adequate amounts of sodium-containing beverages during exercise is particularly useful. Heat cramps appear to occur late in the day after consumption of large volumes of plain water.[37] At the first sign of involuntary muscle twitching or mild muscle cramping, athletes should consume 16 ounces (480 milliliters) of a sports drink that has been supplemented with a teaspoon of table salt.[38] This should then be followed by a steady intake of sodium-supplemented sports drinks for the remainder of the exercise session. To help meet the needs of athletes who experience frequent cramping, companies have developed products that provide a measured amount of sodium, potassium, calcium, and magnesium for adding to a given volume of sports beverage.

Table 3.7   Indications of Cramp-Prone Athletes

- History of heat cramps
- Consume inadequate sodium (eat a salt-restricted diet)
- Sweat profusely early in activity
- Have poor hydration habits during exercise
- Sweat is heavy in salt; stings eyes; tastes salty
- Visible (chalky) salt on body and clothing
- Not adapted to a hot and humid environment
- Family history of cystic fibrosis

Heat Exhaustion

The symptoms of heat exhaustion include weakness, cold and clammy skin, a feeling of faintness, fatigue, nausea, and a weak pulse. It is also possible, when the individual has a severe body water depletion, that sweating has stopped and the skin feels dry. The likely cause of these symptoms is an inadequate blood flow to the brain, with the sufferer typically on the ground but semiconscious. Symptoms usually respond well to rapid cooling, so heat-exhaustion victims should be cooled through whatever means are available. Applying wet, ice-cold cloths to the body or placing the victim in a cold-water bath are both effective. After a return to full consciousness, the athlete can be given sips of cool fluid, but this should not be forced because it may cause nausea. There is no rational reason for a heat-exhausted athlete to try to return to physical activity on the same day. Instead, the person should spend the remainder of the day staying cool and hydrating with sodium-containing fluids, such as sports beverages. Caution: Under no circumstances should an athlete who has stopped sweating continue exercising because this may cause a rapid and dangerous rise in core temperature.

Heatstroke (Sunstroke)

Heatstroke is an extremely dangerous condition, typified by high body temperature (usually above 105 degrees Fahrenheit, or 40.5 degrees Celsius), hot and dry skin, and a rapid pulse. It is also possible for the athlete to be coming in and out of consciousness. The first responder should call 911 (hospitals are best equipped to deal with this life-threatening condition) and then do whatever possible to cool the athlete (fanning, cold water, sponge bath, loosening clothing, cold-water bath). Until the athlete returns to consciousness, do not give fluids.

Heatstroke is caused by a combination of several factors, as shown in table 3.8.[39]

Table 3.8   Risk Factors for Heatstroke

Increased endogenous heat load	Drugs reported to predispose to heatstroke (*continued*)
Overexertion	Diuretics
Drugs (e.g., sympathomimetics, caffeine)	Furosemide
	Hydrochlorothiazide
Increased exogenous heat load	Bumetanide
Temperature	Phenothiazines
Sun exposure	Prochlorperazine
	Chlorpromazine hydrochloride
Decreased heat dissipation	Promethazine hydrochloride
Exogenous	Butyrophenones
Humidity	Haloperidol
Occlusive or excessive clothing	Cyclic antidepressants
Endogenous	Amitriptyline hydrochloride
Dehydration	Imipramine hydrochloride
Lack of acclimatization	Nortriptyline hydrochloride
Healed burns	Protriptyline hydrochloride
Rashes	Monoamine oxidase inhibitors
Drugs (e.g., phenothiazines,	Phenelzine
antihistamines, alcohol)	Tranylcypromine sulfate
	Alcohol
Drugs reported to predispose to heatstroke	Lysergic acid diethylamide (LSD)
Sympathomimetics	Lithium
Amphetamines	
Epinephrine	**Other**
Ephedrine	Concurrent illness (e.g., upper respiratory
Cocaine	infection, gastroenteritis)
Norepinephrine	Prior heatstroke
Anticholinergics	
Atropine sulfat	
Scopolamine HBr	
Benztropine mesylate	
Belladonna and synthetic alkaloids	
Antihistamines	

Hyponatremia

Exercising for long periods may cause low blood sodium (hyponatremia), a potentially fatal condition.[40] Low blood sodium can occur if you drink excessive amounts of water and dilute the sodium content of your blood. This may lead to rapid and dangerous swelling of the brain. Inadequate sodium intake also may play a role. Low blood sodium is most likely to occur during prolonged exercise in dehydrated athletes who lose large amounts of sodium through sweating. It is also possible in athletes who habitually restrict sodium consumption in the foods and beverages they consume. In general, unless it is contraindicated because of a medical condition and the athlete is under the careful supervision of a physician, adding salt to meals and beverages is a desirable strategy for avoiding low blood electrolytes and reducing hyponatremia risk.

Signs and symptoms of low blood sodium include the following:

- Headache
- Confusion
- Nausea
- Cramping
- Bloated stomach

- Swollen fingers and ankles
- Pulmonary edema
- Seizures
- Coma

Just before the 2003 Boston Marathon, *USA Track & Field* announced fluid-replacement guidelines for long-distance runners that are designed to lower hyponatremia risk.[41] Earlier guidelines encouraged runners to drink as much as possible to "stay ahead" of their thirst, but the new guidelines advise runners to drink only as much fluid as they lose through sweat during a race. This recommendation suggests that athletes consume 100 percent of fluids lost through sweat and no more. Higher levels of consumption, particularly of plain water, could cause a drop in blood sodium concentration, leading to hyponatremia. Athletes at increased risk of hyponatremia include those who

- take NSAIDs;
- are on a low-sodium diet;
- drink water or other no-sodium beverages during exercise;
- aren't acclimatized to warm weather or are poorly trained; and
- run slowly, taking longer than 4 hours to complete endurance events.

The highest risk of hyponatremia appears to be in athletes who produce a large volume of sweat with a relatively high concentration of sodium and who consume large volumes of plain water (which contains no sodium).[42] Sports beverages contain approximately 20 milliequivalents (mEq) of sodium chloride (table salt), but even higher levels of sodium are recommended by a number of researchers who have assessed plasma changes during prolonged exercise in the heat.[43, 44] These researchers have recommended 20 to 50 milliequivalents per liter, but it appears that most athletes with normal sweat rates and normal sweat sodium concentrations who consume commercial sports beverages and avoid consumption of plain water during endurance events are protected.[45]

If you eat during exercise, salty foods such as pretzels are a good choice. Sports drinks also are a good source of sodium, water, and carbohydrate. Dehydration during prolonged exercise is still far more common than low blood sodium. It is important, therefore, to start exercise well hydrated and to drink appropriate amounts of fluid during exercise.[46]

Hydration Strategies

No level of low body water is acceptable for achieving optimal athletic performance and endurance, so athletes must develop personal strategies for maintaining optimal body water while exercising. Imagine a full glass of water represents your body in a state of optimal hydration. When not exercising, it's like having a pinhole in the bottom of the glass. The water level will drop, but only at a very slow rate and at a pace that makes it easy for you to maintain an optimal hydration state. Because the water level drops so slowly, drinking an occasional glass of water or other fluid is an adequate means of maintaining hydration state. Now consider what happens when you exercise, which is equivalent to putting a pencil hole in the bottom of the glass: The rate of water loss is much faster. Within even a short period of time, the amount of water loss could be enough to affect exercise performance and endurance. Waiting to drink in this situation is not a reasonable option. If the frequency of drinking when not exercising is once every 2 hours, then the frequency of drinking during exercise should be once every 10 to 15 minutes. Water is lost so quickly during exercise that it becomes difficult, if not impossible, to replace the amount of water being lost and virtually impossible to increase body water while exercising. Waiting too long between drinks causes body water to decrease such that it cannot be adequately replaced. If you wait to drink you may be able to maintain the body's water level at its current state, but that state will be too low.

Without fluid intake, blood volume will quickly drop, sweat rates will drop, and body heat will rise quickly and dangerously, at the rate of approximately 1.8 degrees Fahrenheit (1 degree Celsius) every 5 to 7 minutes. (See table 3.9 for the effects of dehydration on aerobic performance.) Because it is so difficult to consume sufficient

Table 3.9   Effects of Dehydration on Aerobic Endurance Performance

- Hypohydration of >2% leads to decrements in performance.
- Cardiovascular function and temperature regulation are adversely affected.
- Maximal aerobic performance decreases 4 to 8%, with a 3% weight loss during exercise in neutral environments.
- Dehydration and GI distress are evident.
- Fluid and electrolyte balance in muscle cells is disturbed.
- Adverse effects of hyperthermia on mental processes contribute to central fatigue.

fluids during hard physical work, athletes should develop a fixed drinking schedule. With a loss of 1 liter of water per hour, athletes should find a way to drink 4 cups of water per hour. Athletes losing 2 liters of water per hour need to drink more than 8 cups of water per hour. Of course, it's difficult to know precisely how much water is being lost during activity, but a simple technique can help an athlete estimate how much is lost. One liter of water weighs approximately 2 pounds, and 1 pint of water weighs approximately 1 pound. By knowing these relationships, athletes can estimate how much fluid should be consumed during physical activity by doing the following:

1. Write down what time it is just before the exercise session.
2. Write down body weight in pounds. (Preferably, this should be nude weight.)
3. Do the normal exercise, and monitor how much fluid is consumed during the exercise period.
4. Immediately after exercise, take off the sweaty clothing and towel dry. Once dry, write down body weight in pounds. (Again, this should be nude weight.)
5. Write down the current time.
6. Calculate the amount of fluid lost by subtracting ending weight from beginning weight.
7. Calculate exercise time by subtracting ending time from beginning time.
8. The amount of extra fluid that should be consumed during the activity is equivalent to 1 pint (16 ounces) of additional fluid for each pound lost, provided in 10- to 20-minute increments.

Example: If John weighs 4 pounds less after a 2-hour football practice, he should consume an additional 4 pints (8 cups) of fluid during that practice. He was already consuming 2 cups of fluid, so John's total fluid consumption should be 10 cups of fluid per 2-hour practice. In 2 hours there are 12 10-minute time increments, so John has 12 opportunities to consume 10 cups of fluid. Therefore, John should consume 6.5 ounces of fluid, or a bit more than 3/4 of a cup ($10 \div 12 = .8$), every 10 minutes or 13 ounces of fluid (about 1.5 cups) every 20 minutes.

Fluid Intake Before Exercise

It is critical for athletes to be in a state of optimal hydration before the initiation of exercise or competition. All the evidence suggests that even a minor level of underhydration (as little as 2 percent of body weight) can cause a measurable difference in endurance and performance, and the greater the underhydration, the greater the negative impact.[47, 48] Furthermore, it can take 24 hours or longer to bring a dehydrated athlete back to a well-hydrated state. Therefore, waiting until just before practice or competition to bring an athlete to a well-hydrated state or simply failing to take any steps to make certain the athlete is in an optimally hydrated state will doom that athlete to having a poor practice or competition outcome.

In some sports, athletes try to achieve a particular "look" or try to make a particular weight. The classic body profile in rhythmic gymnastics is long, graceful lines with, essentially, no secondary sexual characteristics. It is common for rhythmic gymnasts to restrict water intake before a competition because they think it will help give them the desired look. Wrestlers have a well-established regimen for fluid restriction to achieve a particular weight class. They then have about 24 hours to rehydrate themselves before the competition. Besides the inherent health dangers (there are well-documented deaths associated with this strategy), it is unlikely that dehydrated wrestlers would be able to adequately rehydrate themselves in just 24 hours. Therefore, performance is likely to be affected.

On the other side of the continuum, some athletes try to superhydrate with fluid before exercise. This is typically a strategy of long-distance runners, whose water loss during competition is likely to be greater than their ability to replace it. The runner with the best hydration state near the end of the competition clearly has a major advantage over less-hydrated competitors. When athletes constantly superhydrate they may develop a greater blood (plasma) volume, with resultant lower core temperatures and heart rates during activity, suggesting the potential for improved endurance and performance.[49, 50] Consumption of large fluid volumes is also associated with frequent urination, but this may be somewhat mediated by consumption of sodium-containing fluids.[51] In addition, superhydration is associated with higher sweat rates and a lower heart rate during exercise.[52]

Glycerol is a simple three-carbon lipid that is metabolized like a carbohydrate (see figure 3.4). It is occasionally used by endurance athletes to aid superhydration because it acts as a humectant (i.e., it attracts water).

Limited evidence suggests that adding glycerol at the rate of 1 gram per kilogram of body mass to preexercise fluids improves endurance performance in extremely hot and humid environments. This improvement occurs because glycerol enables a retention of more of the consumed fluids.[53, 54] However, individual athletes have described the

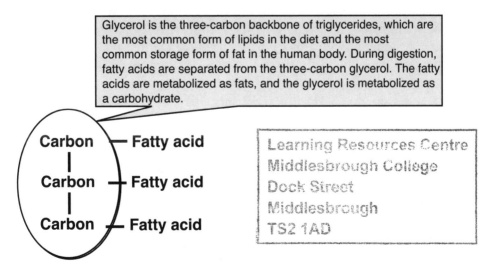

Glycerol is the three-carbon backbone of triglycerides, which are the most common form of lipids in the diet and the most common storage form of fat in the human body. During digestion, fatty acids are separated from the three-carbon glycerol. The fatty acids are metabolized as fats, and the glycerol is metabolized as a carbohydrate.

Carbon — Fatty acid
Carbon — Fatty acid
Carbon — Fatty acid

Figure 3.4   Glycerol (also referred to as "glycerine").

acceptability of this protocol differently. Some athletes find that superhydrating with glycerol makes them feel stiff and uncomfortable, while others are more comfortable with this sensation.[55] Athletes using glycerol should make every effort to maintain electrolyte balance so as not to increase the risk of hyponatremia.[56, 57]

In general, athletes should follow these hydration guidelines before exercise:

1. The sensation of thirst should not be relied on as an indicator of fluid need. Thirst should be considered an "emergency" sensation that occurs when the body has already lost 1.5 to 2.0 liters of water. Because the thirst sensation is likely to be delayed during exercise, waiting for thirst results in excessive water loss and a downward shift in total body water.

2. Athletes should become accustomed to consuming fluids without the thirst sensation. As a practical matter, this is made easier if athletes carry fluids with them, wherever they are and wherever they go. Fluid consumption is much more likely to occur if the fluid is readily available without the need to go looking for it, especially if the athlete doesn't feel thirsty.

3. Athletes should consume enough fluids before exercise to produce clear urine (a sign the athlete is well hydrated). Dark urine is a sign that the athlete is producing a low-volume, concentrated urine that results from the need to retain as much fluid as possible—a clear sign of underhydration.

4. Approximately 1 to 1.5 hours before exercise, the athlete should consume a large volume of fluid (up to .5 liters) within a relatively short time period to ensure adequate hydration and to improve gastric emptying. After this, athletes should sip on fluids (approximately .5 cups every 10 minutes) to maintain hydration state before exercise or competition begins. Athletes should consume fluid as frequently and in as high a volume as can be tolerated to replace water losses.

5. Athletes seeking to superhydrate should not try this technique without careful monitoring, especially if it is done using glycerol. Superhydration should never be attempted by individuals who have compromised cardiovascular systems. It is also something that shouldn't be tried for the first time just before a competition. As a practical matter, the safest way to superhydrate is to frequently consume fluids.

6. Athletes should avoid foods and drinks that may have a diuretic (water-losing) impact. For instance, caffeine and related substances commonly found in coffee, tea, chocolate, and sodas could increase the rate of urinary water excretion if consumed in large quantities. Therefore, these substances could be counterproductive in terms of optimizing hydration state before exercise.

Fluid Intake During Exercise

Athletes consuming fluids during exercise derive clear benefits, including better maintenance of exercise performance and a slowing of the exercise-induced rise in heart rate and body temperature. In addition, blood flow to the skin is improved or maintained. The degree to which the cardiovascular and heat-maintenance capacity is maintained is directly related to the degree to which dehydration can be avoided. It is clear that a failure to consume sufficient fluids during exercise is a major risk factor in the onset of heat exhaustion.[58] The best strategy for athletes to follow to avoid heat exhaustion and maintain athletic performance is to drink fluids during exercise (see figures 3.5 and 3.6).[59-61]

Most studies evaluating the interaction between hydration adequacy and athletic performance have used either plain water or sports beverages that contain, in differing degrees, carbohydrate and electrolytes (see table 3.10, page 97). The results of these studies are similar in confirming the importance of fluid consumption during exercise (see table 3.11, page 98). However, the inclusion of carbohydrate and electrolytes in the fluids affords an athlete certain advantages over plain water. Recent studies suggest that inclusion of carbohydrate in the rehydration solution improves the athlete's ability to maintain or increase work output during exercise and increases the time to exhaustion.[62-65]

Consumed carbohydrate helps athletes avoid depletion of muscle glycogen and provides fuel for muscles when muscle glycogen is low. Carbohydrate also helps maintain mental function, which is critical for maintaining endurance performance. Mental fatigue leads to muscle fatigue, even if muscles have plenty of glycogen and fluids.

Heart rate (beats per minute) with[*] and without fluids during two hours of exercise at 70% $\dot{V}O_2$max in trained men

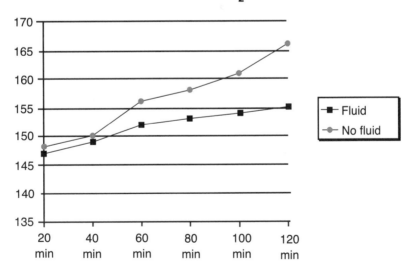

*Fluid ingestion at a rate that prevented loss of body mass

Figure 3.5   Comparison of heart rate in athletes consuming fluids and not consuming fluids during exercise.

Reprinted, by permission, from M. Hargreaves, 1996, "Physiological benefits of fluid and energy replacement during exercise," *Aust J Nutr Diet* 53(4 Suppl): S3-S7.

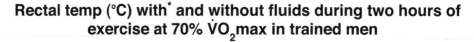

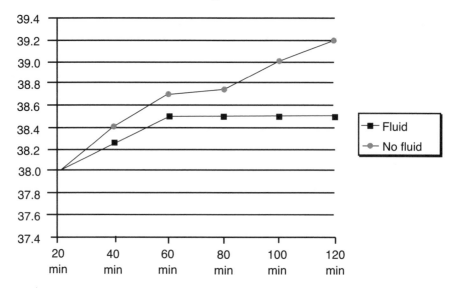

*Fluid ingestion at a rate that prevented loss of body mass

Figure 3.6 Comparison of core temperature in athletes consuming fluids and not consuming fluids during exercise.

Reprinted, by permission, from M. Hargreaves, 1996, "Physiological benefits of fluid and energy replacement during exercise," *Aust J Nutr Diet* 53(4 Suppl): S3-S7.

Different activities result in different rates of carbohydrate utilization, but consuming carbohydrate-containing fluid consistently helps maintain athletic performance, regardless of the sport. For instance, in strenuous cycling the rate of muscle glycogen use is not affected when a carbohydrate solution is ingested;[66] in long-distance running, the rate of muscle glycogen usage is reduced when a carbohydrate-containing fluid is consumed;[67] and in stop–go intermittent exercise, a reduction in muscle glycogen usage is seen with the consumption of a carbohydrate-containing fluid.[68, 69] In each of these scenarios, carbohydrate depletion is generally considered to be the cause of performance degradation. However, there is good evidence that consuming a carbohydrate-containing beverage may also be important for improving athletic performance in high-intensity activities where carbohydrate is not expected to be depleted because of the relatively short duration of the activity.[70-72]

These data all suggest that athletes should adjust to consuming a carbohydrate-containing fluid during exercise. However, the concentration of carbohydrate and the type of carbohydrate are important considerations. Although there are no major differences between the effects of glucose, sucrose, maltodextrins, and starch on exercise performance,[73-75] beverages containing mainly fructose may cause intestinal distress.[76, 77] Maltodextrins are less sweet than sucrose and fructose, so they may be

Table 3.10 Carbohydrate and Electrolyte Content of Common Beverages

Beverage	Carbohydrate composition	Carbohydrate concentration		Sodium (mg)	Potassium (mg)
		%	Grams		
Accelerade (Pacific Health Labs)	Sucrose, glucose, maltodextrin	7	17	127	40
All Sport (Monarch Bev. Co.)	High-fructose corn syrup	9	21	55	55
Carboflex (Unipro, Inc.)	Maltodextrin	24	55	–	–
Coca-Cola (Coca-Cola Co.)	High-fructose corn syrup, sucrose	11	26	9.2	tr
Cytomax (Cytosport)	Fructose corn syrup, sucrose	8	19	10	150
Diet sodas	(None)	–	–	trace	trace
Gatorade Energy Drink (Gatorade Co.)	Maltodextrin, glucose, fructose	23	53	133	70
Gatorade Thirst Quencher (Gatorade Co.)	Sucrose, glucose, fructose	6	14	110	25
Met-Rx (Met-Rx, Inc.)	Fructose, glucose	8	19	10	150
Orange juice	Fructose, sucrose	11	26	2.7	510
PowerAde (Coca-Cola Co.)	High-fructose corn syrup, maltodextrin	8	19	55	30
PowerBar Endurance (PowerBar)	Maltodextrin, dextrose, fructose	7	17	160	10
PowerBar Performance Recovery (PowerBar)	Maltodextrin, dextrose, fructose	8.5	20	250	10
Ultima (Ultima Replenisher)	Maltodextrin	1.7	4	8	16
Ultra Fuel (Twin Labs)	Maltodextrin, glucose, fructose	21	50	–	–
Water	(None)	–	–	trace	trace

Table 3.11 **Performance Benefits of Water and Carbohydrate (Based on 50 min of exercise at 80% $\dot{V}O_2$max)**

- 6.7% improved performance with large volume of fluid compared with ingestion of small volume of fluid
- 6.3% improved performance with ingestion of carbohydrate compared with no carbohydrate
- 12.4% improved performance with combination of large fluid volume with carbohydrate compared with small volume of fluid without carbohydrate

Reprinted, by permission, from P.R. Below, R. Mora-Rodriguez, J. Alonso-Gonzalez and E.F. Coyle, 1995, "Fluid and carbohydrate ingestion independently improve performance during 1 hr of intense exercise," *Med Sci Sports Exerc.* 27: 200-210.

used to add carbohydrate energy to solutions without making them unpalatably sweet tasting.[78] With these exceptions aside, carbohydrate energy, regardless of whether in liquid or solid form and almost regardless of the type of carbohydrate, will aid athletic performance.[79] However, since providing carbohydrate in liquid form enables athletes to address two issues at once (energy and fluid), carbohydrate liquids are preferred.

The volume of carbohydrate provided during exercise is an important consideration as well; providing too much too fast may induce gastrointestinal distress and, at least temporarily, draw needed fluids away from muscle and skin to dilute this excessively concentrated solution in the gut. By contrast, providing a fluid that contains just a scant amount of carbohydrate may induce no performance benefit. Athletes should try to consume approximately 1 gram of carbohydrate per minute of exercise. This intake level can be achieved by drinking solutions that contain between 6 and 8 percent carbohydrate[80] at a volume of .6 to 1.2 liters per hour.[81, 82] Some sports beverages have carbohydrate levels precisely within this range, while others have concentrations outside this range (refer back to table 3.10). Concentrations above 8 percent may cause a delay in gastric emptying and do not necessarily lead to a faster or better carbohydrate metabolism during exercise.[83] Another real advantage of consuming a 6 to 8 percent carbohydrate solution is that it has a faster rate of intestinal absorption than does water alone. This means that fluid status can be more efficiently maintained, and the delivery of carbohydrate to the blood and muscles is enhanced. Doctors commonly prescribe Pedialyte (sugar water) for babies with diarrhea because it induces faster water absorption than does water alone and can more quickly rehydrate the baby.

See table 3.12 for suggested fluid-replacement schedules during exercise.

Fluid Intake After Exercise

Athletes who have exercised intensely for an hour or longer are likely to experience some degree of underhydration. For those athletes who exercise most days (i.e., most elite athletes), postexercise fluid consumption becomes a critically important part of the exercise regimen because it helps the athlete begin each subsequent day of activity in a well-hydrated state. The important point to consider is this: It takes time to dehydrate. The less time there is to dehydrate, the lower the likelihood that the athlete will be optimally hydrated by the beginning of the next exercise session.

Table 3.12 Opportunities for Fluid Replacement in Different Sports During Competition

Event and duration	Opportunities for fluid breaks	Fluid and carbohydrate requirements
Events lasting less than 30 min • Sprints • Jumping • Throwing • Gymnastics	Consume fluids between events but not within 15 min of event.	Not needed during the event but required between events during the course of the entire competition.
Intermediate events lasting less than 60 min • 10K run • Rowing • Aerobics class • Tennis lesson • Track cycling	Consume fluids between events. Runners should consume some fluid at least every 5 km (3.1 mi) (more often if hot and humid). All athletes in this category should bring a beverage container.	Fluid replacement is needed before, during, and after event, and carbohydrate is needed before and after event. However, carbohydrate will aid fluid uptake during event, so beverages should contain carbohydrate.
Endurance events • Marathon • 80 km cycling • Olympic distance triathlon • Tennis (5 sets)	Marathon runners should consume some fluid at least every 5 km (3.1 mi) (more often if hot and humid). Triathletes should consume fluids every 10 km (6.2 mi) during cycling and every 2 to 4 km (1.2 to 2.5 mi) during running. Tennis players should take as much time as allowable during court changes and after 3rd set to take fluids.	Fluid, electrolyte (sodium), and carbohydrate replacement are all recommended during these events. The amounts needed will vary based on environmental conditions, initial glycogen stores, and exercise intensity (e.g., difficulty of the match).
Ultraendurance events • Ironman • English Channel swim • Road cycling • Stage races such as Tour de France	Consume fluids at every opportunity, with a plan to consume fluids once every 10 min. Where fluids are not made available by race organizers (as may occur with cycling races), a fluid-consumption plan with carried fluids must be in place.	Fluid, electrolyte (sodium), and carbohydrate replacement are all recommended during these events. The amounts needed will vary based on environmental conditions, initial glycogen stores, and exercise intensity.
Team sports lasting around 90 min • Hockey • Basketball • Football • Volleyball • Baseball • Soccer	Consume fluids at breaks that naturally occur, but no less frequently than once every 15 min. Ideally, fluids should be consumed every 10 min. Naturally occurring longer breaks (halftime, between innings, between quarters) should be considered an opportunity to replenish fluids.	Fluid, electrolyte (sodium), and carbohydrate replacement are all recommended during these events. The amounts needed will vary based on environmental conditions, initial glycogen stores, and exercise intensity.

Adapted, by permission, from H. O'Connor, 1996, "Practical aspects of fluid replacement," *Aust J Nutr Diet* 53 (4 Suppl): S27-S34.

Athletes rarely consume fluids during exercise at a rate of more than 70 percent of sweat loss, and most athletes replace sweat losses at a rate significantly lower than this.[84, 85] Therefore, most athletes require strategies to achieve adequate hydration before the next exercise session begins. Despite this clear need for fluids, athletes often remain underhydrated even when fluids are readily available to them.[86] This voluntary dehydration suggests that athletes should be placed on a fixed fluid-replacement schedule that will increase the likelihood of maintaining hydration. A way of encouraging this is to make certain that cool, good-tasting fluids are easily available to the athlete as soon as the exercise session is over.[87]

Commercial sports drinks containing both carbohydrate and sodium are more effective than plain water at restoring water balance.[88] To maximize dehydration, however, it appears that a level of sodium greater than that provided in most sports drinks is desirable.[89] This added sodium can be obtained through the normal consumption of foods, many of which have added salt (sodium).[90]

In general, athletes should follow these rules for fluid consumption after exercise:

1. A large volume of fluid (as much as can be tolerated, perhaps .5 liter) should be consumed immediately after exercise. This large fluid volume enlarges the stomach and increases the rate at which fluids leave the stomach and enter the small intestine to be absorbed.

2. After the initial consumption of a large fluid volume, athletes should consume approximately 1/4 liter of fluid every 15 minutes to achieve a fluid intake of approximately 3 liters of fluid in 3 hours. The larger the athlete and the greater the sweat loss experienced during activity, the greater the amount of fluid that must be consumed.

3. Fluids should contain both carbohydrate and sodium because both are useful in returning the athlete to a well-hydrated state. In addition, the carbohydrate content of the beverage helps in returning stored glycogen (energy) to muscles in preparation for the next exercise session.

4. Sports drinks typically provide approximately 10 to 25 millimoles of electrolytes (mainly sodium) per liter of fluid. However, the optimal sodium concentration for fluid retention is approximately 50 millimoles of electrolytes per liter of fluid.[91] Since adding more sodium to fluids may make the fluid unpalatable and cause the athlete to consume less fluid, the athlete should be encouraged to consume some salted snacks (such as pretzels or saltine crackers) during the period immediately after exercise.

5. The loss in body weight that results from exercise should be the key to determining the total amount of fluid that must be replaced before the next exercise session. As a general guide, 1 pint (16 ounces) of retained fluid is equal to 1 pound of body weight. Since not all consumed water is retained, twice as much fluid may need to be consumed to replace the fluid equivalent in weight loss.

6. Fluids containing caffeine and related substances (coffee, tea, colas, chocolate) should be avoided because they increase urinary water loss.

4 | Ergogenic Aids

The term *ergogenic aid* refers to a substance that can increase the capacity for bodily or mental labor, especially by eliminating fatigue symptoms. Nutritional ergogenic aids refer to substances that enhance performance and are either nutrients, metabolic by-products of nutrients, food (plant) extracts, or substances commonly found in foods (e.g., caffeine and creatine) that are provided in amounts more concentrated than commonly found in the natural food supply. The non-nutritional ergogenic aids, including anabolic steroids and their analogues, continue to be used by athletes, but because they are nearly universally banned by sports organizing bodies (NCAA, IOC, USOC, and so on), they are not the focus of this chapter. Instead, this chapter focuses on the legal nutritional ergogenic aids, for which there is an increasing body of scientific information.

Companies selling ergogenic aids often target different athlete populations, with some focusing on strength and power sports while others focus on improving aerobic endurance. This chapter provides critical information on the theory behind each aid, its efficacy, and its safety (although long-term safety studies have rarely, if ever, been performed). In addition, where there may be some potential for performance enhancement by consuming an ergogenic aid, this chapter includes the best strategy for its use. Before reading this chapter, it is important that you consider this fact: The vast majority of substances advertised as having ergogenic properties do not, and those that do work would lose their ergogenic properties if the athlete consumed a regular energy and nutrient intake that satisfied need. Most important, the ergogenesis derived from a properly balanced diet is not only legal but also far less expensive and much more likely to be safe than that provided in bottles and pills.

In short, ergogenic aids claim to enhance performance. The nutritional ergogenic aids are so defined because they work by entering a well-established nutritional metabolic pathway or because they consist of one or more known nutrients. For instance, taking extra carbohydrate to improve performance makes the carbohydrate, by definition, a nutritional ergogenic aid. Also, taking creatine monohydrate to improve sprint performance makes creatine a nutritional ergogenic aid because creatine is a normal constituent of food, and its consumption causes creatine to enter a known metabolic pathway.[1-4] Non-nutritional ergogenic aids represent products (often of unknown origin because producers don't clearly specify what they consist of) that are neither nutrients nor other substances with nutritional properties. The best known non-nutritional ergogenic aids are anabolic steroids.

In most cases, the performance-enhancement claims attributed to ergogenic aids exceed reality. Since many of the products are considered foods, nutrients, or nutrient-based products, there are few controls for government agencies to police these claims. The only truly credible sources of information come from published scientific works and the Office of Dietary Supplements of the National Institutes of Health. Where improvements are seen, it is often due to a placebo effect: People believe it will help, so it actually helps even though there is no biological basis for the improvement. In other cases, improvements occur because the product is providing a chemical missing from the foods that an athlete commonly consumes. For instance, bodybuilders often take protein powders or amino acid powders to aid in the enlargement of muscle mass. However, studies clearly indicate that the rate of protein usage by the body is well below the level consumed by those who take these protein powders. The body's limit for using protein to build muscle and maintain tissues is much lower than the amount of protein commonly consumed through food and protein supplements. The upper limit for protein usage is below 2 grams per kilogram of body weight, and those who take protein supplements often take more than 3 grams of protein per kilogram of body weight. The excess protein is burned as a fuel or stored as fat, but it can't be used to build more muscle. It is also known that bodybuilders frequently consume an inadequate level of energy. This energy inadequacy makes it difficult for them to support their larger muscle mass.[5] The reason the extra protein appears to be ergogenic is more likely to be because of the calories provided than because of its potential tissue-building effect.

Numerous ergogenic aids are available, ranging from known nutrients to supposed nutrients (such as vitamin B_{15}, which has no official definition, varies in content by manufacturer because of no standardization of active ingredient(s), and is not a recognized vitamin) to herbs with no known chemical content or known active ingredients. There is so much misinformation in the marketplace and in the locker room about

A Brief History of Ergogenic Aids

"The first Olympic games took place in Greece in 776 BC. From sources documenting specific training and dietary regimens for athletes in ancient times, we know that some of them ate hallucinogenic mushrooms and sesame seeds to enhance performance. Although the modern Olympic games commenced in 1896, scientific and medical interest in the diet and training of Olympic athletes did not begin until 1922. . . . In 1889, Charles Edward Brown-Séquard, a French physiologist, claimed to have reversed his own aging process by self-injecting testicular extracts. Testosterone, the primary male hormone, was first synthesized in 1935, and in the 1940s, athletes began taking anabolic steroids to increase their muscle mass. Throughout the 1950s and 1960s, amphetamines and anabolic steroids were used extensively. Concerned about that trend, the International Olympic Committee (IOC) banned their use by Olympic athletes in the early 1960s. Formal drug testing began with the 1968 Olympics. In 1988, Canadian Olympic sprinter Ben Johnson was stripped of his gold medal after testing revealed he had used an oral anabolic steroid; this was the first time a gold medallist in track and field was disqualified from the Olympics for using illegal drugs..." [From: Silver, Marc D. Use of ergogenic aids by athletes. Journal of the American Academy of Orthopaedic Surgeons 2001; 9(1): 61-63.]

these products that the buyer should beware. In general, athletes would do better to avoid the focus on a magic bullet to improve performance and should take a more realistic approach by consuming a balanced intake of foods that provide sufficient energy and nutrients to support growth, activity, and tissue maintenance.

Categories of Ergogenic Aids

Ergogenic aids fall into several categories, including mechanical aids, pharmacological aids, physiological aids, nutritional aids, and psychological aids (see table 4.1). Some ergogenic aids, such as blood doping, erythropoietin (EPO), anabolic steroids, and human growth hormone, are widely banned by sports organizing committees and the International Olympic Committee (IOC). For a comprehensive and up-to-date list of widely restricted and banned ergogenic aids, along with prohibited methods for achieving performance enhancement, visit the following Web site: www.wada-ama.org/en/.

Despite widely publicized problems associated with the ingestion of many substances with ergogenic properties, athletes continue to play Russian roulette with their bodies. The side effects from taking anabolic steroids, for instance, may be irreversible and include hypertension; dysplasia resulting in tendon ruptures; liver tumors; psychosis (steroid rage); hirsutism; clitoral hypertrophy and lower voice in women; breast development, testicular atrophy, and impotence in men; and premature closure of the bone epiphyses, causing shorter stature in adolescents.[6] In addition,

Table 4.1 **Categories and Examples of Ergogenic Aids (Both Allowed and Prohibited)**

Category	Examples
Mechanical aids	Free weights to develop strength; lightweight racing shoes; nasal strips to improve airflow to the lungs; running parachutes for resistance to develop strength
Pharmacological aids	Androgenic steroid hormones (and their precursors); high-dose nutrient supplements (vitamins and minerals); quasi-nutrient substances that impart a pharmacological effect (i.e., beyond the nutritional effect you would expect from a normal intake)
Physiological aids	Blood doping; sauna; massage and other forms of physiotherapy
Nutritional aids	Carbohydrate loading; sports drinks; caffeine intake and the consumption of other substances commonly available in the food supply
Psychological aids	Hypnosis; relaxation techniques; imagery techniques; motivational techniques

most ergogenic aids are taken to counter ongoing dietary shortcomings that would be cheaper, safer, and more effectively corrected with simple changes in food and fluid consumption. For instance, the amino acid delivery from protein and amino acid supplements is more than 10 times more expensive than the consumption of a small piece of chicken or meat, and the latter is known to be safe. Of course, the legality of obtaining and consuming certain substances should also be considered. Although widely available, anabolic steroids are prescription medications that may legally be prescribed only by a doctor for a patient who presents with defined clinical symptoms. The issue of safety should not be taken lightly. Products containing combinations of caffeine and ephedrine have resulted in numerous deaths, leading to the banning of ephedra and related substances from U.S. and other markets.[7] See table 4.3 at the end of this chapter for a summary of ergogenic aids, their potential benefits and side effects, and their legality.

Given the widespread advertisements purporting the ergogenic benefits of various substances, it is difficult for coaches and athletes to discern what works and what doesn't, what's safe and what isn't. In an issue of The Clipboard, a Gatorade Sports Science Institute publication, sports nutritionist Ellen Coleman summarizes some critical points to consider in evaluating these products (Adapted from: Coleman, E. How to Evaluate Supplements. The Clipboard. www.gssiweb.com. 12-3-2004):

- The supplement should carry USP (United States Pharmacopeia) on the label. The USP symbol indicates the supplement has passed standard tests for solubility, disintegration, potency, and purity.

- Make sure the product is made by nationally known food and drug manufacturers. Reputable manufacturers follow strict quality-control procedures. Companies failing to answer questions or address complaints should not have your business.
- The supplement should be supported by research. Reputable companies provide research findings from peer-reviewed journals to support claims.
- Look for accurate and appropriate claims. If statements about the supplement are unclear or the label makes preposterous claims, it is unlikely the company follows good quality-control procedures. Claims that sound too good to be true probably are.

A major problem with dietary supplements is that it is difficult to be sure of their content. According to Maughan (2001), the dietary supplements athletes take might cause them to fail a doping test because they may contain nandrolone (an anabolic steroid) or other banned substances.[8] Maughan cites numerous reports of athletes failing drug tests because herbal supplements they believed to be safe and legal actually contained banned substances. Clearly, athletes should ask themselves if the risks of taking a supplement outweigh the potential benefits. They may believe they are doing nothing contrary to sports organizing committee rules (e.g., the IOC or USOC), but there is increasingly a zero tolerance for banned substances. If a banned substance is found in an athlete's body, the athlete is "guilty" even if it got there without his or her knowledge or consent.

Carbohydrate As Ergogenic Aid

Since carbohydrate is typically the limiting energy substrate in exercise (i.e., it will run out before fat or protein runs out), it is critical to begin a bout of physical activity with enough stored carbohydrate to see the athlete through the session; doing so will aid exercise endurance, regardless of the exercise modality. In high-intensity exercise, carbohydrate is the primary fuel used by the muscles. In low-intensity exercise of long duration, fat may be the primary fuel, but fat requires carbohydrate for complete oxidation.[9] In addition, the storage capacity for fat is far greater than that of carbohydrate, even in the leanest athletes. In either form of exercise, carbohydrate depletion results in a dramatically reduced exercise performance.[10, 11] It is the intent of carbohydrate-loading techniques, therefore, to store the maximal amount of carbohydrate the tissues can hold. (See chapter 6 for more information on carbohydrate-loading techniques.)

Not all sports and activities are suitable for carbohydrate loading. Keep in mind that for every gram of stored glycogen, the body stores approximately 3 grams of water. Tissues that are packed full of glycogen and water are likely to cause some degree of muscle stiffness. In sports such as gymnastics and diving where flexibility is important, carbohydrate loading may cause difficulties. It also appears that carbohydrate loading may be less beneficial for women than for men. In a study comparing higher carbohydrate intakes in men and women, men showed both a glycogen and performance improvement, whereas women, because of a higher lipid and lower

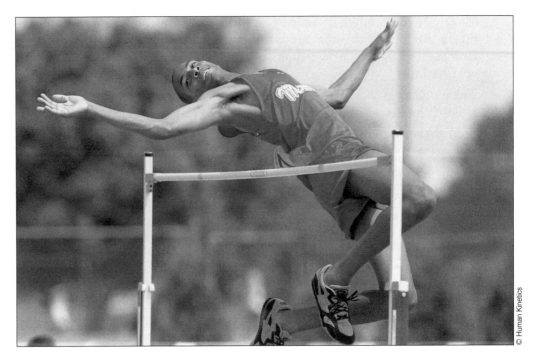

© Human Kinetics

In sports or events where jump height is a factor, as in the high jump, athletes may benefit more from a 250-calorie carboyhdrate supplement than they will from a creatine supplement.

protein and carbohydrate oxidation rate than men, did not experience the same level of improvement.[12]

The type of carbohydrate does appear to make a difference. Glucose polymer products (including commercially available sports gels and polycose) and maltodextrins (which are found in numerous sports beverages) are easily digested into glucose and appear to be more effective for glycogen production than are other carbohydrates. However, starches from pasta, bread, rice, and other cereals are also effective at maximizing glycogen storage.[13, 14]

Different forms of carbohydrates have different rates of digestion and provide varying rates of glucose release into the blood. In a study assessing the rise of blood glucose after a high-carbohydrate meal 2.5 hours before a 90-minute bicycle ride, subjects were given a candy bar with either a high glycemic (HG) index or a low glycemic (LG) index; a no-food control was also used. Both blood glucose and insulin were higher in the LG group than in either of the other two conditions. Blood free fatty acids (FFAs) were highest in the control group, while the LG trial showed higher FFAs than did the HG trial during the ride. This study suggests that a low glycemic index food will provide more sustained energy (and thus improved endurance) during prolonged exercise.[15]

Ingesting a glucose polymer solution before exercise results in a smaller reduction in power than does a noncaloric placebo during 1 hour of maximal exercise. When the same amount of glucose polymer is taken in 15-minute intervals during exercise, there is no observed benefit. This suggests that consumption of a glucose polymer is performance enhancing if consumed before exercise but is without any ergogenic benefit if taken during exercise.[16]

How quickly an athlete can recover from exhaustive exercise by reestablishing muscle glycogen is also an important performance factor, particularly in sports where athletes compete on sequential days. Glycogen depletion may occur in 2 to 3 hours of high-intensity exercise (60 to 80 percent of $\dot{V}O_2$max) and even faster in maximum-intensity activity. Besides reducing performance, low muscle glycogen may predispose athletes to higher injury risk. In activities such as soccer and hockey, where competition frequency and exercise intensity make glycogen depletion more likely, consumption of carbohydrate during a competition or practice is a logical strategy to avoid glycogen depletion. Many athletes in these and related sports continue to miss an important ergogenic opportunity by consuming only water during an event.[17]

After exercise, it seems logical to consume a carbohydrate food (1 gram per kilogram of body weight is recommended) to reduce protein breakdown and aid in protein synthesis. Failure to consume carbohydrate after exercise results in a higher than necessary level of muscle breakdown, thereby reducing the benefit that might be derived from resistance training.[18]

Creatine Monohydrate

Creatine—a compound made from the amino acids arginine, glycine, and methionine—joins with phosphorus to make phosphocreatine. Phosphocreatine serves as a storage depot for maintaining adenosine triphosphate (ATP) levels during high-intensity activities, such as sprinting, that can quickly deplete ATP (see figure 4.1). ATP is the high-energy fuel used by cells. It is believed that athletes who saturate their muscles with creatine will enhance their capacity to maintain the high-energy compound ATP and delay fatigue in high-intensity activity.[19]

Besides our cellular synthesis of creatine from three amino acids, we can also obtain creatine from meat. (*Note:* The Greek root of the word *creatine* is *creas*, which means meat.) However, normal cooking can easily reduce the creatine level of foods by denaturing this simple polypeptide. Well-done meats, therefore, retain a relatively small preformed creatine content.

Many athletes regularly consume creatine in the form of creatine monohydrate, and clear evidence suggests that these supplements can enhance anaerobic power and anaerobic endurance.[20-22] Some limited evidence also suggests a performance benefit.[23] It is possible, however, that the benefit derived from taking creatine monohydrate may be due to the inadequate energy (caloric) intake commonly seen in athletes.[24] In a recent study on repeated jump height, a 250-calorie supplement

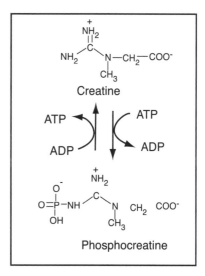

Figure 4.1   Creation of ATP from Phosphocreatine.

of carbohydrate was found to be more effective at sustaining maximal jump height than was a standard creatine monohydrate supplement. In addition, the carbohydrate sustained jump height without an associated weight gain, whereas the creatine monohydrate consumption was associated with a significant increase in weight.[25] As previously mentioned, inadequate energy intake is one of the major problems that athletes face. It is possible that athletes with an adequate energy intake would not benefit from these supplements, although this has never been adequately tested.

Athletes consuming creatine monohydrate typically dose themselves with 10 to 28 grams, divided into four doses over the day. For instance, if the goal is to take 10 grams per day, individual doses should be 2.5 grams four times daily. The smaller the athlete, the smaller the daily dose.

There is evidence that taking daily creatine supplements causes a saturation of creatine in muscle tissue after 5 days.[26] Therefore, creatine should not be consumed for longer than 5 days, followed by about a 5-day break in supplementation. Taking creatine supplements only 5 days per month may even be sufficient to saturate muscle tissue.[27, 28] Creatine storage in muscle also causes a retention of water, with a concomitant increase in weight.[29]

The long-term safety of creatine monohydrate supplementation has never been tested on children, adolescents, or adults. There is also no solid evidence to suggest that creatine supplementation is unsafe for healthy adults, and there is no information on its safety if taken by children or over long periods of time. Athletes must determine whether creatine supplementation is appropriate for them. Before an athlete tries creatine supplementation, it may be prudent to first be certain that an adequate level of energy (calories) is being consumed.

Glycerol

Glycerol (also referred to as glycerine) is a three-carbon simple lipid that is metabolized like carbohydrate. The three-carbon structure of glycerol holds dietary fatty acids together to form triglycerides. Glycerol is a powerful humectant, with a potent capacity to attract a large volume of water. A number of endurance athletes use glycerol as a means of superhydration because of this capacity to hold water, as well as glycerol's ability to be easily and cleanly metabolized for energy. Adding a small amount of glycerol to water enables an athlete to store more water and, in doing so, may aid the athlete in endurance competitions that take place in extremely hot and humid environments. (See chapter 3 for more information about superhydration.)

Maximizing body water may induce a level of stiffness that some athletes find uncomfortable. Indeed, athletes who consume glycerol-laced fluids before an event often complain that they feel, at least initially, stiff and sluggish. But many of these same athletes claim that the benefits of having extra water at the end of a race far outweigh the feeling of sluggishness at the beginning of the race. While other athletes are dehydrated and overheating, these athletes say they feel more fresh when it counts the most.

A word of caution: Although many endurance athletes use glycerated water to enhance their hydration state, this product has never been adequately tested for safety. Because glycerol is a normal component of the diet and is easily metabolized, it is unlikely that small amounts of glycerol, by itself, would cause any difficulty. With higher doses, headaches and blurred vision may occur.[30] Furthermore, it is unclear how much additional stress is placed on the cardiovascular system when additional water is stored in the system.

The IOC bans diuretics because of the detrimental effects of dehydration and because diuretics have been used to lower the concentration of biological markers of steroids and other banned substances in the urine. Glycerol was once classified as a diuretic, but in 1997 the U.S. Olympic Committee (USOC) removed the ban on glycerol because it was widely understood that diuresis is not likely at glycerol doses of between 1.0 and 1.5 grams per kilogram.

There is no widespread consensus on how to best consume glycerated water. The protocol established for a 155-pound (70 kilogram) athlete ingesting approximately 2 liters of fluid 2.5 hours before activity is as follows:[31]

- Drink 5 milliliters per kilogram of a 20 percent glycerol solution.
- Thirty minutes later: Drink 5 milliliters per kilogram of water.
- Fifteen minutes later: Drink 5 milliliters per kilogram of water.
- Fifteen minutes later: Drink 1 milliliter per kilogram of a 20 percent glycerol solution and 5 milliliters per kilogram of water.
- Thirty minutes later: Drink 5 milliliters per kilogram of water.
- Begin exercise 1 hour later.

For events lasting more than 2 hours, consuming 400 to 800 milliliters per hour of a 5 percent glycerol solution before and during the event may also be beneficial, although there is more compelling evidence that consumption of a 6 to 8 percent carbohydrate solution during competition is ergogenic.

Bicarbonate (Sodium Bicarbonate or Bicarbonate of Soda)

Researchers have theorized that sodium bicarbonate buffers the acidity from lactic acid that is created by anaerobic metabolism. If so, this would allow for a prolonged maintenance of force or power.[32] Many activities involve mainly anaerobic metabolic processes, and it would appear that some athletes could benefit from sodium bicarbonate consumption. Study results, however, are mixed and generally indicate that well-hydrated athletes do not derive the performance benefit theorized from bicarbonate ingestion.

The sodium in the sodium bicarbonate may actually be more useful than the bicarbonate (the acid buffer). Sodium is an electrolyte that helps increase or maintain blood volume, creating a larger buffering space (i.e., more fluid) for muscles to excrete the extra acidity created by high-intensity activity. Think of sugar as the acid produced from anaerobic activity and a glass of water as the blood volume, and you can see what might happen. If the glass of water is half full and you drop a cube of sugar in it, the concentration of sugar would be higher than if you put the same amount of sugar in a full glass of water. The potential negative side effects from taking sodium bicarbonate, however—including the potential for severe gastrointestinal distress and nausea—should give athletes reason to be cautious before taking this potential ergogenic aid.

In a 1993 study of 10 collegiate varsity rowers, subjects consumed 300 milligrams of sodium bicarbonate ($NaHCO_3$) per kilogram of lean body mass 1 hour before a 2,000-meter time trial. Power, total work produced, and speed in the event were all significantly improved when compared with the consumption of a non-ergogenic placebo.[33] In another study, six trained males ingested 300 milligrams of $NaHCO_3$ per kilogram of lean body mass and were assessed before, during, and after exhaustive resistance training. The $NaHCO_3$ produced no apparent improvement.[34] In an assessment of male and female runners who competed in a series of four 1,600-meter races scheduled 3 days apart, subjects ingested 400 milligrams of $NaHCO_3$ per kilogram, 500 milligrams of sodium citrate per kilogram, or a placebo (calcium carbonate) 2 hours before three of the races; one race was used as a control. The sodium bicarbonate and sodium citrate had no effect on racing time, and most of the runners complained of uncomfortable side effects. Bicarbonate loading was associated with uncomfortable side effects in the majority of athletes.[35]

Proteins and Amino Acids

Amino acids are the building blocks of proteins. Various numbers of amino acids held together in diverse sequences result in proteins with different characteristics. The protein in hair, for instance, has a particular sequence of amino acids, and the protein in muscle has another sequence of amino acids. When proteins are broken apart, the result is a pool of amino acids derived from the amino acid building blocks of the protein.

Many athletes consume protein or amino acid supplements, believing they promote muscle building. However, dietary assessments of athletes strongly suggest that any benefit of the supplement comes from helping athletes meet their caloric needs rather than independently supporting a larger muscle mass. Because this is most likely the case, most athletes would find it easier, cheaper, and safer to eat more food to obtain the needed calories than to take the protein or amino acid supplements. Studies generally agree that humans use, anabolically, only about 1.5 grams of protein per kilogram of body weight.[36, 37] Protein requirement can be thought of as directly related to the amount of fat-free mass a person has, plus a very small amount used to supply energy. Taken together, this amounts to a requirement range for athletes between 1.0 and 1.5 grams per kilogram of body weight. Consuming more than this amount ensures that the remaining protein will be catabolized as a source of fuel or stored as fat. Burning protein as a source of fuel is undesirable because it creates toxic nitrogenous waste (e.g., ammonia, urea) that must be excreted. This mandatory urinary excretion causes an increase in water loss and increases the chance for dehydration.

Caffeine

Caffeine, one of several methylxanthines found in coffee, tea, cola, chocolate, and a variety of other foods and beverages (see table 4.2), has been shown to help endurance-type performance in people who are unaccustomed to consuming caffeinated products.[38] Caffeine is a central nervous system stimulant and a muscle relaxant. It has recently been removed from the IOC's banned substance list. In a number of studies, caffeine ingestion significantly increased free fatty acid (FFA) concentration in plasma.[39] The increased availability of FFAs enhances the ability of cells to use

Table 4.2   Caffeine Content of Widely Available Foods, Beverages, and Over-the-Counter Drugs

Product	Caffeine content
Coffee, drip, regular (5 oz, 150 ml)	106-164 mg
Coffee, percolated, regular (5 oz, 150 ml)	93-134 mg
Coffee, instant, regular (5 oz, 150 ml)	47-68 mg
Coffee, decaffeinated (5 oz, 150 ml)	2-5 mg
Coffee, Starbucks coffee grande (16 oz, 480 ml)	550 mg
Tea, black (1 cup, 240 ml)	25-110 mg
Tea, oolong (1 cup, 240 ml)	12-55 mg
Tea, green (1 cup, 240 ml)	8-36 mg
Tea, iced (12 oz, 360 ml)	67-76 mg
Soda, Mountain Dew (12 oz, 360 ml)	54 mg
Soda, Coca-Cola (12 oz, 360 ml)	46 mg
Soda, Dr. Pepper (12 oz, 360 ml)	40 mg
Soda, Pepsi-Cola (12 oz, 360 ml)	38 mg
Chocolate, milk chocolate (1 oz, 28 g)	6 mg
Chocolate, cocoa beverage mix (6 oz, 168 g)	2-8 mg
Chocolate, sweet chocolate (1 oz, 28 g)	20 mg
No-Doz tablet (1 dose)	200 mg
Anacin (1 dose)	64 mg
Excedrin (1 dose)	130 mg
Bufferin (1 dose)	0 mg

Adapted, by permission, from D.M. Ahrendt, 2001, "Ergogenic aids: Counseling the athlete," *American Family Physician* 63(5): 913-922.

these fats as a fuel in endurance-type, low-intensity activities. Since humans adapt to caffeine intake, frequent and regular consumption results in a reduced dose effect. Put simply, the more you consume, the more you need to consume to achieve the same ergogenic effect. Overconsumption of caffeine is associated with irritability, insomnia, diarrhea, and anxiety. In addition, a large volume of caffeine intake may induce a diuresis that could exacerbate the state of dehydration.

Caffeine consumed at doses of between 3 and 9 milligrams per kilogram or a total of approximately 250 milligrams appears to aid performance in long-endurance activity and may also improve performance in more intense short-duration exercise.[38, 40] It remains unclear as to why caffeine has this apparent ergogenic benefit, although it has been hypothesized that it may stimulate the sympathetic nervous system and enhance utilization of fatty acids, thereby sparing limited glycogen stores.[41, 42] A central nervous system stimulant, caffeine may stimulate the brain into a lower level of fatigue to allow a continuation of performance at a higher level. Now that the IOC no longer bans caffeine, it is likely that athletes will incorporate caffeine into a more regular and higher usage pattern. Except for the dependence problem it creates with regular use (discontinuation produces irritability, headache, and mood shifts), it is a relatively safe substance to consume.[43]

Carnitine (Typically L-Carnitine)

L-carnitine is a common name for beta-hydroxy butyrate, a quaternary amine that was first discovered in muscles in the early 1900 . It is mainly involved in transporting long-chain fatty acids that reside inside cells into the mitochondria of the cells, where they are metabolized. Carnitine increases blood flow by improving fatty acid oxidation in the artery walls, and it detoxifies ammonia, a by-product of protein breakdown that is associated with early fatigue.[44] We synthesize carnitine from the amino acids lysine and methionine, and it is found in abundant quantities in all meats and dairy products, so a deficiency is unlikely. If a deficiency occurs, it is most likely in vegetarians who avoid consumption of dairy products. With an adequate intake of meats or dairy products, there is little reason to take this relatively expensive supplement. Although never tested, it is possible that pure vegans might benefit from L-carnitine supplementation if they perform high-intensity exercise.

Carnitine is thought to spare muscle glycogen breakdown and decrease lactic acid production, but studies of carnitine generally show no benefit for low-intensity endurance activities.[45] Some studies, however, have demonstrated a benefit in high-intensity activities when consumed either just before the activity or for several days. The typical dose is between 1 and 2 grams per day, but the safety of L-carnitine supplementation has not been adequately tested. The type of carnitine taken is also important. There are reports that DL-carnitine supplementation (a less expensive form of carnitine) may cause muscle weakness.[46] Therefore, if an athlete insists on taking this supplement, only the L-carnitine form should be considered.

Omega-3 Fatty Acids

Omega-3 fatty acids are available as over-the-counter supplements, but they can also be easily obtained through regular consumption of cold-water fish such as salmon, herring, and sardines. These fatty acids may be useful for reducing muscle soreness, and they may have several other benefits, including the following:[47]

- Improved delivery of oxygen and nutrients to muscles and other tissues. Omega-3 fatty acids reduce red blood cell "stickiness," thereby improving the flow of red blood cells to tissues. (*Note:* Excess consumption of omega-3 fatty acids may inhibit normal blood clotting, resulting in excess bleeding should an injury occur.)
- Improved aerobic metabolism due to better delivery of oxygen.
- Higher release of somatotropin (growth hormone) in response to normal stimuli (exercise, sleep, hunger). This may have an anabolic effect and may improve muscular recovery.
- Reduced inflammation of tissues resulting from muscular fatigue and over-exertion, allowing for faster recovery.

Despite these potential benefits, results from the scientific literature do not indicate that an endurance performance benefit is derived from omega-3 fatty acid supplementation.[48, 49]

Medium-Chain Triglycerides

Medium-chain triglycerides (MCTs) are found in coconut oil and palm kernel oil, which are among the most saturated fatty acids in human nutrition. MCTs have carbon lengths of 6 to 12 carbon atoms, while the majority of the triglycerides consumed have considerably longer carbon chains. This difference, plus their water solubility, allows these particular fats to be absorbed and metabolized differently. The liver readily takes them up, where they can be rapidly oxidized for cellular energy.[50] In addition, MCT oils do not require L-carnitine to deliver energy to cell mitochondria for metabolism (other fats require L-carnitine).[51] These oils offer several potential benefits for athletes:[47]

- Provide a quick source of energy
- Help mobilize body fat stores for energy
- Increase the metabolic rate
- Spare lean body mass (muscle)

Widely available in drugstores and health food stores, MCT oils have a long history of safety. They have been used for many years as a source of energy for those on enteral (tube) feedings. Studies assessing the impact of MCTs on performance, however, have not found a benefit even though there is an apparent increase in serum free fatty acid concentration as a result of ingestion.[52-54]

Ginseng

Ginseng has been used for centuries in Asian cultures to reduce fatigue. In a limited number of studies, components of ginseng have been shown to spare glycogen usage and increase the oxidation of fatty acids.[47] Exercised animals that have been injected with a ginseng extract have shown reduced fatigue.[55] However, human studies evaluating various doses of ginseng root for periods of up to 2 months have shown no clear ergogenic benefit. There is only limited evidence that providing a supplement of ginseng extract may improve endurance performance by increasing oxygen delivery to the muscles. Ginseng ingested at either 8 or 16 milligrams per kilogram of body weight for 7 days did not improve either submaximal or maximal cycling performance.[56]

Ergogenic Choices

An almost never-ending array of products advertise their performance-enhancing properties. For the most part, however, there is little evidence that well-nourished athletes derive any of the advertised benefits from the consumption of these products. (On the other hand, those manufacturing and selling the products derive a great deal of benefit.) Athletes should carefully consider the adequacy of their own diets before attempting to use ergogenic aids. These products are expensive, few of them have ever been adequately tested for safety, their contents are often unknown, and the actual amount of the active ingredient is uncertain. Furthermore, the chance that these supplements may be laced with banned substances is real. See table 4.3 for a summary of the most common ergogenic aids and their effects.

Athletes choosing to use an ergogenic aid should proceed cautiously. Speak with an appropriately credentialed health professional (e.g., a doctor, dietitian, or pharmacist) to obtain as much information on the product as possible, and determine if there is a simple dietary fix that would make the supplement unnecessary. When any supplement is consumed for the first time, carefully observe whether gastrointestinal distress or nausea occur, and document your sense of well-being after taking it. Most ergogenic aids are powerful chemicals that are easily handled if taken in the small amounts that naturally appear in the foods we eat. However, when they are taken in the large doses often prescribed to achieve an ergogenic benefit, the impact on your body may be entirely different and unexpected.

Of all the ergogenic aids mentioned in this chapter, it is very clear that carbohydrates hold the greatest promise for improving both endurance and power performance. Before trying anything else, athletes should consider a regular consumption of carbohydrates with plenty of fluids. This is, perhaps, the single most important thing an athlete can do to ensure both an adequate total energy intake and an appropriate consumption of the energy substrate most easily depleted.

Table 4.3 **Summary of Substances Commonly Used by Athletes Because of a Belief in Their Ergogenic Properties**

Substance	Potential action	Research findings	Side effects	Legality
Alcohol	Lowers anxiety	No benefit	Significantly negative	Banned in shooting events
Amino acids: arginine, ornithine, lysine	Stimulate growth hormone; enhance muscle development	No benefit	None known	Legal
Amphetamines	Lower fatigue and appetite	Mixed results; some positive	Significantly dangerous	Illegal
Anabolic steroids	Increase lean mass, exercise motivation, and strength	Clear benefit	Significantly dangerous	Illegal
Androstenediol	Same as anabolic steroids	Limited studies	Unknown	Banned by IOC
Androstenedione	Same as anabolic steroids	No benefit	Significantly negative	Banned by IOC, NCAA
Antioxidants	Enhance muscle recovery; reduce muscle breakdown	Mixed results; no clear benefit	Mild	Legal
Aspartates	Increase use of free fatty acids, thereby sparing muscle glycogen	Mixed results	Mild	Legal
Aspirin	Decreases pain associated with muscle fatigue and muscle breakdown	No benefit	Mild; potential for GI bleeding with large doses	Legal
Bee pollen	Increases strength and endurance	No benefit	Potential for allergic reaction	Legal

(continued)

Table 4.3 *(continued)*

Substance	Potential action	Research findings	Side effects	Legality
Beta-blockers	Lower anxiety	Improves fine motor control; reduces aerobic capacity	Significantly negative	Banned by IOC
Blood doping	Increases aerobic capacity	Clear benefit	Significantly dangerous (increases blood viscosity)	Illegal
Boron	Increases endogenous steroid production	No benefit	Mild	Legal
Branched-chain amino acids (BCAAs)	Reduces central nervous system fatigue	Mixed results	Mild	Legal
Caffeine	Increases muscle contractility; improves aerobic endurance; improves fat metabolism	Clear benefit	Mild	Legal
Calcium	Increases muscle contractility; improves glycogen metabolism	No benefit	Mild	Legal
Carbohydrates	Improve performance; lower fatigue	Clear benefit	Mild	Legal
Carnitine	Increases fat metabolism	No benefit	None	Legal
Choline	Improves endurance	Mixed results	None	Legal

Substance	Potential action	Research findings	Side effects	Legality
Chromium	Increases lean mass	No benefit unless preexisting deficiency	Safe up to 400 mcg/day; dangerous above this level	Legal
Chrysin	Increases endogenous steroid production	No benefit	None	Legal
Cocaine	Stimulates CNS; delays fatigue	Mixed results	Significantly negative; dangerous	Illegal
Coenzyme Q-10 (ubiquinone)	Delays fatigue; antioxidant	No benefit	None	Legal
Coenzyme Q-12	Improves aerobic capacity; speeds muscle repair	No benefit	None	Legal
Creatine	Improves repeated high-intensity activity endurance	Benefit, but no safety data available	None in short term; unknown in long term	Legal
DHEA	Improves endogenous steroid production	No benefit in healthy athletes	Potentially dangerous	Banned by IOC and other groups
Diuretics	Lower body mass to lower resistance	Limited benefit	Potentially dangerous	Banned by IOC
Ephedrine and related substances	Stimulate CNS; delay fatigue; encourage weight loss	No benefit	Potentially dangerous	Banned by IOC and other organizations; illegal to sell in USA and several other countries

(continued)

Table 4.3   *(continued)*

Substance	Potential action	Research findings	Side effects	Legality
Ephedrine plus caffeine	Increases energy; stimulates weight loss	Some benefit	Potentially dangerous; fatal at higher doses	Banned by IOC and other organizations; illegal to sell in USA and several other countries
Erythropoietin (EPO)	Increases aerobic capacity	Clear benefit	Significantly negative; dangerous	Illegal
Fluids	Increase endurance	Clear benefit	Some danger of hyponatremia	Legal
Folic acid	Increases aerobic capacity	No benefit	None	Legal
GHB	Stimulates growth hormone release and muscle growth	No clear benefit	Significantly negative (dose related); abuse potential	Illegal
Ginseng	Increases endurance; improves muscle recovery	No clear benefit	Mild; abuse syndrome reported	Legal
Glucosamine	Serves as NSAID alternative; enhances muscle recovery	Limited benefit	None	Legal
Glutamine	Boosts immunity and growth hormone levels	May boost immunity	None	Legal
Glycerol	Improves hydration and endurance	Some benefit	Mild	Legal
HMB	Decreases muscle breakdown; enhances recovery	Limited studies; some strength benefits	None	Legal

Substance	Potential action	Research findings	Side effects	Legality
Human growth hormone	Has anabolic effect on muscle growth; increases fat metabolism	Limited benefit	Significantly negative; dangerous	Illegal
Inosine	Enhances energy production; improves aerobic capacity	No benefit	Mild	Legal
Iron	Increases aerobic capacity	No benefit unless preexisting deficiency	Mild; toxic at high doses	Legal
Leucine	Decreases muscle breakdown; spares muscle glycogen stores	Limited studies; no benefit	None	Legal
Ma huang (herbal ephedrine)	Same as ephedrine: Stimulates CNS; delays fatigue; promotes weight loss	No benefit	Potentially dangerous	Banned by IOC and other organizations
Magnesium	Enhances muscle growth	No benefit unless preexisting deficiency	Mild at high doses	Legal
Niacin	Increases energy and endurance	No benefit unless preexisting deficiency	Mild at high doses; extremely high chronic doses associated with hepatitis	Legal

(continued)

Table 4.3 *(continued)*

Substance	Potential action	Research findings	Side effects	Legality
Oxygen	Increases aerobic capacity; improves recovery	No benefit	Mild	Legal
Phosphates	Increase ATP production, energy, and muscle endurance	Mixed results	Mild at high doses	Legal
Phytosterols	Stimulate release of endogenous steroids and growth hormone	No benefit	Little data; allergic reaction possible	Legal
Protein	Optimizes muscular growth and repair	Slightly increased need for protein with increased activity	None	Legal
Pyruvate	Increases lean body mass	No benefit	None	Legal
D-ribose	Increases cellular ATP and muscle power	No human research	None known	Legal
Selenium	Enhances antioxidant functions	Limited studies; no benefit	Mild at high doses	Legal
Sodium bicarbonate	Buffers lactic acid production; delays fatigue	Some benefit	Mild; dangerous at high doses	Legal
Tryptophan	Decreases pain perception; increases endurance	Mixed results; no benefit in trained athletes	Mild; potentially dangerous	Legal
Vanadyl sulfate	Increases glycogen synthesis; enhances muscle recovery	No benefit	Mild	Legal

Substance	Potential action	Research findings	Side effects	Legality
Vitamin B_1 (thiamin)	Enhances energy production; increases aerobic capacity; improves concentration	No benefit unless preexisting deficiency	None	Legal
Vitamin B_2 (riboflavin)	Increases aerobic endurance	No benefit unless preexisting deficiency	None	Legal
Vitamin B_6 (pyridoxine)	Enhances muscle growth; decreases anxiety	No benefit unless preexisting deficiency	None	Legal
Vitamin B_{12} (cyanocobalamin)	Enhances muscle growth	No benefit unless preexisting deficiency	None	Legal
Vitamin B_{15} (dimethylglycine)	Increases muscle energy production	No benefit; may make things worse	None proven, but concerns raised	Legal
Vitamin C	Acts as antioxidant; increases aerobic capacity and energy production	No benefit unless preexisting deficiency	Mild at high doses	Legal
Vitamin E	Acts as antioxidant; improves aerobic capacity	Some positive findings	Mild	Legal
Yohimbine	Increases endogenous steroid production	No benefit	Mild	Legal
Zinc	Enhances muscle growth; increases aerobic capacity	No benefit unless preexisting deficiency	Mild	Legal

Adapted, by permission, from D.M. Ahrendt, 2001, "Ergogenic aids: Counseling the athlete," *American Family Physician* 63(5): 913-922.

Part II

Nutritional Aspects of Optimal Performance

Digestion and Absorption

5

Athletes need more energy nutrients, more fluids, and more vitamins and minerals than nonathletes need, and all of these essential substances must go through the gastrointestinal (GI) tract to be digested and absorbed for delivery to organs and muscles. It is critical that athletes be familiar with numerous issues relating to the delivery of nutrients and fluids through the gastrointestinal tract. For instance, understanding gastric emptying enables athletes to adopt the best strategies for delivering the greatest amount of energy and fluids without inducing nausea or vomiting. Understanding the digestion and absorption of nutrients and fluids helps athletes develop optimal methods for delivering needed nutrients and fluids to working muscles while maintaining blood volume (a critical issue for performance). The best food-consumption strategies, based on GI tract function, enhance performance and minimize the potentially damaging effects of poorly timed meals. In cases where iron or calcium supplements are required, understanding GI tract absorption of these minerals will help athletes plan the best way to incorporate them into their dietary intake.

This chapter presents issues to consider when delivering the nutrients and fluids that are in such high need for athletes. The goal is to deliver the most needed nutrients while lowering the risk of gastrointestinal distress, particularly when training and during competition. The information is presented in a way that helps readers understand GI function in exercise and nonexercise situations so they'll acquire the tools to make the best eating and drinking decisions in a variety of situations.

The Gastrointestinal (GI) Tract

Food is the carrier of nutrients, and it is the job of the GI tract to break down (i.e., digest) food into its nutrient components and bring these nutrients into the blood and lymph for delivery to cells (e.g., absorption and transport). We are amazingly efficient at digesting and absorbing nutrients and transporting the absorbed nutrients to body tissue—a process that begins when you place food in your mouth and continues through the stomach and intestines. On this trip through the GI tract, food is mechanically ripped apart, attacked by chemicals to aid in the release of nutrients, exposed to radical changes in acidity, and compacted for removal of what is left.

Mouth and Esophagus

Mouth and esophagus health is important for athletes because problems with either inevitably lead to food intake restrictions that limit nutrient consumption and, ultimately, lead to malnutrition. Given the predisposition of athletes to consume a relatively high level of simple carbohydrates in snacks and sports beverages, which have a high cariogenic potential, frequent visits to a dentist to ensure healthy teeth and gums are advised. In addition, the high abdominal forces inherent in many sporting activities (e.g., weightlifting) may predispose athletes to hiatal hernias that lead to esophagitis. An acutely irritated esophagus is painful, makes swallowing difficult, and inevitably leads to food restrictions.

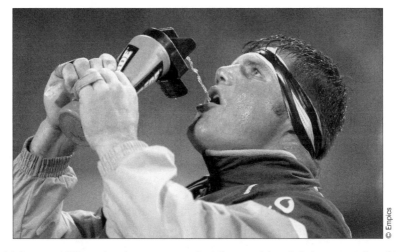

Food and drinks taste differently when consumed while exercising. It is important for athletes to test beverages during training to prepare for intake during competition.

Placing food in your mouth initiates a series of events that begin the digestive process. Chewing breaks apart food so it can be more completely mixed with digestive enzymes, and salivary amylase begins the digestion of carbohydrates (mainly the conversion of cooked starch to dextrins and maltose). The secretion of saliva and amylase occurs from the thought, sight, smell, and taste of food. All the food placed in the mouth is covered with saliva, which contains the glycoprotein mucin. This mucin has excellent lubricating properties that help foods slide into the stomach through the esophagus without irritation. The pH of the mouth is approximately neutral (between 6.0 and 7.0; see table 5.1), which does not change in the esophagus.

Table 5.1 The pH Ranges in the GI Tract

Location	pH
Mouth	6.0-7.0 (neutral)
Esophagus	6.9-7.1 (neutral)
Stomach	2.0-2.5 (very acidic)
Small intestine	6.9-7.1 (neutral)
Large intestine	6.9-7.1 (neutral)

Note: pH of 1 = battery acid

The feel and taste of foods and drinks in the mouth have much to do with whether they are acceptable to an athlete. These food and drink properties, commonly referred to as their organoleptic properties, may be altered during exercise, which is an important consideration for the athlete. Therefore, taste testing a sports beverage while lying on a couch and watching television is not an appropriate strategy for determining how palatable this sports beverage will be during exercise. Put simply, food and drink taste and feel differently while you're exercising than while you're not. If you're a cyclist wishing to try a carbohydrate gel for your next race, try it after you've been cycling for a while or you could be in for a big surprise during the event. In summary, always try a food, whether it's a sports beverage or snack, during the activity for which its use is intended.

Stomach

Food passes from the esophagus to the stomach, where additional digestive processes take place. A rapid shift in pH occurs from ~6.0 to 7.0 to between pH 2.0 and 2.5. This highly acidic stomach environment initiates a series of events that promote protein digestion, while continuing the mixing action that was initiated in the mouth. Specialized cells in the stomach also produce *intrinsic factor*, which is needed for the absorption of vitamin B_{12}. A persistent failure to absorb vitamin B_{12} eventually results in a condition called *pernicious anemia*.

Risk factors for an acute irritation of the stomach, referred to as gastritis, are generally considered to be excessive use of nonsteroidal anti-inflammatory drugs (NSAIDs), excessive use of alcohol, and increasing age. The common cause of gastritis in athletes would most likely be regular NSAID use, which may irritate the stomach lining. NSAIDs come in prescription (e.g., Naprosyn) and over-the-counter forms (e.g., aspirin or ibuprofen). These common pain relievers reduce a protective substance in your stomach called prostaglandin. When taken infrequently and short term, NSAIDs usually don't cause many stomach problems, especially if taken with antacids or food. However, regular use may result in gastritis and, eventually, in stomach ulcers as well. Other factors could be associated with gastritis in athletes:

- Severe physical and psychological stress
- Alcohol abuse
- Infection from Helicobacter pylori (H. pylori)[1]
- Cocaine use

Gastric Emptying

Gastric emptying refers to the speed at which food and drink leave the stomach. High-fat, high-protein meals take longer to digest and require more processing time in the stomach. Therefore, precompetition or pretraining meals should be consumed with gastric emptying time in mind. With the goal of exercising with no solid food in the stomach, higher-protein and higher-fat meals should be eaten a minimum of 2.5 hours before physical activity, while low-fiber, starchy carbohydrate meals should be eaten a minimum of 1.5 hours before physical activity. Exercising with food in the stomach may lead to nausea and vomiting. Furthermore, the sensation of fullness may inhibit adequate fluid consumption, which could lead to dehydration and heat stress. Cyclists may better tolerate solid foods in the stomach while exercising, but in general, all athletes should be wary of eating meals too close to the time of exercise. The following known factors affect gastric emptying:[2, 3]

- Ingested volume (higher volumes result in faster gastric emptying)
- Energy concentration (higher concentrations result in slower gastric emptying)
- Type of carbohydrate (glucose results in slower gastric emptying than other mono- and disaccharides)
- Osmolality (higher osmolar solutions result in slower gastric emptying)
- pH (deviations from neutral pH slow gastric emptying)
- Exercise intensity (higher intensities result in slower gastric emptying)
- Stress (severe psychological stress slows gastric emptying)

See chapter 3 for additional information on gastric emptying and related issues.

Small Intestine

The small intestine has three distinct compartments: the duodenum (closest to the stomach), jejunum (middle), and ileum (closest to the large intestine). The liquid mass of consumed food formed by the stomach is passed into the small intestine for additional digestive processing and, for the first time in the GI tract, absorption into the blood and lymph. The pyloric valve separates the stomach from the small intestine. The small portion of the small intestine proximal to the pyloric valve is the primary absorption site for the bivalent minerals, including iron, calcium, magnesium, and zinc (all of which are important to athletes).

Bivalent minerals are competitively absorbed because the site of absorption is relatively small. Therefore, an excessively high intake of one bivalent mineral may occupy the entire absorption site and make the absorption of other bivalent minerals difficult. The principle of nutrient balance is critical (i.e., more than enough is not better than just enough). For instance, female athletes are often appropriately concerned about iron status, but a frequent high-dose intake of iron may mitigate the absorption of calcium, magnesium, and zinc to create a series of other nutrition problems. Put simply, the strategy for bivalent mineral intake is crucial for optimizing nutrition health and, because these minerals are so closely tied to muscle function and bone health, athletic performance.

A short distance from the proximal duodenum where bivalent minerals are absorbed, the bile duct and pancreatic duct enter the small intestine.[4] The pancreas is stimulated by secretin, which travels up the pancreatic duct to cause the release of pancreatic juice into the duodenum. Because of its large volume (between 20 and 27 ounces daily, or 600 and 800 milliliters) and high pH (~8.0), pancreatic juice neutralizes the acidity of the food mass that has left the stomach. The pancreas also releases several digestive enzymes, including

- pancreatic amylase to digest starch into dextrins and maltose;
- pancreatic proteases to digest larger proteins into smaller polypeptides; and
- pancreatic lipase to digest fats into monoglycerides, individual fatty acids, and glycerol.

Of course, the pancreas also produces powerful hormones (insulin by the beta cells and glucagon by the alpha cells). Insulin will be discussed fully in following chapters.

The liver manufactures bile, which is stored in the gallbladder until it is required. Cholecystokinin, which is produced in the small intestine, travels up the bile duct to stimulate the gallbladder to release its stored bile into the small intestine. Bile is a powerful emulsifying agent that helps in the digestion of fats.[5] The daily bile volume is between 17 and 37 ounces (500 and 1,100 milliliters), helping to explain our efficiency at digesting and absorbing fats.[6]

The mucosal (border) cells of the small intestine (mainly in the duodenum) produce enzymes that break down disaccharides into their component monosaccharides. Specifically, these disaccharidases do the following:

- Sucrase breaks down sucrose to glucose and fructose.
- Maltase breaks down maltose to two molecules of glucose.
- Lactase breaks down lactose to glucose and galactose.

These seemingly minor digestive enzymes are important for athletes to consider, particularly as they relate to the composition of sports beverages. For instance, a sports beverage deriving 100 percent of its energy from pure glucose (the ultimate energy source for cells) would induce delayed gastric emptying and, once absorbed, would produce a sudden, high, and relatively short-lived rise in blood sugar (glucose). On the other hand, an isocaloric sports beverage containing a combination of sucrose and glucose would have some inherent advantages in maintaining blood sugar for a longer period of time. The lower concentration of glucose in the beverage would not significantly delay gastric emptying, so there would be a more rapid infusion of glucose into the blood without achieving such a high peak. The sucrose would be digested into its component glucose and fructose, a process that takes some time. The glucose from this breakdown would follow the glucose already absorbed, and the fructose would be converted to glucose in the liver (still more time required) before infusion into the blood. The end result is a lower glucose peak but a much more sustained infusion of glucose into the blood, helping the athlete feel energized for a longer time.

Nutrients are absorbed mainly in the duodenum and jejunum, but some absorption also takes place in the ileum and the large intestine:

- Minerals are mainly absorbed in the proximal duodenum.
- Monosaccharides and water-soluble vitamins are mainly absorbed in the jejunum.
- Fat-soluble vitamins, amino acids, fats, vitamin B_{12},[7] and bile salts are absorbed mainly in the ileum.

The interior surface of the small intestine is composed of microvilli that dramatically enlarge its absorptive surface, accounting for an extraordinary efficiency in absorbing consumed energy substrates: 98 percent of all digestible carbohydrate is absorbed; 95 percent of all fat is absorbed; and 92 percent of all protein is absorbed.

Large Intestine

The large intestine is made of six parts, including the cecum, ascending (right) colon, transverse colon, descending (left) colon, sigmoid colon, and rectum. The small intestine connects to the large intestine at the cecum, which is actually the beginning part of the ascending colon. A small projection attached to the cecum, called the appendix, serves no well-understood function. However, the appendix is predisposed to becoming infected, a condition referred to as appendicitis. The main function of the large intestine is to reabsorb water from the stool and eliminate the remaining relatively dry waste. Food and drink consumption and intestinal secretions result in approximately 5 gallons (19 L) of fluid being placed in the large intestine daily. A failure to adequately resorb this fluid would result in dehydration. The following factors keep a GI tract healthy:

- Adequate dietary fiber (viscous: soluble)
- Adequate dietary fiber (nonviscous: insoluble)
- Optimal bacterial flora
- Adequate fluids

- Regular movement; physical activity
- Balanced diet with adequate folate
- Reduced intake of simple sugars
- Avoidance of bacterial contamination
- Avoidance of antibiotics (disrupt microflora)

The large intestine is populated by bacteria, many of which are essential for human nutrition. Some of these bacteria manufacture vitamin K (an important substance for blood clotting). The bacterial flora is also important for normal large intestine function by creating gas that aids peristalsis and by aiding in the digestion of certain materials. Certain consumed foods may create a healthy bacterial flora, which can help overwhelm "bad" bacteria that try to populate the gut. For instance, live-culture yogurt often contains *Lactobacillus bulgaricus* and *Streptococcus thermophilus*,[8] which convert pasteurized milk to yogurt during fermentation. In addition, some yogurts contain *Lactobacillus acidophilus* and *Bifidobacterium bifidum*. The amount of intestinal bacteria varies depending on diet and use of antibiotics but can make up more than half the weight of fecal material. An infection with "bad" bacteria creates an irritation that causes an increase in mucus production and a failure to resorb water from stool, leading to diarrhea. Of course, the use of antibiotics disturbs the bacterial flora in the gut and often leads to abnormal gut function until the "healthy" bacteria return.

Common problems of the large intestine include constipation, diarrhea, diverticulosis or diverticulitis, and colon cancer. Constipation, diverticular disease, and colon cancer risks are increased with low fiber intakes. Currently, Americans consume approximately half of the 20 to 35 grams of dietary fiber recommended to reduce disease risk and maintain healthy gut function. To obtain the recommended level of fiber, athletes would need to consume at least five servings of fresh fruits and vegetables and three servings of whole grain products daily, as well as legumes occasionally. Because of the gas and bloating caused by higher fiber intakes, athletes could experience performance difficulties unless the fiber intake is timed correctly so it does not interfere with training or competition. The issue of food timing is comprehensively discussed later in this book.

GI Concerns for Athletes

Frequent fluctuations in hydration state could cause digestion and absorption difficulties for athletes, requiring a constant vigilance to make certain that fluid consumption matches need. The stress associated with competition and overtraining is also a concern; GI dysfunction (e.g., nausea, gastritis, colitis) is a common outcome with persistent stress and a lack of adequate rest. Once stress-related GI problems occur, nutrient intake drops. This gives rise to numerous other nutrient-deficiency disorders that can be adequately dealt with only when the athlete returns to a more stress-free and rested state.

Common causes of GI distress in athletes include the following:

- Dehydration
- Consumption of fructose-only beverages during exercise
- Consumption of carbonated beverages during exercise
- Febrile disease
- Excessive use of common ergogenic aids
- Fatigue from overtraining
- High doses of vitamin and mineral preparations
- Psychological and physiological stress

Before Exercise

In the period immediately before training or competition, nutritionally balanced meals are not needed and may even be counterproductive. The goal for athletes in the preexercise period is to make certain that blood sugar is maintained, that hydration state is optimal, and that the stomach is empty. To do this, the focus should be on starchy, low-fiber carbohydrates and fluids for the last meal before exercise, followed by a sports beverage sipping protocol that maintains blood glucose and volume up to the beginning of the training or competition. Eating the final meal too soon may cause blood sugar to become low just before the exercise period, and eating the final meal too close to the activity may leave food in the stomach.

During Exercise

Perhaps the most common error during physical activity is to delay drinking fluids until the sensation of thirst manifests itself. Besides the fact that drinking at this point is not likely to adequately hydrate working muscles during the activity (see chapter 3), the natural response to thirst is to drink a large volume of fluid at one time. Because the thirst sensation suggests that the athlete is already dehydrated, gastric emptying will be delayed, which will make the athlete feel nauseated. In general, care should be taken to never allow thirst to occur during exercise so that consumed fluids will rapidly leave the stomach and be delivered quickly to needy muscles. Additionally, no solid foods or high-concentration carbohydrate beverages (e.g., beverages with a carbohydrate concentration that exceeds 8 percent) should be consumed during physical activity unless the athlete knows that these foods and beverages do not cause GI distress.

After Exercise

The greater the degree of dehydration, the greater the fluid requirement. However, since dehydration causes a delay in gastric emptying, dehydrated athletes should be

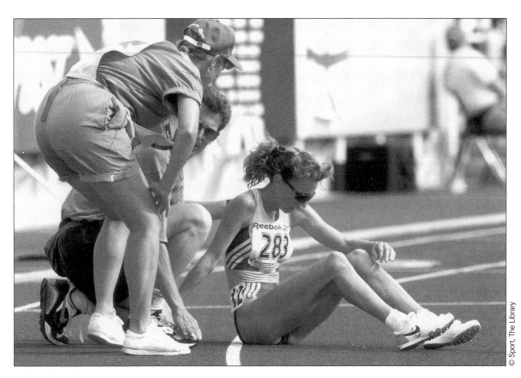

Athletes should not consume food or beverages high in carbohydrate while exercising, as GI distress could result and be a detriment to performance.

wary of taking in large volumes of fluid at one time. Instead, athletes should continually sip on fluids until they feel the dehydration resolving itself. For athletes involved in sequential day practices or competition, the immediate postexercise period is an opportunity to replenish depleted glycogen stores. The enzyme glycogen synthetase is highest when glycogen stores are most depleted. This enzyme converts glucose to glycogen, so consuming high-carbohydrate foods, as tolerated, immediately after exercise is a desirable practice. This practice is inhibited by the relative degree of dehydration experienced by the athlete. The greater the degree of dehydration, the smaller the amount of food tolerated (because of delayed gastric emptying).

6 Timing of Energy and Fluid Intake

The traditional view of energy and nutrient delivery is to provide recommendations in units of 24 hours. Although these guidelines may be useful for some people, they are inadequate for athletes wishing to optimize fuel and fluid delivery to enhance performance. Put simply, the *dynamics* of energy and fluid intake should match the *dynamics* of energy and fluid usage. Any delivery system that deviates widely from this principle can't help athletes train and perform at their best. Studies have shown that matching intake and expenditure dynamics helps athletes maintain lean mass, reduce body fat levels, improve sense of well-being, and enhance athletic performance. This chapter provides a critical summary of studies that have looked at within-day energy balance and eating frequency and the underlying physiological and nutrition principles that show the importance of reducing the magnitude of energy surpluses and deficits during the day. In addition, the chapter provides practical strategies for how athletes involved in morning and afternoon, afternoon and evening, or one-time daily training regimens can sustain an optimal within-day energy and fluid balance.

Exercise has two major effects on the requirement for nutrients. It results in an increase in the rate of energy usage and, because of the greater heat production associated with higher levels of energy metabolism, an increase in the rate of water lost as sweat. Athletes must increase energy substrate and fluid consumption to meet this additional nutrition burden, yet nutrition surveys suggest that athletes don't eat enough and don't drink enough.[1-3] Moreover, it appears that energy consumption is not well timed, which negatively affects both body composition and performance.[4-6]

The outcome of this widespread athletic malnutrition is all too well understood: an excessive reliance on supplements and ergogenic aids to overcome the deficits created by inadequate energy and fluid consumption. Athletes will likely achieve better results by paying attention to food and drink intake than by following any other course of action. Focusing on food and drink is a less expensive, more dependable, and safer strategy for improving athletic performance than relying on supplements and ergogenic aids, which may have indefinite content and unpredictable quality.

Fuel for the Final 5 Kilometers

"This is the first time I learn how Deena is looking as she runs up the hills into Athens. She had run strongly through all her workouts on Crete and resented the need to taper. Chatting to Benardot on Crete, she said she has never felt so strong in her life, noting she has adjusted her eating patterns to follow his advice. While at the resort, the nutritionist analyzed the eating patterns of all three women marathoners. All eat well and are getting the requisite calories. Deena, however, is closest to the ideal pattern of balancing her intake of calories with her expenditure of energy throughout the day. She eats frequently and adventurously, shunning few foods. . . . Inside the stadium, all is wild. Everyone is on their feet. Noguchi enters, a tiny runner gamely hanging on for the final 500 meters. Close behind is Kenya's Catherine Ndereba, who has led Deena the whole way. Deena bursts in a minute behind, having run the 5K between 35K and 40K in 16:20, the fastest 5K of the entire race by any runner—this after 21K of hills in 90-degree heat." [Julia Emmons. "They Practice on Mountains: An Olympic Marathon Coach's View of the 2004 Olympics." *Marathon and Beyond* 2005; 9(1): 53-66.]

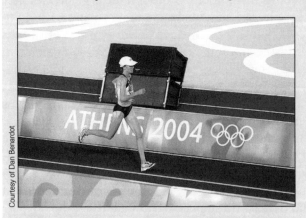

Courtesy of Dan Benardot

Deena Kastor heads toward the finish line in Athens.

Note: Deena Kastor won the bronze medal at the 2004 Olympic Games in Athens, the first American woman to win an Olympic marathon medal in 20 years.

Intake for Performance Enhancement

Much of the discussion on energy intake focuses on the optimal distribution of the energy substrates: carbohydrate, protein, and fat. Despite the popular recommendations for high-protein, low-carbohydrate diets, there is no question that focusing on a diet high in complex carbohydrates, moderate in protein, and relatively low in fat is performance enhancing. But this discussion has little meaning in the face of energy intake inadequacy. Put simply, it doesn't matter if high-octane fuel is put in the system if there isn't enough fuel to get you where you want to go.

Weight and lean-mass stability are the best indicators that energy intake matches need. A failure to consume sufficient energy leads to either a reduction in weight or a reduction in lean mass (or both) as the body tries to compensate for this deficiency. For most athletes, a lower relative lean mass and higher relative fat mass is not desirable and is a physiological marker associated with decreased performance. In what must be considered a terribly unwise reaction to this relatively higher fat mass, athletes commonly reduce energy intake still further to reduce the excess fat. The impact of this constant ratcheting down of energy intake is weight loss with a greater loss of lean mass than fat mass, with fat constituting an ever-higher proportion of body weight.[7, 8] If caloric intake is inadequate, the body reduces the metabolic mass (i.e., the muscle mass) to make a downward adjustment in the metabolic rate and the need for calories.

It is possible that this cycle of lowering energy intake to adapt to a constantly rising relative fat mass is predictive of the eating disorders seen too often in athletes where appearance plays a factor in a sport's subjective scoring.[9] To emphasize this point, it should be noted that anorexia nervosa victims at death show a terrible loss of weight and a terrible loss of lean mass (the weight of the heart is typically 50 percent of normal) but have a relatively high body fat percentage. Severely deficient caloric intakes, therefore, lead to a greater wasting away of lean mass than of fat mass.[10] The concept that a significant reduction in calories (i.e., dieting) results in an improved body profile and body composition simply does not stand up to scrutiny. Although a short-term lowering of body weight may be temporarily associated with enhanced performance, the long-term effect of such low-calorie diets is to lower the intake of needed nutrients (a problem that can manifest itself in disease frequency and increased risk for low bone density); to lower the muscle mass (as an adjustment to the inadequate caloric intake); and to regain the weight, which is made up of less lean tissue and more fat. To make matters worse, the lowering of lean mass makes eating normally without weight gain more difficult.

A microeconomic view of the energy balance issue may shed some light on how athletes should eat to achieve an optimal body composition that enhances performance. A study of four groups of national-level female athletes (rhythmic gymnasts, artistic gymnasts, middle-distance runners, and long-distance runners) found that those who deviated most widely from perfect energy balance during the day had the highest body fat levels, regardless of whether the energy deviations represented surpluses or deficits (see figure 6.1).[11] In fact, the rhythmic gymnasts, who as a group had the most pronounced energy deficits (nearly –800 kcal), had the highest body fat percent of all the groups assessed, while middle-distance runners had the best within-day energy balance and the lowest body fat percents.

This strongly suggests that the common eating pattern of athletes, which is typified by infrequent meals with a heavy emphasis on a large end-of-day meal, is not useful for meeting athletic goals because it is guaranteed to create large energy deficits during the day. Although this energy deficit may be made up for at the end of the day to put an athlete in an energy-balanced state, this eating pattern is typified by weight stability but higher than desirable body fat levels.

The reason for the higher body fat level becomes clear when you consider how blood sugar fluxes (after a meal, it rises, levels off, and drops over a period of 3 hours). With delayed eating, blood sugar drops and the amino acid alanine is recruited from muscle tissue to be converted to glucose by the liver. Although this stabilizes blood sugar, it does so at the cost of the muscle mass. In addition, both low blood sugar and large meals are associated with hyperinsulinemia, which encourages the manufacture of fat. So, delayed eating followed by an excessively large meal, which is typical of the athletic eating paradigm, is an ideal way to lower muscle mass and increase fat mass . . . not what athletes want to do. Frequent eating reduces the size of within-day energy deficits and surpluses and helps stabilize blood sugar.

Many studies assessing eating frequency have come to the same conclusion: The more frequent the eating pattern, the lower the body fat and the higher the muscle mass.[12-14] In addition, frequent eating patterns provide a simple, workable strategy for increasing energy intake while simultaneously reducing GI discomfort associated with larger meals.[12]

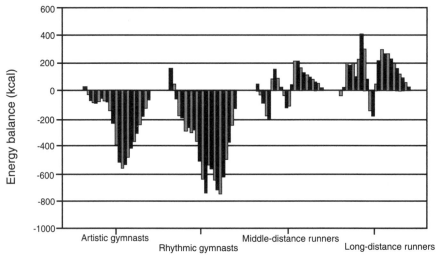

Figure 6.1 Body composition and within-day energy balance.

Reprinted, by permission, from B. Deutz, D. Benardot, D. Martin and M. Cody, 2000, "Relationship between energy deficits and body composition in elite female gymnasts and runners," *Med Sci Sports Exerc* 32(3): 659-668.

A study assessing the impact of meal frequency on body composition and weight in boxers found that, even with isocaloric intakes (both groups had the same caloric intake for 2 weeks), the group consuming two meals each day experienced a significant reduction in lean body mass, whereas the group consuming six meals each day did not.[6] In another study of wrestlers, athletes who recorded cyclic weight changes, typified by long periods of very low caloric intakes, had lower metabolic rates, suggestive of a loss of lean body mass.[15]

These studies suggest that large within-day energy deficits clearly cause muscle catabolism, which can be avoided by supplying energy in smaller but more frequent meals. This finding is consistent with a recent study of 60 male and female collegiate athletes that assessed the impact of adding a 250-calorie snack or a noncaloric placebo between each major meal and after dinner (i.e., between breakfast and lunch, between lunch and dinner, and after dinner, for 750 calories provided as snacks each day). After 2 weeks of this protocol, the group consuming the caloric snack experienced a significant reduction in body fat, a significant rise in lean body mass, a significant improvement in anaerobic power and anaerobic endurance, no change in weight, and no change in total caloric intake.[16] Weight stayed the same because energy intake did not change (an important principle of energy thermodynamics), a result that presents an interesting point. When snacks were provided with no instructions regarding the other meals, the athletes spontaneously reduced the size of the other meals to compensate for the snacks. A failure to do so would have increased total caloric intake and resulted in a weight gain.

The snacks were removed 2 weeks into the study. The athletes were remeasured 4 weeks later; they had assumed their old eating patterns and returned to baseline values for body fat and muscle mass. The findings of this study make it clear that an athlete's eating pattern will default to his or her usual practice (e.g., two or three meals a day, with the largest meal at the end of the day) unless a new pattern becomes the accepted standard. Indeed, studies have found that the environment (e.g., who the athletes tend to eat with; food availability) plays a major role in eating patterns.[17] Getting athletes to eat more frequently on their own, in opposition to the environmental norm, is extremely difficult.

Animal studies have also found benefits to increasing meal frequency so that large within-day energy deficits and surpluses can be avoided. A study using dogs found that providing a set amount of calories in small but frequent meals rather than large infrequent meals significantly reduces the insulin response to food, even in dogs fed a high-carbohydrate meal. In addition to this clear benefit, more meals result in higher thermogenesis (faster energy metabolic rate) and better fat utilization.[18] What does this mean for athletes? A high insulin response to food translates into high fat production, so having a reduced insulin response means less fat production. Having a faster metabolic rate makes it easier for athletes to eat without getting fat because more calories are being burned per unit of time. These factors, plus a more efficient fat utilization, all translate into eating more, taking in more nutrients, maintaining muscle mass, and lowering body fat percentage. A failure to eat frequently, causing a mini-starvation state during the day, has just the opposite effect on metabolic rate. The resulting lower metabolic rate is associated with a higher fat mass and more difficulty eating normally without gaining fat.[19-21] The act of eating more frequently, in and of itself, appears to play a role in the thermic effect of food (the number of calories burned as a result of eating; a higher burn rate is considered good because it is associated with lower body fat). The thermic effect of food is higher in subjects eating at regular, short intervals when compared with subjects eating at irregular, longer intervals.[22]

The benefits of eating frequently enough to reduce the magnitude of within-day energy deficits and surpluses go beyond body composition, weight, and performance. There is also evidence that people with frequent eating patterns have lower serum lipid levels, a risk factor in cardiovascular disease.[23] A study assessing the impact of food restriction during the period of the Ramadan fast found that insulin production was increased, as was the production of leptin (a hormone produced by fat cells), both of which are associated with a greater fat-mass production.[24]

Many athletes concerned about weight have learned to cope with the feeling of low blood sugar by consuming a diet product (diet colas are popular). Although these diet products do nothing to resolve the very real physiological need for energy to maintain an adequate blood sugar, they do provide a central nervous system stimulant (usually caffeine) that masks the sensation of hunger. However, since this strategy maintains the low blood sugar level, the outcome will inevitably be less muscle and more fat. It is clear from these studies that the only appropriate strategy for weight loss is a subtle energy deficit that results in only a slight deviation from a within-day energy-balanced state.

What are athletes to do? Never get hungry. This is not easy with a typical three-meal-a-day eating pattern, which provides for a refueling stop every 5 to 6 hours, and the typical athlete eating patterns that heavily backload intake make it even more difficult. Since blood sugar is known to rise and fall in 3-hour units, it makes sense to have planned snacks. If an athlete is weight stable, the best way to initiate this process is to eat a bit less at breakfast, eat the remainder at midmorning, and do the same for lunch and dinner. Total caloric intake will remain the same, but the athlete will avoid sharp energy deficits and surpluses during the day. Besides the improved nutrient intake and better body composition associated with this type of eating pattern, athletes can also expect improved mental acuity and enhanced athletic performance. (See chapters 16 through 18 for diet plans that provide examples, at different caloric intakes, of how to avoid large within-day energy surpluses or deficits.)

Considerations for Fluid Intake

Studies have demonstrated that athletes experience a degree of voluntary dehydration, even in the presence of available fluids, that lowers blood volume and negatively affects performance.[25] Given the tremendous amount of heat that must be dissipated during exercise through sweat evaporation, athletes must pursue strategies that will sustain the hydration state. Failure to do so will result in poor performance and may also lead to heat illness.

Temperature regulation represents the balance between heat produced or received (heat-in) and heat removed (heat-out). When the body's temperature regulation system is working correctly, heat-in and heat-out are in perfect balance, and body temperature is maintained.[26] The two primary systems for dissipating, or losing, heat while at rest are (1) moving more blood to the skin to allow heat dissipation through radiation and (2) increasing the rate of sweat production. These two systems account for about 85 percent of the heat lost when a person is at rest, but during exercise virtually all heat loss occurs from the evaporation of sweat.

Working muscles demand more blood flow to deliver nutrients and to remove the metabolic by-products of burned fuel, but at the very same time there is a need to shift blood away from the muscles and toward the skin to increase the sweat rate. With low blood volume, one or both of these systems fail, with a resultant decrease in athletic performance.

Heavy exercise can produce heat that is 20 times greater than the heat produced at rest. Without an efficient means of removing this excess heat, body temperature will rise quickly. The upper limit for human survival is about 110 degrees Fahrenheit (43.3 degrees Celsius), or only 11.4 degrees Fahrenheit (or 6.3 degrees Celsius) higher than normal body temperature. With the potential for body temperature to rise at the rate of about 1 degree Fahrenheit every 5 minutes, it is conceivable that underhydrated athletes could be at heatstroke risk only 57 minutes after the initiation of exercise.[27]

Athletes working hard for 30 minutes would create 450 kilocalories of excess heat that need to be dissipated to maintain body temperature. Since 1 milliliter of sweat can dissipate approximately .5 calories, athletes would lose about 900 milliliters (almost 1 liter) of sweat. In 1 hour of high-intensity activity, approximately 1.8 liters of water would be lost. On sunny and hot days when the heat of the sun is added to the heat produced from muscular work, athletes would need to produce even more sweat to remove more heat. Sweat doesn't evaporate off the skin as easily when it is humid, so even more sweat must be produced in hot and humid weather. Well-trained athletes exercising in a hot and humid environment may lose more than 3 liters of fluid per hour.[28]

No level of low body water is acceptable for achieving optimal athletic performance and endurance, so athletes should have a strategy for maintaining optimal body water during exercise. The problem is that athletes often rely on thirst as the marker of when to drink. Since the thirst sensation occurs only after a loss of 1 to 2 liters of body water, thirst is an inappropriate indicator of when to drink.[29] Instead, the athlete should strategize on how to never get thirsty. Ideally, this strategy should involve helping athletes determine how much fluid is lost during typical bouts of physical activity and developing a fixed fluid-consumption schedule from that information (typically 3 to 8 ounces every 10 to 15 minutes of a sodium-containing 6 to 8 percent carbohydrate solution.)

Considerations for Energy Intake

The question most frequently asked by athletes concerns what to eat before competition. Although this is important, it is of relatively small importance when compared with how the athlete should eat most of the time. It is impossible to properly prepare

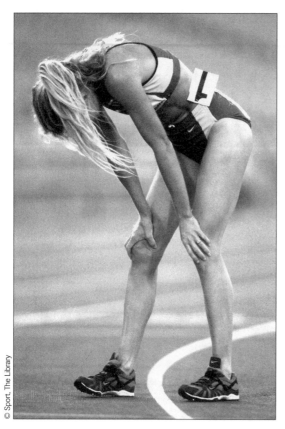

© Sport, The Library

Failure to consume enough energy during training can lead to a poor outcome at competition.

for a competition by consuming some pancakes several hours before the feet are placed in the starting blocks. It takes a consistent and long-term effort in conditioning and good nutrition. There is no way an athlete with iron deficiency can magically cure the condition by consuming some red meat the day before an event. It may take 6 months on a proper diet to reach a state of normal iron status. Therefore, the first and most important step in preparing for competition is to consistently eat enough energy and nutrients to support the body's energy and nutrient requirements. Failure to do so will inevitably lead to a poor competition outcome, no matter what you do just before the competition.

In addition to consuming enough energy and nutrients, it's equally important to eat foods when the body can benefit the most from them. The timing of meals is also important to make certain the muscles have enough energy and nutrients to grow and get stronger during training sessions rather than get burned for energy because the athlete hasn't eaten enough. Put simply, it's important to get enough and get it on time. This isn't easy to accomplish because athletes have terribly hectic schedules, and it takes strategic thinking and good scheduling to ensure food is consumed when it's needed. Although careful meal planning may not seem as important as having a well-developed training plan, both should be considered equally important. They should also be thought of collectively to make certain the training plan can be properly supported with the foods that are consumed.

If the general food intake is supportive of the training plan, what should an athlete do differently on the days leading up to a competition? The sequence of events for the seven days before a competition should meet three major goals:

1. The athlete should gradually become rested. This may be a problem for many athletes and coaches because athletes (either with or without the encouragement of the coach) often increase the training schedule during the week leading up to a competition. Overtraining is a big problem and may increase the risks of getting sick or getting injured. It certainly doesn't help an athlete do his or her best at the upcoming competition.

2. The athlete should gradually build up muscle glycogen (energy) stores. The main purpose of gradually reducing the intensity and duration of training sessions before the competition is to be sure the athlete can begin the competition with full muscle glycogen stores. The storage capacity for glycogen is relatively small, and athletes are heavily reliant on stored glycogen for muscular work (it's the limiting fuel for muscular work, regardless of the type of exercise the athlete is doing). Therefore, it's important to eat plenty of carbohydrates and reduce work so glycogen stores are full going into the competition.

3. The athlete should become well hydrated. When athletes work hard it is difficult (if not impossible) to maintain an optimal hydration state. It takes time to return lost body water, and athletes should give themselves the opportunity to do so by reducing the training intensity and duration and by drinking plenty of fluids. An additional benefit of becoming well hydrated is that glycogen storage is enhanced. The gradual tapering of training during the 7 days before competition makes it easier for the athlete to start the competition in a well-hydrated and optimally energized state.

Of course, many sports don't provide athletes the luxury of tapering activity on a 7-day cycle. Basketball and hockey players play several games each week during the season, and baseball players play nearly every day. Although their schedules don't permit 7-day activity tapering, the principles behind tapered activity, glycogen storage, and optimal hydration should be remembered and, when possible, adhered to. For athletes with daily schedules that eliminate the possibility of tapering, consumption of high-carbohydrate diets and maintenance of optimal hydration become even more important components of athletic performance. Athletes with these schedules should develop eating and drinking plans that are as solid as their training and competition plans.

All too often athletes prepare for a big competition by increasing their training regimen as the competition draws nearer. This is a big mistake. Coaches working in high-skill sports, such as figure skating and gymnastics, may ask their athletes to perform multiple run-throughs of their routines the day before competition just to be sure they can do them. The message this sends to an athlete (i.e., "I don't believe you're ready, and we're going to keep practicing until you get it right") is counterproductive. There is nothing more confidence building for athletes than entering the competition well rested and knowing the coach is secure in their ability to do a good job. This is true whether an athlete is a professional or a tee ball player in little league baseball.

Carbohydrate Ingestion Before Exercise

A high-carbohydrate meal that is completed approximately 90 minutes before physical activity has been shown to improve endurance performance. After this preexercise meal, athletes should consume carbohydrates right up to the beginning of the training session or competition to avoid low blood glucose. Two strategies can be followed:

1. Ingestion of a carbohydrate-containing sports beverage using a sipping strategy, where approximately 2 to 4 ounces (60 to 120 milliliters) of beverage is consumed every 10 to 15 minutes.

2. Snacking on low-fiber, starchy foods (such as saltine crackers) every 15 minutes, washed down with ample quantities of water.

Athletes should avoid eating patterns that could stimulate a reactive hypoglycemia, which is caused by ingestion of large quantities of foods with a high glycemic index, but should also avoid the hypoglycemia that could occur from consuming no carbohydrates or from delayed eating. Snacking and sipping procedures appear to be well tolerated and help maintain blood glucose.

Carbohydrate Maintenance During Exercise

Avoiding low blood glucose and avoiding depletion of muscle glycogen stores are both critical for maintaining exercise performance. Consumption of carbohydrate-containing beverages (e.g., sports beverages) and food during exercise delays fatigue and improves performance, even if the consumption occurs late in the exercise session. This strategy delays fatigue through the following mechanisms:

1. Maintains blood glucose, which preserves liver glycogen
2. Maintains branched-chain amino acid (BCAA) levels, which avoids central fatigue by maintaining the ratio of tryptophan and BCAAs
3. Inhibits the production of cortisol, which is catabolic to muscle tissue
4. Reduces the usage of muscle glycogen by providing a constant source of glucose from the blood to working muscle cells

During exercise, carbohydrate is best obtained through a 6 to 7 percent carbohydrate solution, with 4 to 8 ounces (120 to 240 milliliters) taken every 10 to 20 minutes (the amount to consume depends on sweat rate; see chapter 3). A number of different carbohydrate solutions are available to athletes, each with a different concentration and composition of carbohydrate. Issues of gastrointestinal distress and osmolarity should be considered. Of equal 6 percent concentrations of glucose, fructose, or sucrose, the fructose has been shown to cause more gastrointestinal distress. Therefore, athletes should carefully check their tolerance of fructose-only beverages before consuming them in critical situations. (Most sports beverages contain multiple carbohydrate types.)

Few sports beverages are milk based or use lactose as a predominant form of carbohydrate because of the relatively common problem of lactose intolerance. This condition, caused by an inadequate production of the enzyme lactase, results in diarrhea, gas, and abdominal pain. Given the possibility of lactose intolerance in some athletes, it is prudent for athletes to avoid lactose-containing products immediately before and during physical activity.[30]

Glucose polymers have the advantage of being able to deliver more carbohydrate in a lower osmolar solution.[31] Isocaloric with simple sugars, glucose polymers improve gastric emptying and enhance absorption. Athletes involved in extremely high-intensity activity for a long duration may need a high volume of carbohydrate calories during physical activity, and glucose polymers may provide a good solution for these athletes.

Carbohydrate Replenishment After Exercise

Glycogen and fluids are usually, to a degree, depleted after exercise, and protein requirements are also higher to aid in muscle recovery. The protein and fluid issues are discussed in other sections of this book. The carbohydrate and glycogen issues are presented here.

One of the main postexercise goals is to replenish glycogen to prepare the athlete for the next bout of exercise. As glycogen becomes depleted, the enzyme glycogen synthetase becomes elevated in the blood. Providing glucose or sucrose (but not fructose) while glycogen synthetase is elevated efficiently replaces muscle glycogen stores.[32] Glycogen synthetase reaches its peak at the point of greatest glycogen depletion, which is immediately after exercise. Therefore, athletes should consume carbohydrates as soon as physical activity ends. Ideally, the carbohydrate consumed for the first 2 hours after exercise should be high glycemic, followed by medium-glycemic carbohydrates for another 2 hours and finally medium to high-glycemic carbohydrates for the remainder of the day. Athletes should plan on consuming 200 to 400 kilocalories from carbohydrate (50 to 100 grams) immediately after physical activity, followed by sufficient carbohydrates to fulfill the guidelines presented in table 1.6 (Carbohydrate Requirement for Athletes, page 15).

Carbohydrate Loading

Consumption of carbohydrates before exercise improves carbohydrate stores and reduces the chance for premature fatigue, regardless of whether the sport is high endurance and low intensity, intermittent (as in many team sports), or high intensity and low endurance.[33-38]

Carbohydrate loading is a strategy commonly followed by many athletes before an endurance competition to increase muscle glycogen storage. The general technique is to gradually increase carbohydrate and fluid intake each day,[39] beginning the week before competition, while exercise is tapered downward.[40] This reasonable, safe strategy maximizes glycogen storage. (See figure 6.2 for a comparison of the techniques commonly followed to maximize glycogen storage.)

An older strategy for carbohydrate loading involved depleting carbohydrates by exercising intensely while consuming low-carbohydrate foods.[41] This was followed by the technique described in the previous paragraph. This older carbohydrate-loading technique is dangerous (depletion of glycogen stores may cause a sudden and dangerous drop in blood pressure), and there is no evidence that it better optimizes glycogen stores.

Seven-Day Taper

The following tables provide an example of how the principles for maximizing carbohydrate storage can be put to work. They illustrate what and how athletes might eat if they typically train twice daily. You'll notice that the food is spread out over six

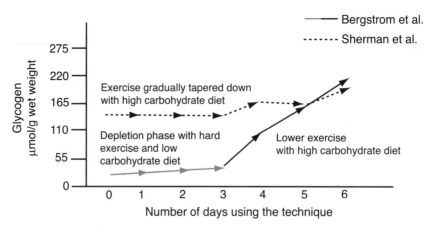

Figure 6.2 Comparison of the Bergstrom et al. (1967) and Sherman et al. (1983) glycogen loading techniques. (*Note:* The Bergstrom et al. depletion phase is potentially dangerous and is not recommended.)

smaller meals rather than two or three larger ones. You'll also notice that the caloric level of the meals does not emphasize dinner at the end of the day. Although dinner is important, training takes place before dinner, so ample energy must be available when the athlete needs it the most. Breakfast comes before the morning workout; when an athlete wakes up, blood sugar is marginal and the liver is virtually depleted of energy, so maintaining blood sugar is virtually impossible. Eating some food before the morning workout ensures that the muscles will benefit from the training and makes the athlete feel better. Nobody feels good with low blood sugar.

As indicated by the tables, foods should be consumed long enough before the training session so an athlete feels no discomfort from training because there is food in the stomach. In addition, the meal plan always includes some carbohydrates immediately after a workout. This helps ensure an effective replenishment of the glycogen that was used up during the training. Waiting too long after training to eat can diminish the efficiency of muscle glycogen replacement.

Seven Days Before Competition

One week before competition is the time for a complete, total, and exhaustive workout. The athlete should practice all skills completely and repetitively, focusing on his or her weakest area. If a basketball player has trouble making foul shots during the game, then a good deal of time should be spent shooting from the foul line after all the other practice regimens have been followed. He or she should get a sense of what it's like to feel a bit tired, just like in a game. In other words, 7 days before the competition is not a time for being timid about the workout. Give your body a sufficiently good workout so you know you've really gone through the paces. (See table 6.1 for a sample schedule for competition-minus-7-days.)

During this workout, all the protocols discussed earlier in this book should be followed. It's important to drink plenty of carbohydrate-containing fluids during

Table 6.1   Sample Exercise and Eating Schedule for Competition-Minus-7-Days

Time of day	Activity	Food
7:00 A.M. to 8:00 A.M.	• Light breakfast (*before* getting dressed for workout) • Dress for A.M. workout	• 2 slices white bread toast • 1 cup fruit juice • 1 cup sports beverage [Average 300 calories]
8:00 A.M. to 9:30 A.M.	• Stretch (30 minutes) • 1 hour vigorous run, bike, or equipment-based activity	• 1 cup sports beverage during stretch (sipped over 30 minutes) • 16 ounces sports beverage during 1 hour activity (sipped at the rate of 4 ounces every 15 minutes) [About 150 calories]
9:30 A.M. to 10:00 A.M.	• Postexercise breakfast (*before* getting washed and dressed)	• 1 boiled egg • 4 slices of toast with 2 tablespoons of jam • 1 fresh orange • 1 bowl (1 cup) of whole-grain cereal with 6 ounces of 1% milk • 12 ounces fruit juice [About 900 calories]
10:00 A.M. to 12:30 P.M.	• Shower and dress • Relaxed activities (read, walk, light work around the house, desk work, etc.)	• Sip on 12 ounces of fluids (any kind except those containing caffeine or alcohol) [About 75 calories if a sports beverage]
12:30 P.M. to 1:00 P.M.	• Lunch	• Large bowl (2.5 cups) of pasta with marinara sauce • 3 slices of French bread • 12 ounces of fruit juice [About 1,200 calories]
1:00 P.M. to 2:45 P.M.	• Postlunch relaxation (read, desk work, slow walking, driving, etc.)	• Sip on 12 ounces of water [0 calories]
2:45 P.M. to 3:30 P.M.	• Preparation for afternoon workout (get dressed for exercise, etc.)	• Sip on 12 ounces of sports beverage [About 75 calories]
3:30 P.M. to 7:00 P.M.	• Late-afternoon workout • Practice skills • Work on conditioning • Work on endurance • Work up a sweat!	• Sip on 16 ounces of sports beverage per hour (4 ounces each 15 minutes) • Take your nude weight prior to exercise and after exercise to see if you have consumed an appropriate amount of fluid. For each pound of weight loss, you should have consumed an additional 16 ounces of beverage. [About 350 calories]

(continued)

Table 6.1 *(continued)*

Time of day	Activity	Food
7:00 P.M. to 7:30 P.M.	• Postexercise nutritional replenishment	• 1 banana • 12 ounces of sports beverage • 2 slices of bread [About 315 calories]
7:30 P.M. to 8:00 P.M.	• Shower and dress	• Don't drink the shower water unless you're really thirsty!
8:00 P.M. to 9:00 P.M.	• Dinner	• Large baked potato • Broccoli (1 spear) • Small lean steak (4 ounces) • Orange juice (1 cup) • Rice pudding (1 cup) [About 1,050 calories]
9:00 P.M. to 10:00 P.M.	• Relaxation activities	• 1 cup of water or sports beverage (sipped) [About 75 calories if a sports beverage]
10:00 P.M. to 7:00 A.M.	• Sleep, glorious sleep!	• No eating or drinking permitted!

Intake totals:

4,500 calories
79% of calories from carbohydrate
11% of calories from protein
10% of calories from fat

Note: The food intake in this example would meet the needs of a 190-pound (86.4-kilogram) athlete with a very intensive exercise schedule. In this example, the energy requirement for competition-minus-7-days is estimated as 50 calories per kilogram of body weight. Importantly, it is high in fluids, high in carbohydrates, low in fat, and moderate in protein. This type of intake supports glycogen (energy) storage in the muscles and liver. Athletes weighing less than this would consume proportionately less food, while maintaining the same frequency of intake.

the workout (see chapter 3). It's also important to follow the workout with plenty of carbohydrates. Consuming at least 400 calories from carbohydrate (100 grams) immediately after the training regimen is desirable, followed by at least 800 calories (200 grams) during the next several hours. This is your first attempt at getting your muscles to replace the glycogen that has been lost during the workout.

Six Days Before Competition

Six days before competition represents the first day of tapered exercise plus maintenance of a high-carbohydrate intake with plenty of fluids. Since activity is reduced, total energy intake should also be trimmed to match needs. Activity can be decreased by reducing total time spent in training or by reducing the intensity of the training activities. For instance, a weightlifter could do fewer repetitions or could do the same repetitions with less weight. Regardless of the technique followed, competition-minus-6-days should provide a training schedule that is not as exhaustive as competition-minus-7-days. (See table 6.2.)

Table 6.2   Sample Exercise and Eating Schedule for Competition-Minus-6-Days

Time of day	Activity	Food
7:00 A.M. to 8:00 A.M.	• Light breakfast (*before* getting dressed for workout) • Dress for A.M. workout	• 1 slice white bread toast • 1 cup fruit juice • 1 cup sports beverage [Average 230 calories]
8:00 A.M. to 9:30 A.M.	• Stretch (30 minutes) • 1 hour vigorous run, bike, or equipment-based activity	• 1 cup sports beverage during stretch (sipped over 30 minutes) • 12 ounces sports beverage during 1 hour activity (sipped at the rate of 4 ounces every 15 minutes) [About 125 calories]
9:30 A.M. to 10:00 A.M.	• Postexercise breakfast (*before* getting washed and dressed)	• 1 boiled egg • 2 slices of toast with 2 tablespoons of jam • 1 fresh orange • 1 bowl (1 cup) of whole-grain cereal with 6 ounces of 1% milk • 8 ounces fruit juice [About 690 calories]
10:00 A.M. to 12:30 P.M.	• Shower and dress • Relaxed activities (read, walk, light work around the house, desk work, etc.)	• Sip on 12 ounces of fluids (any kind except those containing caffeine or alcohol) [About 75 calories if a sports beverage]
12:30 P.M. to 1:00 P.M.	• Lunch	• Large bowl (2.5 cups) of pasta with marinara sauce • 2 slices of French bread • 8 ounces of fruit juice [About 1,000 calories]
1:00 P.M. to 2:45 P.M.	• Postlunch relaxation (read, desk work, slow walking, driving, etc.)	• Sip on 12 ounces of water [0 calories]
2:45 P.M. to 3:30 P.M.	• Preparation for afternoon workout (get dressed for exercise, etc.)	• Sip on 12 ounces of sports beverage [About 75 calories]
3:30 P.M. to 7:00 P.M.	• Late-afternoon workout • Practice skills • Lower the conditioning/ endurance training intensity from the day before • Should be an invigorating, but not exhaustive, training regimen	• Sip on 16 ounces of sports beverage per hour (4 ounces each 15 minutes) • Take your nude weight prior to exercise and after exercise to see if you have consumed an appropriate amount of fluid. For each pound of weight loss, you should have consumed an additional 16 ounces of beverage. [About 350 calories]

(continued)

Table 6.2 *(continued)*

Time of day	Activity	Food
7:00 P.M. to 7:30 P.M.	• Postexercise nutritional replenishment	• 1 banana • 12 ounces of sports beverage • 2 slices of bread [About 315 calories]
7:30 P.M. to 8:00 P.M.	• Shower and dress	• Don't drink the shower water unless you're really thirsty!
8:00 P.M. to 9:00 P.M.	• Dinner	• Large baked potato • Broccoli (1 spear) • Small lean steak (4 ounces) • Orange juice (1 cup) • Rice pudding (1 cup) [About 1,050 calories]
9:00 P.M. to 10:00 P.M.	• Relaxation activities	• 1 cup of water (sipped)
10:00 P.M. to 7:00 A.M.	• Sleep, glorious sleep!	• No eating or drinking permitted!

Intake totals: 3,900 calories
78.5% of calories from carbohydrate
11.3% of calories from protein
10.2% of calories from fat

Note: The food intake in this example would meet the needs of a 190-pound (86.4-kilogram) athlete with an intensive exercise schedule. In this example, the energy requirement for competition-minus-6-days is estimated as 45 calories per kilogram of body weight. Importantly, it is high in fluids, high in carbohydrates, low in fat, and moderate in protein. This type of intake supports glycogen (energy) storage in the muscles and liver. Athletes weighing less than this would consume proportionately less food, while maintaining the same frequency of intake.

Five Days Before Competition

On the second day of reduced exercise intensity and duration, a consistent high carbohydrate and fluid intake is still maintained. Again, total energy intake should be reduced to match needs. This day, competition-minus-5-days, is characterized by activity that is discernibly less than the athlete is accustomed to doing. (See table 6.3.)

Four Days Before Competition

Four days before the event is a good time for making your final strategic plans for the competition. Your training regimen should focus on key elements of the special skills you have, with an emphasis on practicing skills in a way that keeps you from becoming exhausted. As with the previous days, you should maintain a high carbohydrate and fluid intake to support your needs.

This is also a good time to eat a little extra protein, up to 2 grams per kilogram, to make certain all your tissue-repair needs are covered and to support the manufacture of creatine. For a 190-pound (86 kilogram) athlete, 2 grams of protein per kilogram

Table 6.3   Sample Exercise and Eating Schedule for Competition-Minus-5-Days

Time of day	Activity	Food
7:00 A.M. to 8:00 A.M.	• Light breakfast (*before* getting dressed for workout) • Dress for A.M. workout	• 1 slice white bread toast • 1 cup sports beverage • NO FRUIT JUICE [Average 115 calories]
8:00 A.M. to 9:30 A.M.	• Stretch (30 minutes) • 1 hour moderate-intensity run, bike, or equipment-based activity	• 1 cup sports beverage during stretch (sipped over 30 minutes) • 12 ounces sports beverage during 1 hour activity (4 ounces sipped every 15 minutes) [About 125 calories]
9:30 A.M. to 10:00 A.M.	• Postexercise breakfast (*before* getting washed and dressed)	• 1 boiled egg • 2 slices of toast with 1 teaspoon of jam • 1 fresh orange • 1 bowl (1 cup) of whole-grain cereal with 6 ounces of 1% milk • 4 ounces (1/2 cup) fruit juice [About 600 calories]
10:00 A.M. to 12:30 P.M.	• Shower and dress • Relaxed activities (read, walk, light work around the house, desk work, etc.)	• Sip on 12 ounces of water
12:30 P.M. to 1:00 P.M.	• Lunch	• Large bowl (2.5 cups) of pasta with marinara sauce • 3 slices of French bread • 4 ounces of fruit juice [About 925 calories]
1:00 P.M. to 2:45 P.M.	• Postlunch relaxation (read, desk work, slow walking, driving, etc.)	• Sip on 12 ounces of water
2:45 P.M. to 3:30 P.M.	• Preparation for afternoon workout (get dressed for exercise, etc.) • Stretch (at least 30 minutes)	• Sip on 12 ounces of water
3:30 P.M. to 6:30 P.M.	• Late-afternoon workout • Practice skills • Both time and intensity of training are reduced	• Sip on 16 ounces of sports beverage per hour (4 ounces each 15 minutes) • Take your nude weight prior to exercise and after exercise to see if you have consumed an appropriate amount of fluid. For each pound of weight loss, you should have consumed an additional 16 ounces of beverage. [About 350 calories]

(continued)

Table 6.3 *(continued)*

Time of day	Activity	Food
6:30 P.M. to 7:30 P.M.	• Postexercise nutritional replenishment	• 1 banana • 12 ounces of sports beverage • 1 slice of bread [About 250 calories]
7:30 P.M. to 8:00 P.M.	• Shower and dress	• Don't drink the shower water unless you're really thirsty!
8:00 P.M. to 9:00 P.M.	• Dinner	• Large baked potato • Broccoli (1 spear) • Small lean steak (4 ounces) • 1 glass water • Rice pudding (1 cup) [About 850 calories]
9:00 P.M. to 10:00 P.M.	• Relaxation activities	• 1 cup of water (sipped)
10:00 P.M. to 7:00 A.M.	• Sleep, glorious sleep!	• No eating or drinking permitted!

Intake totals: 3,200 calories
75.61% of calories from carbohydrate
12.54% of calories from protein
11.85% of calories from fat

Note: The food intake in this example would meet the needs of a 190-pound (86.4-kilogram) athlete with a moderate exercise schedule. In this example, the energy requirement for competition-minus-5-days is estimated as 40 calories per kilogram of body weight. Importantly, it is high in fluids, high in carbohydrates, low in fat, and moderate in protein. This type of intake supports glycogen (energy) storage in the muscles and liver. Athletes weighing less than this would consume proportionately less food, while maintaining the same frequency of intake.

of body weight amounts to 172 grams of protein. The examples in chapter 1 provided 1.26 grams of protein per kilogram of body weight, an amount that is well within the general requirements for athletes (1 to 2 grams per day). Therefore, providing a little extra protein merely provides some assurance that protein intake is not a limiting factor in performance.

Three Days Before Competition

Similar to 4 days before competition, 3 days before competition places a continued emphasis on low- to moderate-intensity exercise, a high carbohydrate intake, and a low fat intake, along with a slightly greater emphasis (up to 2 grams per kilogram) on protein. Other activities during the day should also be reduced, with more time made available for both physical and psychological relaxation. The athlete should absolutely avoid becoming overheated or exhausted from any activity. Use table 6.4 as a sample exercise and eating schedule for competition-minus-4-days and competition-minus-3-days.

Table 6.4   Sample Exercise and Eating Schedule for Competition-Minus-4-Days and Minus-3-Days

Time of day	Activity	Food
7:00 A.M. to 8:00 A.M.	• Light breakfast (*before* getting dressed for workout) • Dress for A.M. workout	• 1 slice white bread toast • 1 cup sports beverage [Average 115 calories]
8:00 A.M. to 9:30 A.M.	• Stretch (30 minutes) • 1 hour low-to-moderate-intensity run, bike, or equipment-based activity	• 1 cup sports beverage during stretch (sipped over 30 minutes) • 12 ounces sports beverage during 1 hour activity (4 ounces sipped every 15 minutes) [About 125 calories]
9:30 A.M. to 10:00 A.M.	• Postexercise breakfast (*before* getting washed and dressed)	• 2 boiled eggs • 2 slices of toast with 1 teaspoon of jam • 1 fresh orange • 1 bowl (1 cup) of whole-grain cereal with 6 ounces of 1% milk • 4 ounces (1/2 cup) fruit juice [About 530 calories]
10:00 A.M. to 12:30 P.M.	• Shower and dress • Relaxed activities (read, walk, light work around the house, desk work, etc.)	• Sip on 12 ounces of water
12:30 P.M. to 1:00 P.M.	• Lunch	• Medium bowl (1.5 cups) of pasta with marinara sauce • 2 slices of French bread • 1 banana (in place of 4 ounces of fruit juice) [About 800 calories]
1:00 P.M. to 2:45 P.M.	• Postlunch relaxation (read, desk work, slow walking, driving, etc.)	• Sip on 12 ounces of water
2:45 P.M. to 3:30 P.M.	• Preparation for afternoon workout (get dressed for exercise, etc.) • Stretch (at least 30 minutes)	• Sip on 12 ounces of water
3:30 P.M. to 5:30 P.M.	• Late-afternoon workout • Practice skills • Both time and intensity of training are reduced	• Sip on 16 ounces of sports beverage per hour (4 ounces each 15 minutes) • Take your nude weight prior to exercise and after exercise to see if you have consumed an appropriate amount of fluid. For each pound of weight loss, you should have consumed an additional 16 ounces of beverage. [About 350 calories]

(continued)

Table 6.4   *(continued)*

Time of day	Activity	Food
5:30 P.M. to 7:30 P.M.	• Postexercise nutritional replenishment	• 1 banana • 12 ounces of sports beverage • Omit bread [About 175 calories]
7:30 P.M. to 8:00 P.M.	• Shower and dress	• Don't drink the shower water unless you're really thirsty!
8:00 P.M. to 9:00 P.M.	• Dinner	• Medium baked potato • Broccoli (1 stalk) • Small lean steak (4 ounces) • 1 glass water • Rice pudding (1 cup) [About 800 calories]
9:00 P.M. to 10:00 P.M.	• Relaxation activities	• 1 cup of water (sipped)
10:00 P.M. to 7:00 A.M.	• Sleep, glorious sleep!	• No eating or drinking permitted!

Intake totals: 3,000 calories
65.0% of calories from carbohydrate
20.0% of calories from protein
15.0% of calories from fat

Note: The food intake in this example would meet the needs of a 190-pound (86.4-kilogram) athlete with a light-to-moderate exercise schedule. The energy requirement for competition-minus-4-days and minus-3-days is estimated as 35 calories per kilogram of body weight. Importantly, it is high in fluids, high in carbohydrates, low in fat, and moderately high in protein. This type of intake supports glycogen (energy) storage in the muscles and liver. Athletes weighing less than this would consume proportionately less food, while maintaining the same frequency of intake.

Two Days Before Competition

Two days before an event is an excellent time to get more rest, and a good way to achieve this goal is to eliminate the morning training schedule. The afternoon training should be reduced to no more than 1.5 hours, with a moderate to low intensity. The focus should be on reviewing skills and reinforcing the mental strategy it will take to compete effectively. Of course, carbohydrate and fluid intake should remain high. (See table 6.5.)

One Day Before Competition

The day before competition should be characterized by plenty of rest (both physical and mental) and relaxation. Athletes and coaches should be restrained from running through multiple full routines, a full-speed run, or a full "game intensity" practice. Walking parts of the course, getting familiar with the competition venue, or watching films of your opponents are OK activities but only if you know they won't make you anxious and unable to relax. Sport psychologists I have worked with have indicated

Table 6.5 Sample Exercise and Eating Schedule for Competition-Minus-2-Days

Time of day	Activity	Food
← Sleep Late! No Morning Exercise →		
9:30 A.M. to 10:00 A.M.	• Postexercise breakfast (*before* getting washed and dressed)	• 2 boiled eggs • 2 slices of toast with 1 teaspoon of jam • 1 fresh orange or banana • 1 bowl (1 cup) of whole-grain cereal with 6 ounces of 1% milk • 1 slice white bread toast • 1 cup sports beverage [About 650 calories]
10:00 A.M. to 12:30 P.M.	• Shower and dress • Relaxed activities (read, walk, light work around the house, desk work, etc.)	• Sip on 12 ounces of water
12:30 P.M. to 1:00 P.M.	• Lunch	• Medium bowl (1.5 cups) of pasta with marinara sauce • 2 slices of French bread • 1 banana [About 800 calories]
1:00 P.M. to 2:45 P.M.	• Postlunch relaxation (read, desk work, slow walking, driving, etc.)	• Sip on 12 ounces of water
2:45 P.M. to 3:30 P.M.	• Preparation for afternoon workout (get dressed for exercise, etc.) • Stretch (at least 30 minutes)	• Sip on 12 ounces of water
3:30 P.M. to 5:00 P.M.	• Late-afternoon workout • Practice skills • Both time and intensity of training are reduced	• Sip on 16 ounces of sports beverage per hour (4 ounces each 15 minutes) • Take your nude weight prior to exercise and after exercise to see if you have consumed an appropriate amount of fluid. For each pound of weight loss, you should have consumed an additional 16 ounces of beverage. [About 350 calories]
5:00 P.M. to 7:30 P.M.	• Postexercise nutritional replenishment	• 1 banana • 12 ounces of sports beverage [About 175 calories]
7:30 P.M. to 8:00 P.M.	• Shower and dress	• Don't drink the shower water unless you're really thirsty!

(continued)

Table 6.5 *(continued)*

Time of day	Activity	Food
8:00 P.M. to 9:00 P.M.	• Dinner	• Medium baked potato • Broccoli (1 stalk) • Small lean steak (4 ounces) • 1 glass water • Rice pudding (1 cup) [About 800 calories]
9:00 P.M. to 10:00 P.M.	• Relaxation activities	• 1 cup of water (sipped)
10:00 P.M. to 7:00 A.M.	• Sleep, glorious sleep!	• No eating or drinking permitted!

Intake totals: 2,800 calories
65.0% of calories from carbohydrate
20.0% of calories from protein
15.0% of calories from fat

Note: The food intake in this example would meet the needs of a 190-pound (86.4-kilogram) athlete with a light-to-moderate exercise schedule. The energy requirement for competition-minus-2-days is estimated as 35 calories per kilogram of body weight. Importantly, it is high in fluids, high in carbohydrates, low in fat, and moderately high in protein (approximately 1.8 grams of protein per kilogram of body weight to assure tissue maintenance and repair needs are met). This type of intake supports glycogen (energy) storage in the muscles and liver. Athletes weighing less than this would consume proportionately less food, while maintaining the same frequency of intake.

it's probably better to watch films of your own successful competitions rather than to watch films of what your opponent might do. By 1 day before competition, you should have already been briefed about who you're competing against and what strategy to follow.

This is almost your last chance to make certain your glycogen stores are at peak values, and you should maintain a steady fluid intake to ensure optimal hydration going into the next day's activities (see table 6.6). The carbohydrates you consume should be high in starch and relatively low in fiber. Pasta, bread, rice, and fruits (without seeds or skins) are excellent choices. Vegetables and legumes tend to have lots of fiber but may produce gas (causing you to become uncomfortable and bloated). Vegetables in the cabbage family (cabbage, brussels sprouts, kohlrabi) are particularly notorious for their gas-creating capabilities.

Competition Day

It is particularly important that athletes avoid doing anything they are unaccustomed to doing, or eating anything they are unaccustomed to eating, on the day of an event. Athletes should have a checklist prepared of what is needed and where it is. Competition day is not the time for running around the house screaming, "Where did I put my running shoes!" Leave nothing to chance, and have a backup plan for everything that might go awry (e.g., transportation).

Table 6.6 Sample Exercise and Eating Schedule for Competition-Minus-1-Day

Time of day	Activity	Food
← Sleep Late! No Morning Exercise →		
9:30 A.M. to 10:00 A.M.	• Breakfast [*Note:* Avoid eating high-fiber cereals if they cause you to bloat or give you gas. If this occurs, puffed rice or cornflakes may be good alternatives.]	• 2 boiled eggs • 2 slices of toast with 1 teaspoon of jam • 1 fresh orange or banana • 1 bowl (1 cup) of cereal with 6 ounces of 1% milk • 1 slice white bread toast • 1 cup sports beverage [About 650 calories]
10:00 A.M. to 12:30 P.M.	• Shower and dress • Relaxed activities (read, walk, light work around the house, desk work, etc.)	• Sip on 12 ounces of water
12:30 P.M. to 1:00 P.M.	• Lunch	• Medium bowl (1.5 cups) of Spanish rice • 2 slices of French bread • 1 banana [About 800 calories]
1:00 P.M. to 2:45 P.M.	• Postlunch relaxation (read, desk work, slow walking, driving, etc.)	• Sip on 12 ounces of water
2:45 P.M. to 3:30 P.M.	• Preparation for afternoon workout (get dressed for exercise, etc.) • Stretch (at least 30 minutes)	• Sip on 12 ounces of water
3:30 P.M. to 5:00 P.M.	• Late-afternoon workout should be very mild. Walking around your neighborhood or becoming familiar with the competition venue are good activities. • Both time and intensity of training are low.	• Sip on 16 ounces of sports beverage per hour (4 ounces each 15 minutes) • Take your nude weight prior to exercise and after exercise to see if you have consumed an appropriate amount of fluid. For each pound of weight loss, you should have consumed an additional 16 ounces of beverage. [About 350 calories]
5:00 P.M. to 7:30 P.M.	• Postactivity nutritional replenishment	• 1 banana • 12 ounces of sports beverage [About 175 calories]
7:30 P.M. to 8:00 P.M.	• Shower and dress	• Have fluids available in a bottle to sip on to avoid thirst

(continued)

Table 6.6   *(continued)*

Time of day	Activity	Food
8:00 P.M. to 9:00 P.M.	• Dinner [*Note.* Avoid eating high-fiber vegetables that could cause bloating and gas. Cabbage, broccoli, cauliflower, and raw spinach are particularly known for causing gas.]	• Medium baked potato (do not eat the skin) • Cooked carrots (3/4 cup) • Medium chicken breast without skin (baked) • 1 glass water • Rice pudding (1 cup) [About 800 calories]
9:00 P.M. to 10:00 P.M.	• Relaxation activities	• 1 cup of water (sipped)
10:00 P.M. to 7:00 A.M.	• Sleep, glorious sleep!	• No eating or drinking permitted!

Intake totals: 2,800 calories
65.0% of calories from carbohydrate
20.0% of calories from protein
15.0% of calories from fat

Note: The food intake in this example would meet the needs of a 190-pound (86.4-kilogram) athlete with a light activity schedule. The energy requirement for competition-minus-1-day is estimated as 35 calories per kilogram of body weight. Importantly, it is high in fluids, high in carbohydrates, low in fat, and moderately high in protein (approximately 1.8 grams of protein per kilogram of body weight to assure tissue maintenance and repair needs are met). This type of intake supports glycogen (energy) storage in the muscles and liver. Athletes weighing less than this would consume proportionately less food, while maintaining the same frequency of intake.

Eating and drinking appropriately on competition day is important, so make certain you have the right foods and drinks immediately available (don't leave it to chance). Take charge of knowing what you need, and take charge of getting it. Imagine drinking sports beverage X during practice all year, then getting up the morning of the competition to discover that your spouse couldn't find sports beverage X at the store, so he bought sports beverage Y instead. Avoid being put in any situation that will cause you stress on competition day.

Early-Morning Competition   If the competition is early in the morning, you should get out of bed 2 to 3 hours beforehand. If you have difficulty getting up early in the morning, practice it for several days before the competition. Give yourself enough time to eat some carbohydrates, drink some fluids, and get to the competition. Finish eating at least 1.5 hours before the start of your competition (assuming you are eating mainly starchy carbohydrates). Different athletes process foods differently, so knowing the best time differential between eating and the competition is important. Some athletes feel best when they finish eating 2 hours before competition, while others feel best finishing 3 hours before an event. Each athlete should know what works for him or her. The athlete should make whatever minor adjustments are needed if he or she eats with a team; make certain everything is right for you! After eating, maintain a sipping protocol on sports beverages for the entire time leading up to the competition. The athlete should not be placed in a position of feeling rushed.

When that happens, the food inevitably gets the short end of what should be done, and the athlete suffers, either through poor endurance or GI distress, during the entire competition.

Late-Morning or Early-Afternoon Competition   People often feel tired and hungry in the late morning and early afternoon because the food they ate for breakfast has stopped providing energy by this time. Therefore, it's important for athletes to eat something every 2.5 to 3.5 hours. For an 11:00 a.m. competition, wake up and have breakfast at 6:30 a.m., and eat again at 9:00 a.m. After the 9:00 a.m. meal, initiate your constant fluid-sipping protocol until competition time. For an early-afternoon competition (at 1:00 p.m.), have your last meal at 10:30 a.m., then begin your fluid-sipping protocol. Going into competition hungry is a sure formula for failure.

Midafternoon or Early-Evening Competition   It's difficult to compete in the midafternoon or early evening, especially if it's an outdoor sport and it's hot. Athletes typically go off schedule with a midafternoon competition. The best thing to do is spend the morning eating and drinking as usual (breakfast, midmorning snack, lunch), and then begin the countdown to the competition by having some starchy carbohydrates (e.g., a banana, toast, or crackers) and some fluids about 1.5 to 2.0 hours before the competition starts. The fluid-sipping protocol should then be initiated until competition time. The excitement of the competition can make athletes forget they're hungry. Therefore, it's a good idea to develop a well-rehearsed eating, snacking, and drinking schedule—and stick to it.

Late-Evening Competition   The late evening is also a difficult time to compete; the body wants to sleep, but the competition is keeping it awake. Therefore, sleeping late and eating something every 2.5 to 3.0 hours will help keep your energy level up until it's time to compete. Keep checking your hydration state (urine should basically be clear). Remember that a successful late-evening competition is sweet and will help you get a good and restful night's sleep!

Seven Day Wrap-Up

The main idea behind getting ready for competition is to set your body up so that it has a full tank of both carbohydrate (as glycogen) and fluid. The muscles and psyche should be well rested, and the athlete should be getting clear messages of confidence from the coach. Getting sufficient rest before competition can't be overemphasized. When athletes are involved in sports that require frequent competition, sufficient rest is critical. Anything that keeps you from getting a good night's sleep and being well rested will cause performance difficulties. The keys to good preparation for competition include the following:

1. Get plenty of rest.
2. Begin tapering physical activity 6 or 7 days before competition.
3. Eat enough carbohydrates to maximize glycogen stores.

4. Drink sufficient fluids to maximize fluid stores.

5. Eat frequently, approximately once every 3 hours, to maintain blood glucose and muscle glycogen levels and to feel good.

6. Consume enough energy before activity to ensure there's enough fuel in the system to support the activity and to avoid burning muscle as a fuel.

7. Practice the eating and drinking schedule of your competition day in advance so you know what makes you feel good.

8. Don't do anything on competition day that you haven't practiced doing beforehand.

9. Be ready with everything you'll need (sports beverages, snacks, and so on) long before the competition day arrives.

Both hunger and thirst are emergency sensations marking the onset of performance-reducing problems. As such, they should be avoided through a planned eating and drinking timetable that is integral to an athlete's training schedule and lifestyle. Perhaps no other two factors have the potential for making such an enormous positive impact on health and performance. Put simply, athletes interested in performing up to their conditioned abilities and skill levels should never get hungry and never get thirsty.

Efficient Delivery of Oxygen

7

It is difficult to imagine how an athlete could be successful without fully functional mechanisms for pulling in enough oxygen, transporting oxygen through the blood to working cells, using the delivered oxygen efficiently by having sufficient oxidative enzymes in mitochondria, efficiently excreting oxygen by-products (carbon dioxide), and dealing with the side effects of excess oxygen exposure through adequate anti-oxidant intake. Every one of these functions has an important nutrition component, with iron playing the critical role for oxygen delivery and carbon dioxide removal; vitamins B_{12} and folic acid playing a role in red blood cell formation; and the antioxidant nutrients beta-carotene, vitamin C, vitamin E, and selenium protecting cells from oxidation reactions. Strenuous physical activity, in and of itself, may increase the rate of energy utilization 20 to 100 times above the energy expended in a resting state, and the nutrient–oxygen relationship is a critical factor in ensuring that this can continue to happen.[1] This chapter reviews the nutrient relationship in the utilization of oxygen, as well as the critical relationship between oxygen, nutrition, and human performance.

Oxygen Uptake

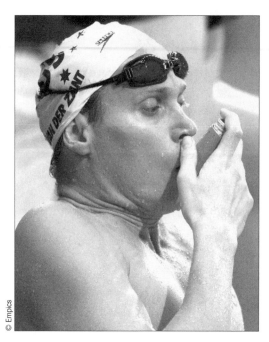

© Empics

Many elite athletes suffer from EIA, but it is treatable.

Air is breathed in through the nostrils and mouth before entering the left and right bronchi of the lungs. Gas exchange in the lungs occurs in the 150 million alveoli humans have in each bronchi. The average adult male can inhale approximately 4 liters (close to 4 quarts) of air with each breath, from which the oxygen is diffused into the alveoli, passes into the blood through capillaries, and enters the hemoglobin in red blood cells. At the same time, carbon dioxide in the blood passes to the alveoli and is exhaled. The oxygen content of air is approximately 21 percent, and the oxygen content of expired air is approximately 15 percent, indicating that only a small proportion of the oxygen in air is captured by the lungs. The typical water content of air is .5 percent, while the water content of expired air is approximately 6 percent, demonstrating why rapid respiration is a major route of water loss in athletes.

The rate of cellular respiration increases with exercise intensity, with vigorous high-intensity exercise causing a 25-fold increase in the demand for oxygen in working muscles. This increase in oxygen requirement is satisfied by an increase in the rate and depth of breathing. However, it is the rising rate of carbon dioxide, rather than the higher demand for oxygen, that triggers the increased breathing rate. A higher carbon dioxide level causes the medulla to stimulate the motor nerves controlling the intercostal and diaphragm muscles to increase their activity.

Diseases that affect the lungs, such as pneumonia, asthma, emphysema, bronchitis, chronic obstructive pulmonary disease, and lung cancer, compromise an individual's ability to obtain sufficient oxygen and excrete sufficient carbon dioxide. An area of particular interest to athletes is exercise-induced asthma (EIA), which affects a significant proportion of the athlete population. The prevalence of EIA in athletes is not fully established, but there are published reports of a 55 percent prevalence in cross-country skiers and a lower (12 percent) prevalence in basketball players.[2, 3]

EIA is an airway obstruction that occurs as a result of exercise (either during or after); includes cough, wheezing, and a tightness in the chest; and may occur in people who do not suffer from chronic asthma.[4] The recommended nonpharmacologic treatment for EIA includes the following:[5]

1. Become well conditioned for the activity that induces EIA. Well-conditioned athletes can exercise at lower breathing rates at any given work intensity and are therefore less likely to suffer from EIA.

2. Avoid exercising in cold and dry air. If the sport mandates exercising outside in these conditions (as in cross-country skiing), athletes should cover the mouth and nose with a scarf or ski mask to warm and humidify the breathed air.

3. A warm-up period is important, with the intensity of the warm-up dependent on how each athlete responds to EIA.

4. A cool-down period may diminish the severity of EIA by slowing airway changes.

5. Exercise on days when chronic asthma symptoms that may result from allergies or other conditions (if they exist) are controlled.

Oxygen Delivery and Cellular Utilization

Several elements, vitamins, and protein carriers provide, as a major function, the delivery and cellular utilization of oxygen. These elements work in unison to capture oxygen from the environment, transport oxygen through the blood to cells for metabolic actions, and remove the by-products (including carbon dioxide) of the oxygen-related metabolic activities.

Iron   Iron is a critical element in the delivery of oxygen to working tissues. It is part of red blood cell hemoglobin, muscle myoglobin, and enzymes involved in electron transfer for energy metabolism. The body uses a priority-based system for iron, with hemoglobin at the top of the priority system. If stores of iron become sufficiently low to cause hemoglobin to drop, iron in myoglobin and iron-containing enzymes are scavenged so as to maintain red blood cell hemoglobin. Because of this, it is possible for an athlete to experience a reduction in performance even if hemoglobin and hematocrit (the two most common measures of iron status) appear to be in the normal range. It is important, therefore, that ferritin (stored iron) also be measured as a normal component of a blood test intended to screen for iron status (see table 7.1).

A typical iron-deficiency anemia is referred to as *microcytic* (small cell), *hypochromic* (dark in color). It is characterized by an inadequate number of red blood cells and existing cells that are smaller than normal due to low hemoglobin levels.

Transferrin   Transferrin is a blood protein that carries iron through the blood to the bone marrow, spleen, and liver for either the storage of iron as ferritin or the manufacture of new red blood cells. It is a protein with a relatively short half-life that can be a marker for recent protein status, and it is used for this purpose. Low blood transferrin may be an indicator of protein or calorie malnutrition, resulting in inadequate synthesis of transferrin by the liver, or it can result from excess protein loss through the kidneys (proteinuria). A systemic infection or cancer can also lower the blood transferrin level. A high blood transferrin is a marker of iron deficiency. If an athlete has a low blood transferrin level, the production of hemoglobin can be impaired and can lead to anemia, even if there is ample iron in the body.

Ceruloplasmin   Ceruloplasmin is a copper-containing protein involved in handing over iron from transferrin to hemoglobin in the formation of new red blood cells,

Table 7.1 Terms Related to Iron Status

Ferritin	Ferritin is an iron-storage protein found in the liver, spleen, and bone marrow, with only a small amount in the blood. The amount in the blood is thought to be proportionate to the amount stored in the liver, spleen, and bone marrow, so a blood ferritin test is an indicator of the amount of stored iron. The lower the ferritin level, even within the "normal" range, the more likely a patient is iron deficient. Normal ferritin values: • Adult males: 20 to 300 ng/ml • Adult females: 20 to 120 ng/ml *Note:* ng/ml = nanograms per milliliter
Hematocrit	Hematocrit is the proportion of whole blood that is composed of red blood cells and is often referred to as the number of red blood cells per unit of blood. Normal hematocrit values: • Adult males: 42 to 52% • Adult females: 36 to 48%
Hemochromatosis	Hemochromatosis is an iron overload disease caused by uninhibited iron absorption. It can result in liver damage if the iron concentration is not lowered.
Hemoglobin	Hemoglobin is the iron-containing, oxygen-carrying protein in red blood cells.
Hemosiderosis	Hemosiderosis is a disease condition that results from excess iron in the body, often from blood transfusions. It is often seen in individuals with thalassemia.
Serum iron	Serum iron represents the total amount of iron in the blood serum. Normal serum iron values: • Adult males: 75 to 175 mcg/dl • Adult females: 65 to 165 mcg/dl
Total iron binding capacity (TIBC)	The TIBC test measures the amount of iron the blood could carry if transferrin were fully saturated with iron molecules. Since transferrin is produced by the liver, the TIBC can be used to monitor liver function and protein-status nutrition.
Transferrin	The transferrin test is a direct measurement of the protein transferrin (also called siderophilin) in the blood. The saturation level of transferrin can be calculated by dividing the serum iron level by TIBC. Normal transferrin values: • Adult males: 200 to 400 mg/dl • Adult females: 200 to 400 mg/dl Normal transferrin saturation values are between 30 and 40%.

or in removing iron from old red blood cells for inclusion in new ones. A copper deficiency results in low ceruloplasmin and can result in anemia that presents much like iron-deficiency (microcytic, hypochromic) anemia, possibly leading to a misdiagnosis. A ceruloplasmin deficiency is associated with iron accumulation in the pancreas, liver, and brain, resulting in neurological disorders.

Vitamin B$_{12}$ Vitamin B$_{12}$ is a cobalt-containing vitamin that is also referred to as cobalamin. Two of its primary functions are the formation of red blood cells and the preservation of a healthy nervous system. The absence of vitamin B$_{12}$ when red blood cells are being formed results in cells that have a weak membrane. These cells, called megaloblasts, are fragile and live half as long as a normal red blood cell (60 days versus 120 days). The shortened life of these cells requires a constantly faster production of red cells to maintain normal oxygen-carrying capacity. However, this fast level of red cell production cannot be maintained, resulting in anemia. The anemia resulting from vitamin B$_{12}$ deficiency is referred to as pernicious anemia because it develops slowly over several years. Pernicious anemia is a megaloblastic, hypochromic anemia, meaning that the red blood cells are large and misshapen and are low in color (the hemoglobin is spread out over a larger cell area, diluting the color.) Besides the reduced oxygen-carrying capacity from the anemia, pernicious anemia is associated with neurological symptoms and nerve degeneration. A small amount of vitamin B$_{12}$ is needed (the amount in one egg is likely to be sufficient for more than a month), but since it comes almost exclusively from meat sources, vegetarian athletes are at risk.

Folic Acid   Folic acid, vitamin B$_{12}$, and vitamin C are all involved in protein metabolism. In conjunction with vitamin B$_{12}$, folate is needed for the production of red blood cells. Folate is also involved in nerve tissue development and is known to eliminate neural tube defects in newborns. The anemia associated with inadequate folate is similar to that produced by a deficiency of vitamin B$_{12}$ (megaloblastic, hypochromic anemia), and the reduced oxygen-carrying capacity that results is equally severe. However, while vitamin B$_{12}$ is obtained from animal sources, folic acid is best obtained from fresh fruits, fresh vegetables, and legumes.

The Oxygen–Nutrient Performance Relationship

There is no question that physical activity can alter blood-iron status and that blood-iron status can also alter physical activity performance. One study assessing 747 athletes and 104 untrained controls found that endurance athletes had lower hemoglobin and hematocrit levels than either power- or mixed-trained athletes, suggesting that the difference may be due to dilutional pseudoanemia and, perhaps, a greater degree of foot-strike hemolysis (see shaded section on next page).[6]

Athletes with higher exercise durations and workloads also appear to store less iron (ferritin). These findings imply that athletes are indeed at higher risk of compromised iron status than are nonathletes, and higher exercise durations within the athlete pool create even greater iron-status risk. Endurance athletes who put in large numbers of training hours (and miles) are therefore at highest risk of poor

Dilutional pseudoanemia

When athletes begin an intensive exercise program, they experience a rise in both blood volume and red blood cells. However, because the blood volume increases at a faster rate than the red blood cells, it appears as if they have anemia. Since this condition is transient (eventually the concentration of red cells becomes normal), it is referred to as a *dilutional pseudoanemia* (also known as *sports anemia* or *athletic anemia*).

Foot-strike hemolysis

Repeated foot strike associated with running causes red blood cells to break down. Red cells circulating in capillaries through the bottom of the feet are crushed by the foot strike. The faster red blood cells break down from foot-strike hemolysis, the more difficult it is for athletes to maintain a normal concentration of red blood cells (their bodies can't make the red blood cells fast enough), which may result in anemia.

iron status even though they rely most on aerobic metabolic processes to achieve their endurance.

Restrictive intakes, as are common among athletes involved in weight-classification or aesthetic sports, almost always supply inadequate levels of vitamins and minerals. There is real risk, therefore, that a significant proportion of the athlete population has less than optimal oxygen-utilization capacity—a fact that surely inhibits optimal performance. Iron deficiency, even without anemia, reduces muscle work potential, and iron-deficiency anemia makes matters worse because of a further reduction in oxygen-carrying capacity.

Iron-deficiency anemia is likely to be more prevalent among athletes (particularly female athletes) than among nonathlete groups.[7] The effects include reduced athletic performance and impaired immune function. Young female athletes should consider either consuming more iron-rich foods (particularly red meats) or taking iron supplements under the supervision of a doctor.

Iron deficiency occurs in athletes for many reasons, including inadequate intake, hemolysis, and menstrual blood loss in females.[8] However, the most common iron problem in athletes is caused not by blood loss but by an enlargement of the blood volume without a concomitant increase in the constituents of the blood, including red blood cells. This condition, referred to as sports anemia or dilutional pseudo-anemia, is a normal state that occurs when athletes increase training intensity (see figure 7.1).

The underconsumption of other nutrients may also affect oxygen utilization. Magnesium deficiency increases oxygen requirements needed to perform submaximal exercise, thereby reducing endurance performance.[9] Folate and vitamin B_{12} deficiencies result in megaloblastic anemia, a condition that results in malformed red blood cells with a reduced life expectancy. This reduced functional duration makes it difficult for athletes to constantly manufacture red cells, which are also being destroyed

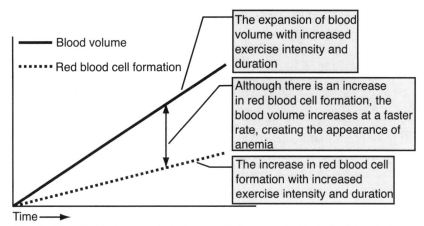

Note: The differential in blood volume and red cell concentration becomes noticeable after 3 to 5 days of an increase in exercise duration or intensity. After a period of time, blood volume ceases to increase and red cell production catches up, removing the appearance of anemia.

Figure 7.1   Dilutional pseudoanemia.

through foot-strike hemolysis. The result is fewer cells that can carry oxygen and remove carbon dioxide, a sure formula for poor athletic performance.

Data from past studies indicate a higher prevalence of hematuria in athletes, with multiple causes that include the following:[10]

- Foot-strike hemolysis
- Renal ischemia
- Hypoxic kidney damage
- Release of a hemolyzing factor
- Bladder or kidney trauma
- Nonsteroidal anti-inflammatory drug intake
- Dehydration
- Increased circulation rate
- Myoglobinuria release
- Peroxidation of red blood cells

A chronic loss of red blood cells in the urine, a condition brought on by frequent high-intensity and long-duration practice sessions, would contribute to anemia, a problem that reduces competitiveness in any athlete. Athletes should be careful, therefore, to take in sufficient nutrients (particularly iron) to replace that which is lost. Luckily, the erythropoietic process (production of new red blood cells) appears to be remarkably resilient in the face of exercise stress; it is capable of producing a large and adequate number of red blood cells provided a sufficient nutrient base (in particular iron, folate, and vitamin B_{12}) is available.[11] Some athletes try to enhance erythropoiesis by taking erythropoietin (EPO), but this blood-doping technique is illegal and has the potential for increasing blood viscosity, with subsequent thrombosis and potentially fatal results.[12]

Oxidative Stress

Oxidative stress refers to the creation of an increased volume of reactive oxygen species (ROS) because of an inadequate presence of antioxidants.[13] Also referred to as peroxides and free radicals, ROS cause damage to cells because their radical movement inside cells destroys them, producing "clinkers" (dead cells). The body inhibits ROS production through antioxidant vitamins and minerals (see table 7.2). The minerals work to regulate enzyme activity so as to diminish ROS production, while vitamins accept ROS to remove them from the cellular environment, thereby limiting their potential hazards.

Table 7.2   Antioxidant Nutrients

Nutrient	Daily Recommended Intake (age 19 to 30)		Function(s)
	Male	**Female**	
Vitamin C	90 mg/day	75 mg/day	Vitamin C scavenges reactive oxidants in leukocytes and in lung and gastric mucosa, and it reduces lipid peroxidation in cells.
Vitamin E	15 mg/day	15 mg/day	Vitamin E mainly prevents the peroxidation of lipids.
Selenium	55 mcg/day	55 mcg/day	Selenium functions through selenoproteins, which form oxidant defense enzymes. The DRI is based on the amount needed to synthesize selenoprotein glutathione peroxidase.
Beta-carotene	(900 mcg/day)	(700 mcg/day)	12 mcg of beta-carotene can form 1 mcg of retinol (vitamin A). The human nutrient requirement is for vitamin A, not beta-carotene. However, there is no question that beta-carotene is more than just a precursor to the production of vitamin A. Besides being an important biomarker for the intake of fresh fruits and vegetables, it has important antioxidant properties.

Early studies of vitamin E, a fat-soluble antioxidant vitamin found mainly in vegetable oils, initially showed promise in reducing ROS. However, there has been a recent concern that vitamin E supplementation, by itself, may place the pool of antioxidants out of balance, thereby diminishing the overall defenses humans have to prevent ROS. A proposed strategy to avoid this imbalance is to consume a cocktail of antioxidants rather than a single antioxidant vitamin. In doing so, the sensitive balance between the antioxidants can remain intact while there is an increase in antioxidant presence to provide an improved defense against ROS.

Nutrient imbalances can also cause difficulties with immune function. Excess vitamin E can negatively affect the immune system, but inadequate levels of this vitamin, iron, selenium, zinc, calcium, and magnesium can also create immune problems.[14] All this information points to the importance of maintaining a balance of all the nutrients rather than pushing one or two with the hope of inducing a desirable biochemical effect.

Oxidative metabolic processes are constantly working, even during events that are primarily anaerobic. The anaerobic athlete who just completed a 10-second high-intensity sprint has something in common with a gymnast who just completed a 90-second floor routine: the need to breathe a large volume of air (oxygen) to recharge the fuels they will need for the next bout of high-intensity exercise. Iron is a primary element for transporting oxygen to working tissues and carbon dioxide away from working tissues—it is a critical nutrient for athletes. Nevertheless, iron is the most common nutrient deficiency, and athletes may be at even greater risk for iron deficiency than the general public because of the hemolysis and hematuria commonly experienced. Other nutrients are also important to ensure a healthy red blood cell production (vitamin B_{12} and folate) and to ensure all the oxygen brought into the system will not be damaging (the antioxidant nutrients beta-carotene, selenium, vitamin C, and vitamin E).

Oxygen is sufficiently important for athletic performance that athletes of all sizes, sports, and ages should regularly check their iron status via a blood test that measures hemoglobin, hematocrit, and ferritin. Only with the information from such a test will athletes know if they should alter food intake or consume iron or other supplements to ensure that oxygen will not be a negative factor in performance.

Inhibitors of Fuel and Nutrient Utilization

8

Under healthy, normal circumstances, consumed food passes through the gastrointestinal (GI) tract for the processing (mechanical and chemical) and absorption of nutrients. Once absorbed, these nutrients are transformed by tissues and organs into forms that are needed for normal respiratory and metabolic purposes. There are circumstances, however, when this normal and usual process can be corrupted by disease or by the consumption of substances that cause a malabsorption of nutrients, either through a direct irritation of the GI tract or through a chemical sequestering of nutrients that makes them unavailable for absorption. Other substances may corrupt the normal processing of nutrients by tissues, often in the liver, so that the potential metabolic benefits of the consumed foods are not realized. It is also possible that the timing of consumption of one food may conflict with the absorption of nutrients in another food. This chapter discusses the major factors that influence how well we consume, absorb, and use energy substrates, with a secondary focus on strategies that can help athletes get the most out of what they eat.

Factors Influencing Food Consumption

Several factors may influence food consumption and thereby the total nutrient intake of any individual. These factors range from appetite loss, which may result from conditions as varied as transitional depression to consumption of certain drugs; micronutrient deficiency or toxicity, which may alter appetite through the impact it has on taste sensitivity; dieting, which purposefully lowers total food consumption with the hope of achieving a desirable weight loss; and overtraining, which is a major problem for many athletes.

Appetite Loss   A loss of appetite (anorexia), regardless of the cause, interferes with food consumption and may result in malnutrition if it progresses for a sufficient duration of time. Appetite can be affected by both nutrition and non-nutrition factors. A death in the family, for instance, often leads to some reduction in appetite, while a zinc deficiency is also associated with appetite loss. Inadequate consumption of carbohydrates, as is possible on high-protein, high-fat, low-carbohydrate diets, may result in some degree of ketosis, which is associated with nausea and a loss of appetite. Consumption of certain drugs is also known to result in an altered taste perception or an appetite loss, both of which may result in lower energy consumption (see table 8.1). Even something as seemingly unimportant as a small toothache can reduce food intake or, at the very least, reduce the variety of foods consumed so as to create a below-optimal nutrient and energy intake.

Micronutrient Deficiency or Toxicity   Micronutrients also play a role in appetite, creating a problem that is difficult to address. A deficiency of a vitamin, thiamin for instance, results in poor appetite. However, because this deficiency creates poor appetite, it becomes difficult to increase food intake to reverse the deficiency. See table 8.2 for a list of vitamins and minerals that may create a loss of appetite from either an excessive or deficient intake.

Popular Diets   Popular diets are, by design, meant to restrict the intake of foods. Some diets achieve this by eliminating whole food groups, while others encourage the intake of some energy substrates (typically protein and fat) while discouraging the intake of other substrates (typically carbohydrate). Regardless of the diet plan, most diets involve a massive

Table 8.1   Sample of Drugs That May Cause Appetite Loss or an Altered Taste Perception

Loss of appetite	Altered taste perception
Tylenol with codeine	Amphetamines
Tamoxifen	Ampicillin
Colchicine	Benzocaine
Amphogel	Clofibrate
Azulfidine	Griseofulvin
	Lidocaine
	Lithium carbonate
	D-penicillamine

Source: Mahan LK & Escott-Stump S. "Krause's Food, Nutrition, & Diet Therapy," 10th Edition, Philadelphia: W.B. Saunders Company © 2000, pg 401.

Table 8.2 Vitamins That Can Affect Appetite

Vitamin	Inadequate intake	Excessive intake
Thiamin (vitamin B_1)	Poor appetite; mental depression	
Riboflavin (vitamin B_2)	Tongue sores; mouth sores	
Niacin	Poor appetite; weakness	Nausea; liver damage
Vitamin B_6	Tongue sores	
Pantothenic acid	Poor appetite; nausea (extremely rare deficiency)	
Choline		Nausea; GI distress
Vitamin C	Bleeding gums	
Copper		Nausea (extremely rare toxicity)
Zinc	Poor appetite; altered sense of taste; reduced sense of taste	

reduction in calories that ultimately results in a loss of lean mass and a reduction in performance. Sudden and large reductions in caloric intake result in a lowering of fat-free mass (i.e., lean mass), which results in a lowering of metabolic rate. This condition forces people to constantly eat less to adapt to the frequent ratcheting down of metabolic rate. At some point, low-calorie diets become low-nutrient diets, with all of the potential dangers associated with a chronically inadequate nutrient intake.

Overtraining Overtraining can lead to a cascade of problems including sleep loss, increased illness frequency, and appetite loss. The major point to remember here is this: Anything that interferes with food intake is likely to have a major impact on nutrition status and energy intake, both of which will diminish athletic performance and will likely place the athlete at increased disease risk. Athletes who experience sleepless nights, constant fatigue, frequent illness, appetite loss, weight loss, and large mood swings are likely to be overtraining.

Factors Influencing Digestion and Absorption of Nutrients

Any number of factors may result in maldigestion or malabsorption, either of which will diminish nutrient delivery to needy cells. It is important to consider that a problem early in the GI tract (i.e., the mouth or esophagus) is likely to create a cascade of problems later in the GI tract. For instance, the pain associated with esophagitis (an irritation in the esophagus from frequent vomiting, frequent alcohol consumption, or gastric reflux) may inhibit normal drinking patterns to the point of changing normal bowel habits, causing colonic irritation and, of course, dehydration. The most common problem areas include the following:

- Mouth: irritations, dental caries, mouth sores
- Esophagus: irritation of the lower esophageal sphincter from gastric reflux or alcohol
- Stomach: gastritis from alcohol, stress, or overtraining
- Small intestine: malabsorption from celiac disease or Crohn's disease or other inflammation (often from alcohol)
- Large intestine: Crohn's disease irritation, with possible bowel obstruction associated with a fluid and electrolyte imbalance

Diseases of the Mouth   Any condition that affects the mouth can have an impact on food intake. Dental caries, cold sores, sensitive gums, and swollen tongues all have the potential of limiting food intake and, therefore, restricting nutrient and fuel exposure to needy tissues. Regular visits to a dentist will resolve the majority of these problems. However, a B-vitamin deficiency (particularly deficiencies of vitamins B_2 and B_6) may also lead to mouth and tongue problems that inhibit food intakes.

Celiac Disease   Celiac disease is an intestinal intolerance of the protein gluten (found in wheat, barley, rye, and oats). It is associated with dermatitis herpetiformis, which occurs in 70 to 80 percent of people with gluten-induced GI tract damage.[1] Celiac disease has a strong genetic association, so relatives of someone who has celiac disease may also develop the condition.[2] Uncontrolled celiac disease results in intestinal damage, with associated malabsorption, and causes diarrhea, steatorrhea (fat malabsorption), iron-deficiency anemia, other vitamin deficiencies, and eventually weight loss.[3] It may be asymptomatic for years before these symptoms occur, or some signs, such as milk intolerance or iron deficiency, may be present without any of the other signs. Recent studies suggest that celiac disease is underdiagnosed around the world, with incidence rates much higher than previously thought. In people diagnosed with iron-deficiency anemia, for instance, 10 to 15 percent have celiac disease.[4]

Individuals with malabsorption, frequent diarrhea, iron deficiency, or any of the other symptoms of GI dysfunction associated with celiac disease should consider the possibility that they do not tolerate gluten. It is quite possible that at least a proportion of those who report feeling so much better on the Atkins diet (a high-protein, low-carbohydrate diet that restricts bread intake) improve because of the elimination of gluten rather than any of the other purported benefits of the Atkins regimen. For those wishing a firm diagnosis of celiac disease, clinically accepted tests are available, often involving a small bowel biopsy, to confirm the presence of the disease. Patients with celiac disease who remove gluten-containing products from the diet are initially distressed at having this limitation in food consumption, but the improvement in bowel function with gluten restriction often allows them to comfortably consume other foods that may previously have caused GI distress. Virtually all celiac patients feel so much better with the restriction of gluten-containing products that they are self-motivated to continue with a gluten-free diet.[5] In addition, numerous gluten-free bread products on the market, typically made of rice or corn, are excellent substitutes for wheat and rye breads. See table 8.3 for a list of common foods that are high in gluten and foods that have no gluten. There are numerous online resources on gluten-free foods and recipes for readers who wish additional information.

Table 8.3   Sample of Gluten-Containing and Gluten-Free Foods

Gluten-containing	Gluten-free
• Wheat (wholemeal, whole wheat, and wheatmeal flour; wheat bran) • Barley • Rye (rye flour) • All foods made from wheat, rye, semolina, and barley, including barley-based drinks, malted drinks, and beer; pasta, noodles, pastry, pies, wafers, and cakes unless they specifically indicate they are gluten-free • Sauces and soups that contain wheat and, therefore, gluten • Oat cereals that contain wheat • Breaded food products, such as fried chicken	• Arrowroot • Buckwheat • Corn and maize • Potato flour • Rice, rice bran, rice flour • Tapioca • Soya, soya bran, soya flour, soya products • Eggs, milk, cream, butter, cheese, curd cheese • Tea, coffee • Cocoa • Most alcoholic drinks • All fruits and vegetables • Beans (except certain brands of baked beans and beans with a gluten-containing sauce) • Jam, marmalade • Sugar, honey • Salt, pepper, vinegar, herbs, and spices

Note: Wheat products are often used as fillers or thickeners in foods that the consumer may not realize have been processed. The habitual reading of labels is an important means of eliminating foods that contain wheat, barley, and rye (or their derivatives) to be certain of consuming a gluten-free diet.

Reprinted from "Drugs that may result in the loss of appetite or an altered taste perception," Mahan et al., *Krause's Food, Nutrition and Diet Therapy*, p. 401, © 2000, with permission from Elsevier.

Crohn's Disease   Crohn's disease is a regional inflammation of the ileum but may affect the entire small or large intestine. It is associated with abdominal pain and frequent diarrhea, with bowel obstruction a serious problem for the Crohn's patient.[6] This form of irritable bowel syndrome (IBD) causes a thickening of the intestinal wall that reduces the internal transit diameter of the affected portion of the intestines. This reduced interior intestinal diameter is responsible for the bowel obstruction. Crohn's disease equally affects men and women and appears to run in families, although about only 20 percent of Crohn's patients have a relative with the disease. The disease has no known cause, but it is theorized that an immune system reaction against a bacteria or virus causes the inflammation. It appears clear that, unlike some intestinal disorders, Crohn's disease is not related to stress.

For an athlete, Crohn's can have a debilitating effect on the capability to absorb sufficient nutrients, and the associated diarrhea affects fluid and electrolyte balance. The ileum (the main intestinal area affected by Crohn's disease) is the site of vitamin B_{12} absorption. A failed absorption of vitamin B_{12} will eventually lead to megaloblastic, hypochromic anemia, which negatively affects oxygen-carrying capacity.

Athletes who have been diagnosed with Crohn's disease are most commonly treated with an anti-inflammatory drug (commonly containing mesalamine; sulfasalazine is the most common of these drugs), along with treatments that aim to correct the nutrition deficiencies and relieve the pain and diarrhea.[7] Treatment with fluids and electrolytes is common for patients who are suffering from frequent diarrhea. Some drugs also reduce the immune response so as to reduce the cause of the inflammation. An irritated GI tract may require that no solid foods be consumed to allow for a reduction in the inflammation and to reduce the chance for a bowel obstruction. Liquid full-nourishment meals are often consumed during these periods. No foods appear to universally increase the GI inflammation of Crohn's disease, but doctors often ask patients to limit the intake of foods that are not well tolerated in large portions of the population or foods that are known irritants (e.g., milk, alcohol, spicy foods).[8] In the presence of a vitamin B_{12} deficiency, consumption of oral supplements or foods high in vitamin B_{12} (foods of animal origin) does not resolve the deficiency because, regardless of the amount consumed, the absorption of vitamin B_{12} is sufficiently corrupted that it will not enter the blood. Periodic injections of vitamin B_{12}, which bypass the GI tract, are typically needed to correct the vitamin B_{12} deficiency.

Drugs   Certain drugs may also have an impact on the digestion and absorption of nutrients. Antibiotics destroy the intestinal microflora (bacteria) that assist in digestive and absorptive processes and that are even involved in creating certain nutrients, such as vitamin B_{12}. The commonly prescribed antibiotic neomycin, for instance, causes a malabsorption of fat, protein, sodium, potassium, and calcium.[9] Because of the competitive absorption of divalent minerals (calcium, iron, magnesium, and zinc), a high intake of calcium-containing antacids could, for instance, take up most of the absorption site and interfere with the absorption of the other minerals.[10] Nonsteroidal anti-inflammatory drugs (NSAIDs) that are commonly taken by athletes to resolve the bumps, bruises, aches, and pains of athletic endeavors may create a GI irritation that results in blood loss and an iron-deficiency anemia.[11] These are but a few examples of how drugs can result in an altered fuel intake and utilization. Athletes should be fully aware that virtually every drug taken, including over-the-counter drugs, is likely to have a digestive, absorptive, or metabolic impact that could be a detriment to performance. Athletes should therefore consult with an appropriate health care professional rather that pursue self-diagnosis and self-prescription.

Factors Influencing Energy Metabolism

Nutrients that are consumed, digested, and absorbed must still be delivered to the correct tissues for metabolic purposes. A number of factors may inhibit the normal metabolism of nutrients, including nutrient–nutrient interactions, drug–nutrient interactions, and excess alcohol consumption. Of these, regular alcohol consumption is likely to present the greatest difficulties for athletes.

Alcohol Although alcohol is a nutrient that provides 7 calories per gram, it must also be considered an antinutrient because of the way it inhibits the normal metabolism of vitamins and, therefore, the main energy substrates (carbohydrate, protein, and fat) if consumed in excess. Most important, alcohol should not be mistaken for an essential nutrient, which it is not. It is a toxic substance that humans have a limited capacity to detoxify, and in the process, alcohol leaves other toxic substances in its wake.

A regular high intake of alcohol increases disease risk, including cancers of the liver, mouth, throat, and esophagus (these latter three cancers are even more likely if combined with smoking) as well as cirrhosis of the liver (a condition where increasing portions of the liver become fibrotic and are no longer able to function). In addition, alcohol can be an irritant to all segments of the GI tract and, as a result, can cause the malabsorption of nutrients. To make matters worse, alcohol increases the urinary excretion of calcium and magnesium. Magnesium is a cofactor in enzymes transferring phosphate groups, so it is a needed ingredient in energy metabolism. Regular alcohol intake lowers the resorption of magnesium (increasing urinary losses) and also increases magnesium excretion in sweat. The result is an increase in muscle cramps, weakness, and cardiac arrhythmias. Athletes can ill afford creating the magnesium deficiency associated with regular alcohol consumption.[12]

Because liver function is impaired, alcohol may also interfere with the normal metabolism and storage of nutrients. Taken together, alcohol increases nutrient requirements so as to repair the damage it creates and to counteract the malabsorption it produces. Chronic alcohol abuse may weaken the heart; alter brain and nerve function; increase blood lipids (particularly triglycerides); result in a fatty, cirrhotic liver that malfunctions; and cause pancreatitis (which can have a major impact on blood glucose control and digestive processes.) Besides the increased risk of athletic injury induced by alcohol consumption, there is also evidence that more than one drink per day can have a clear impact on performance by negatively affecting reaction time, coordination, and energy metabolism.[13]

Alcohol dehydrogenase, a liver enzyme, is made by the liver to dehydrogenate the active form of vitamin A (retinol, an alcohol). However, with alcohol (ethanol) consumption, the limited production of alcohol dehydrogenase is shunted to dehydrogenate ethanol, thereby leaving the potentially toxic form of vitamin A in the alcohol form. The result is an adverse interaction between alcohol and vitamin A that can result in liver toxicity and increased cancer risk.[14]

The risk of alcohol-related health effects is real in athletes. Although elite athletes consume alcohol half as often as age-equivalent nonathletes, many athletes (particularly those in team sports) still consume far more alcohol than would support good health, good nutrition, and optimal athletic performance.[15] However, non-elite, adolescent athlete groups are more likely to engage in problem drinking than their nonathlete counterparts.[16] Male athletes appear more likely than female athletes to consume alcohol daily.[17] See table 8.4 for a list of the major effects of alcohol on athletic performance.

Nutrients   Nutrient intake and availability has a clear impact on energy metabolism (see figure 8.1). Even a single low nutrient from this list will corrupt the normal metabolic pathways for energy utilization and therefore affect athletic performance. Given the potential hazards of inadequate intake, maldigestion, malabsorption, and altered metabolic processes from drug or alcohol ingestion, it is a credit to the human system that most people are able to supply nutrients to the tissues that need them at the time they're required. However, any chronic insult from poor intake, heavy alcohol abuse, or untreated illness will eventually have a negative impact on performance, a fact that athletes and their coaches should constantly bear in mind.

Table 8.4   Summary of the Effects of Alcohol on Human Performance

Effect	Consequence
1. Increased risk of hypoglycemia	In prolonged exercise, hypoglycemia is more likely because alcohol suppresses liver gluconeogenesis
2. Increased heat loss	Hypoglycemia results in impairment of temperature regulation, particularly in cold environments
3. Reduced performance in middle- and long-distance running	As alcohol intake increases, performance deficits are seen in middle- and long-distance events
4. Reduced vertical jump height	A 6% reduction in vertical jump height and a 10% reduction in 80 m sprint performance
5. Adverse effect on concentration	Central nervous system effect
6. Adverse effect on visual perception	Central nervous system effect
7. Adverse effect on reaction time	Central nervous system effect
8. Adverse effect on coordination	Central nervous system effect
9. Increased risk of dehydration	Alcohol has a diuretic effect
10. Poor postexercise glycogen recovery	Alcohol impairs carbohydrate status of the liver and may also impair muscle glycogen storage
11. Poor postexercise recovery	Alcohol impairs the repair of injured tissues

Reprinted, by permission, from L.M. Burke and R.J. Maughan, 2000, Alcohol in sport. In *Nutrition in sport*, edited by R.J. Maughan (London, England: Blackwell Science), 405-414.

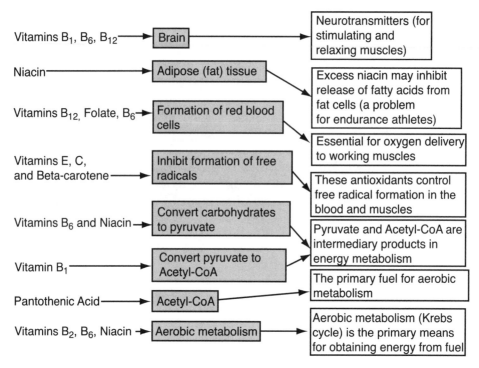

Figure 8.1 Vitamins related to energy metabolism.

Physical activity increases the need for fuel and for the metabolic processes that are involved in its utilization. Anything that either limits the provision of adequate calories to support the cellular requirement or alters the cells' capacity to properly metabolize the provided fuel will have a negative impact on performance. Some factors are within athletes' control, including adequate food consumption, careful consumption of drugs and supplements, and avoidance of regular alcohol consumption; other factors are not within athletes' control, including disease states that may alter food intake or food absorption. This book is filled with information on how to best provide the fuels needed for successfully pursuing athletic endeavors. For those conditions that are not within the direct control of the athlete (e.g., celiac and Crohn's disease and other GI tract disorders), an increasing number of medical solutions are available; athletes should not hesitate to seek medical advice that can ameliorate the impact these conditions have on health and performance. Ultimately, if the fuel doesn't make it to a cell that has the capacity to burn it, athletic endeavors cannot be successfully pursued.

Part III

Factors Affecting Nutritional Needs

9 Travel

Whether traveling for pleasure or competition, serious athletes should try to maintain a regular training and eating regimen. Regardless of where in the world athletes find themselves, it is important for them to follow certain key principles that will help them adapt more quickly to their new environments, reduce the nutrition stresses associated with eating in a nonfamiliar setting, and adjust their circadian rhythms to the local time zone. Only a few scientific studies have addressed this issue, but there are many well-tested practical strategies that athletes can follow to avoid the performance problems associated with jet lag, food intolerance, consumption of unsafe diarrhea-causing foods, and dehydration. This chapter focuses on useful strategies for reducing the potentially negative impact of travel on performance.

Serious athletes inevitably find themselves competing away from home, often in locations with unfamiliar foods. Regardless of how far away athletes travel, planning ahead is essential to ensure final performance matches trained capabilities. Sadly, few athletes and their coaches take the necessary steps to minimize the negative physical and psychological impact of traveling long distances. Perhaps it is because many athletes and coaches believe that home advantage consists of nonmodifiable factors, and the impact of travel is relatively unimportant compared with site familiarity and officials' bias.[1] Others believe, however, that part of the home court advantage includes the impact of travel, particularly if the team or individual athletes must cross multiple time zones without sufficient time to adapt.[2]

Creating a plan that ensures the availability of the right kinds of foods and fluids at the right time is critical when competing at home, and it is no less critical when competing away from home. Perhaps the biggest mistake athletes can make when traveling to a competition is to assume that what they need to eat

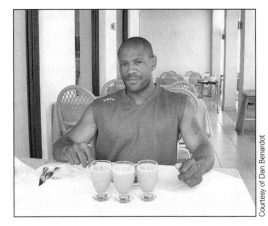

For Olympic athletes like Maurice Green who travel to different countries for competition, keeping consistency in their diet is key to a good performance.

and drink will be there waiting for them. No such assumption should be made. If an athlete doesn't take care of his or her own training and eating plan, no one else will either. Of course, an inadequate knowledge of nutrition makes it impossible for athletes to make the correct dietary choices, particularly if presented with new foods in a new environment. There is no single perfect food that will guarantee an optimal athletic performance, but athletes must know the basic elements of the best foods and fluids to consume.

Both food and adaptation are important considerations. It takes time for an athlete's circadian rhythms to adapt to a new location, so adequate time at the new location is required for these adaptive changes to take place. The desynchronisation of an athlete's normal rhythms results in malaise, loss of appetite, fatigue, and disturbed sleep, all of which can affect performance.[3] The severity of these effects depends, to a large degree, on the number of time zones crossed, the direction of the flight, the age of the athlete, and the steps taken by the athlete before travel to minimize the disruption in normal rhythm.[1, 4] Even a relatively brief air travel that crosses only two time zones can negatively affect team performance.[5] This clearly suggests that, when possible, athletes should arrive at the competition early enough for their circadian rhythms to return to normal before the competition begins.[6] Each athlete has a different capacity to adapt to a new location. Therefore, to the greatest degree possible, the adaptive strategy should be individualized.[7] Studies assessing the impact of jet lag on members of the U.S. women's soccer team traveling to Taiwan, North American students traveling to Western Europe, and European students traveling to North America found that mood state, anaerobic power and capacity, and dynamic strength were all negatively affected. It took 3 or 4 days to eliminate the impact of travel on these performance measures.[8]

Some athletes consider massage or chiropractic adjustment a critical component of a speedy adaptation. However, there is limited evidence that this approach is truly useful. One study of Finnish junior elite athletes investigated whether the impact of jet lag could be reduced with chiropractic adjustment after a trip. Looking at sleep patterns and mood score (via the Profile of Mood States instrument), it was found that the chiropractic care had no impact on the effects of jet lag.[9]

Acclimatization is particularly important for athletes traveling to locations that are hotter and more humid than where training normally occurs. Physiological adjustments to heat take 7 to 14 days, and without adequate heat adaptation, performance will clearly be affected.[1] Planning ahead to ensure optimal access to the right foods and fluids and to allow for sufficient adaptation time is the key to success.

Travel must also be considered a time of increased disease risk. The traveling athlete may be exposed to unfamiliar pathogens (i.e., those for which the body has yet to develop protective systems); and the lack of sleep, increased mental stress, and increased fatigue associated with travel may increase the chance of infection. Strategizing for how to rest and eat properly before, during, and immediately after a trip is a critical component of staying healthy and reducing the risk that a disease state compromises athletic performance.[10] Maintaining personal hygiene and washing the hands frequently can reduce the risk of infection—these habits should become a regular component of the traveling athlete's strategy for keeping healthy.[11]

General Guidelines for Eating on the Road

Most guidelines require advance planning. Just as an athlete must pack his or her uniform, he or she should also give thought to where, when, and how the right foods and beverages can be obtained to satisfy needs. The worst thing that can happen to an athlete while traveling is to become hungry or thirsty and not have anything quickly available to eat or drink. Make sure this doesn't happen by trying to follow these general tips for eating on the road:[12]

- Bring your own snacks. Fresh fruits, fruit juices, crackers, low-fat rice and pasta salads, and low-fat energy bars are nutritious and easy to carry (see table 9.1).
- Watch out for hidden fats. Creamy soups, bread-type flaky pastries, mayonnaise-based salad dressings, and sauces in sandwiches add unnecessary fat to food. However, good alternatives are available. Consuming clear, broth-based soups instead of creamy soups may provide all the nutrients but with considerably less fat. Using lemon juice–based salad dressing rather than mayonnaise-type dressing lowers the fat and makes it possible to eat more salad.
- Consume grilled, baked, boiled, and broiled foods rather than fried or sauteed foods. You must ask for it the way you want it. Make no assumptions about how food will be prepared by the way it is described on the menu. When possible, request lower-fat dairy products and lower-fat salad dressings.
- Order "a la carte" to get exactly what you want. Full dinners often don't fit the way a serious athlete should be eating. For instance, the grilled fish may be exactly what you want, but the full dinner may come with mashed potatoes

Table 9.1   Good Snacks for Athletes to Take With Them When Traveling

Food	Approximate energy substrate distribution[1]		
	% carbohydrate	% protein	% fat
Bagel	76	14	10
Breadsticks	76	13	11
Breakfast cereal, unsweetened (such as Cheerios)	70	15	15
Cheese[2]	7	37	56
Cookies (such as oatmeal)	65	4	31
Crackers (such as saltines or graham crackers)	66	8	26
Cut-up vegetables (such as carrots and celery)	94	4	2
Dried fruit (such as apricots)	93	6	11
Energy bar, breakfast bar, granola bar	91	4	5
Fresh fruit (such as apples, oranges, and grapes)	75	10	15
Fruit juice (such as apple, grape, and orange)	99	0	1
Pretzels	78	10	12
Sports beverages	100	0	0
Trail mix (including nuts, dried fruit, and M&Ms)	43	11	46
Yogurt with fruit[2]	75	17	8

[1]Energy substrate distribution varies with brand name and type
[2]May require refrigeration

that are soaked in gravy, broccoli that is covered with cheese sauce, and a piece of apple pie with ice cream. The serious athlete would be better off with broiled fish, a plain baked potato, broccoli with lemon juice, and fresh fruit for dessert.

- If you travel by air, tell the travel agent you'd like to eat vegetarian. There's a greater chance you'll receive foods that are higher in carbohydrates and lower in fat. However, you need to give the airlines fair warning of your special dietary requirements, so make certain the airlines are notified at least 24 hours in advance of the flight.

- If you travel by air, bring something to drink on the plane with you. There may be a significant delay between the time you take off and when you receive your first drink. Air travel is one of the most dehydrating experiences a person can have. Because of this, passengers often contract sore throats and other upper respiratory illnesses. As a preventative measure, keep sipping on fluids during the flight to keep your mouth and throat moist. Drink bottled water or sports beverages.

• If you're changing time zones, get on the local schedule as soon as possible. Have dinner when the local population is eating rather than at the time you eat at home. You'll still have difficulty getting your eating pattern on track because traveling and changing time zones are tiring and disorienting. To make certain you're completely ready to compete, try to arrive at the competition site early.

Minimizing Jet Lag

Leaving enough time to adjust to long-distance travel is important. Even the most seasoned travelers suffer from jet lag, and most of them don't have to run, jump, hit, kick, flip, or swim when they reach their destinations. Jet lag can impart a feeling of illness, will lower appetite, and can disturb normal sleep.[13] Jet lag comes in two forms: (1) travel involving small but consecutive trips, causing multiple small shifts in usual eating patterns; and (2) travel involving one large trip that crosses multiple time zones, causing a major change in eating and sleeping behaviors. Athletes should never delay eating when the sensation of hunger occurs, so snacks should always be quickly available to fill the gap in time until a regular meal can be obtained. The following recommendations may help alleviate the effects of jet lag:[3]

1. For small, consecutive time-zone changes (called phase shifts):

    • Eat meals at regular times after arriving at the new destination. This will help you get on the local schedule quickly and aid your adjustment to the new time zone.

    • Drink plenty of liquids. Plane cabins are notoriously dry, and dehydration is the cause of many complaints, including headaches and mild constipation.

    • Alternate light meals with heavy meals before the flights. The stress of travel may increase protein requirements slightly, so eat a high-protein breakfast and a low-protein, high-carbohydrate dinner after the phase shift.

    • Avoid caffeine until the end of the flight. Caffeine is a diuretic that can increase water loss in an environment that is already dehydrating. Consume fluids that will help you maintain hydration state (water, sports beverages, fruit juices).

    • Avoid alcohol during and after the flight. Besides the negative metabolic alterations that alcohol causes, it is also a diuretic that can increase water loss. There is *no* reason why serious athletes should drink alcoholic beverages at any time.

- Engage in social activity or exercise after the flight. This will help you get on the local schedule more quickly and will aid in reducing the stress associated with travel.

2. For a large phase shift:

- Arrive at your destination at least 1 day early for each time zone crossed. For flights crossing more than six time zones, a minimum of 4 days and preferably 1 week should be allowed to return to a normal circadian rhythm and a feeling of well-being. Cost and scheduling limitations may keep athletes from arriving as early as needed, so getting on the local schedule as quickly as possible, but with as much rest as possible, is important.

- Exercise and get involved in social activities on your arrival in the new location. It helps to become familiar with your new environment right away. The exercise and social activities will reduce the stress of travel and will help you get on the local schedule more easily.

- Maintain regular sleeping and eating times on arrival to your new destination. The sooner you can eat and sleep on the schedule of your new destination, the more quickly your body will feel as if it can perform well. Eating and sleeping regularly and on schedule are keys to doing well when you travel.

- Continue to eat and drink frequently before, during, and after travel. Creating a snacking schedule at your new location may be difficult because you may not know where to buy good high-carbohydrate snacks. However, maintaining a frequent eating and drinking schedule (eating something about every 3 hours) is an important strategy for helping you adjust to your new environment. Bring some snacks with you to get started, and then find a good source of snacks once you arrive. However, always avoid alcohol.

- Have more protein than usual. The stress associated with travel may slightly increase your protein requirement, so make a conscious effort to consume a little more protein each day. For instance, consuming a higher-protein breakfast (add a boiled egg to your normal intake) could be useful in ensuring that your protein requirement is met. However, the focus of your intake should continue to be carbohydrates.

Travel Location

When traveling to most places in the United States, Canada, and Western Europe, there's a high likelihood familiar foods will be available. Breakfast cereals, for instance, can be found in virtually every grocery store, and there is bread everywhere you go. The preparation of many of the foods is different, however. If you're accustomed to having a cup of coffee in the morning, you may be surprised (perhaps even shocked!) at the variety of ways different cultures treat the coffee bean.

All this information indicates that athletes should do whatever they can to sustain dietary and sleep habits because it is impossible to know what the outcome will be if there is a sudden change in usual lifestyle practices and procedures. A particularly useful gadget to have with you is an in-cup electric water heater that has the appropriate power adapters for the country. These little heaters allow consumption of familiar soups, and athletes can brew familiar-tasting coffee. For a traveling athlete, this is one of the best inventions ever.

Some countries have reputations for unsafe water or food supplies. If there is any doubt whatsoever about the safety of the food or water supply, call your nearest consular office or your travel agency. Employees should be able to provide you with the information you need. Pick up a good travel book for the location you're heading to. A good book will describe the foods that will be available and will tell you about the water supply.

When traveling abroad, take the following items with you even if you think the food and water supply is safe and familiar (you can adjust the quantities depending on your length of stay):

- Power-cord adapters and converters to fit the power supply of the country you're traveling to
- An in-cup electric heater
- A water-filter pump
- A box of saltine crackers
- Powdered sports beverage packets to make 20 quarts of beverage
- Two quarts of bottled water
- A medium-size box of raisins (or other favored dried fruit)
- Five individually packaged low-fat granola bars
- Two nonfat powdered milk packets
- One small box of your favorite cereal

Dealing With the Water Supply   It doesn't matter where the travel destination is, athletes will, for one reason or another, need water. Different water supplies can cause gastrointestinal (GI) difficulties, even if the water supply is perfectly safe. Different levels of bromide or fluoride in the water may, for instance, cause severe gut pain. Of course, drinking bottled water or bottled sports drinks is a good solution if these are available. However, if bottled drinks are not easily available, you need a way to deal with the situation. It is virtually impossible to travel with a significant number of bottled drinks, but athletes should travel with powdered packages of sports beverages and a water filter to purify the water. The best water filters are those capable of removing microscopic parasites and bacteria—check your local camping goods store. These water filters are also at the top of the list of excellent inventions for the traveling athlete. They don't take up much space and work extremely efficiently, giving you the peace of mind you need so you can deal with other more pressing matters.

Eating Locations   Travel inevitably keeps athletes from eating when and where they'd like, so plan ahead for what you might select before you enter an eating establishment. Seeing the dizzying array of foods and menu items can easily influence your order if you're not already committed to your selection. Airports are filled with fast-food restaurants that typically offer high-fat and high-sugar foods. These are not easy places to make the right selections. In general, athletes should stick with foods that aren't fried. However, if you don't have a choice, minimize the fried (fatty) food and maximize the carbohydrate. For instance, instead of a double-patty hamburger, it would be better to order two regular hamburgers because you get twice the bread (carbohydrate).

Try to find pasta, baked potatoes, bread, vegetables, and salads in restaurants. It might be necessary to request a substitution (e.g., a baked potato instead of French fries), but don't be afraid to ask. Restaurants in airports or ports may be less likely to want to satisfy your special needs because they know they'll probably never see you (or your business) again. Nevertheless, it's important that athletes always ask for exactly what they want. Even when ordering baked potatoes, ask for everything on the side rather than on the potato. See table 9.2 for key words to look for when viewing a menu.

Table 9.2   Selecting Items Through a Careful Review of the Menu

Cuisine	Foods to avoid	Foods to seek
General	Fried, crispy, breaded, scampi-style, creamed, buttery, au gratin, gravy	Marinara, steamed, boiled, broiled, tomato sauce, in its own juice, poached, charbroiled
Mexican	Deep-fried shells, fried flour tortillas, refried beans, corn chips, sour cream, guacamole	Low-fat refried beans, chicken or lean beef and bean burritos, baked soft corn tortillas, salsa, rice, baked flour tortillas
Italian	Cream sauces, high-fat dressings, rich desserts	Pasta with marinara sauce, cheese or vegetable pizza, salad with dressing on the side, low-fat Italian ice, low-fat frozen yogurt
Chinese	Deep-fried egg rolls, deep-fried wontons, sweet and sour pork, tempura	Stir-fry and steamed dishes, chicken and vegetables with rice, clear broth soups
Burger places	High-fat dressings in salad bars, mayonnaise, french fries, milkshakes	Low-fat dressings in salad bars, baked potatoes, grilled items
Cafes	Prebuttered items, limit coffee intake	Pancakes, toast, bagels, waffles, fruit, fruit juices, whole grain cereals, breads, muffins

Adapted, by permission, from E.R. Burke and J.R. Berning, 1996, *Training nutrition: The diet and nutrition guide for peak performance* (Carmel, IN: I.L. Cooper), 134.

The key to successful travel is advance planning. Make no assumptions about the availability of foods or drinks that will satisfy your needs. Bring some limited items with you when traveling to be certain you have some key foods and drinks that will keep you happy and nourished. Don't try new foods until after the athletic event, and then only on the recommendation of your local hosts. Experimenting on your own can be dangerous. Find out as much as you can about where you're going by visiting a bookstore or library, or do some research on the Internet. Your travel agent and nearby consular office are also excellent sources of information. Give yourself plenty of time to get acclimatized to the location you're traveling to. It takes about 1 day for each time zone you cross, so for a trip from New York to Paris, you should arrive at least 6 days before the event. If that's not possible, do whatever you can to reduce stress by getting plenty of rest, relaxing with friends, and getting on the local schedule as soon as possible.

10 | High Altitude

Doing physical work at high altitude presents enormous challenges, whether a person climbed to get there or was taken there as a member of a search crew. High altitudes are likely to be cold, often to the extreme, and the terrain is sufficiently harsh that the human system is under constant strain to do physical work. Moving quickly from lower to higher altitude (as often occurs when athletes who live at sea level train at high altitude to enhance oxygen-carrying capacity) may result in headache and nausea, both of which can negatively influence food and fluid consumption. The lower oxygen level of high-altitude air makes fatigue come early, and the difficulty of eating and drinking normally may lead to enough tissue loss that cold tolerance is decreased. Maintaining body fluid balance in extreme cold is just as difficult as maintaining fluid balance in hot and humid environments, with increased urinary flow and voluntary dehydration both contributing to the problem of taking in sufficient fluids to avoid dehydration. Simply preventing drinking fluids from freezing presents a challenge, and cooking takes much longer at higher altitudes than at lower altitudes (so more fuel must be transported). The challenges of performing physical work at high altitude are daunting, but nutrition strategies can help people attain their goals in this environment, whether it's a 3-day 14,400-foot (4,390 meter) climb up Mount Rainier or a week-long trek up the 19,340-foot (5,890 meter) Mount Kilimanjaro. This chapter reviews the physiological and nutritional stresses the human body experiences when working in the often cold setting of a high altitude and presents recommendations for successfully dealing with this environment.

High-Altitude Training

There is less oxygen at higher altitudes, requiring that athletes undergo a degree of adaptation before training regimens and performance can approach sea-level expectations for aerobic (predominantly endurance) activities. Even for anaerobic events, a degree of adaptation is necessary to adjust to the lower oxygen concentration of high altitude so that altitude illness does not impede training. Because the concentration of oxygen is lower at progressively higher altitudes, a stepwise progression to higher and higher altitudes makes sense to allow for an efficient and illness-free adaptive response.

Athletes training at higher altitudes can expect a faster respiration and faster heart rate, which are adaptations to the lower oxygen being pulled into the lungs with each breath. Only a greater red blood cell concentration will mediate this physiological response, an adaptation that may take days, weeks, or months before a more normal breathing rate and heart rate occur. It should be remembered that several nutrition factors are associated with successful production of red blood cells, including adequate caloric intake, sufficient iron to increase the red blood cell concentration, folic acid, and vitamin B_{12}. A healthy diet may satisfy most of these requirements, but care should be taken that iron in particular be consumed at the level of ~18 milligrams per day. This may be more difficult than it

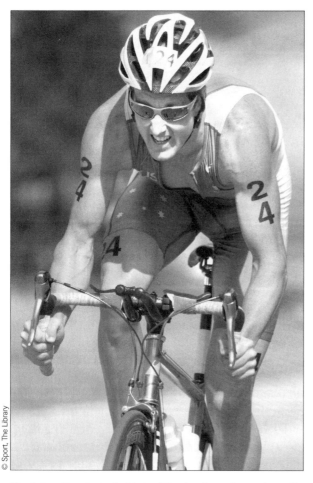

Cyclists often train in high altitudes in order to benefit from the adaptation to lower oxygen levels.

© Sport, The Library

Table 10.1   Common Definitions Regarding Altitude

High altitude	1,500 to 2,500 m (5,000 to 8,200 ft)
Very high altitude	2,500 to 5,500 m (8,200 to 18,000 ft)
Extreme altitude	Above 5,500 m (above 18,000 ft)

seems because athletes often complain of a loss of appetite at high altitude. Table 10.1 defines what should be considered high altitude.

Cold environments cause heat loss through both convection and conduction, although humans do have systems that help maintain core body temperature and increase heat production.[1] This process of thermoregulation helps ensure survivability when exposed to cold temperatures. With cold exposure, the body attempts to lower the amount of heat loss through peripheral vasoconstriction. However, the reduced blood flow to the skin and extremities predisposes individuals to frostbite, particularly of the fingers and toes. To counteract this risk, the body initiates a process referred to as cold-induced vasodilation (CIVD) after approximately 10 minutes of cold exposure. The pulsing of peripheral vasoconstriction and vasodilation results in the preservation of core temperature, but at the cost of fluctuating temperatures of the skin and peripheral tissues.[1]

Humans mainly produce heat when muscles work. Of the calories used by working muscles, approximately 30 to 40 percent actually results in muscular movement, while 60 to 70 percent is lost as heat. Put simply, as warm-blooded animals we are more efficient at creating heat than creating movement. We can also produce heat by shivering, which is an involuntary central nervous system–induced mechanism that is invoked by a 3 to 4 degree drop in body temperature.[2, 3] The increase in muscle contraction from shivering results in a 2.5-fold increase in total energy expenditure, most of which is the result of increased carbohydrate oxidation.[4] Cold stress also increases muscle glycogen utilization as a result of increased plasma catecholamines.[5]

Therefore, consumption of sufficient amounts of carbohydrate is important when exercising in an environment where cold stress and shivering occur.[6] Older individuals who have experienced some degree of muscle loss fare less well in cold environments, mainly because their lower level of muscle mass reduces their capacity to produce heat, whether from work or shivering.[7] However, older age would not automatically increase hypothermic risk if a program of regular exercise were instituted to maintain the lean mass.

Cold-weather exposure creates a significant dehydration risk. Soldiers in cold environments commonly lose up to 8 percent of body weight from dehydration.[8] There are several reasons for this dehydration, including difficulty obtaining adequate amounts of potable water, high levels of water loss (particularly if excess clothing is worn or heavy equipment is being carried), respiratory water loss, and cold-induced diuresis (CID).

Working at high altitude, by itself, increases nutrition risks because the work takes place in a reduced-oxygen environment. Many experienced skiers and mountain climbers are aware of the potential for nausea, confusion, and easy fatigue with high-altitude work. It takes time to adapt to this relatively hypoxic environment, mainly by improving the capacity to deliver oxygen to working tissues. High-altitude exposure increases oxidative stress, a fact that may alter nutrient requirements in favor of more antioxidant intake.[9] It is estimated that most humans are 80 percent acclimatized after 10 days at altitude and approximately 95 percent acclimatized by 45 days at altitude.[10] People can expect certain normal changes when going to a higher altitude. These include faster breathing, more shortness of breath than the person is accustomed to, higher urination frequency, and altered sleep patterns. The lower barometric pressure of high altitude lowers the oxygen concentration of every breath, forcing a more frequent breathing pattern in an attempt to pull in the same level of oxygen. However, it is impossible to take in the same level of oxygen at high altitude when compared with sea level, no matter how fast the breathing pattern. For this reason, physical work will always be more difficult, and fatigue will occur more quickly at high altitude. A failure to properly acclimatize to the altitude is commonly referred to as altitude sickness and may result in additional symptoms:[11]

- Headaches
- Anorexia
- Nausea
- Vomiting
- Malaise

Factors that can increase the risk of developing altitude sickness include the following:

- A fast rate of ascent
- A long stay at altitude
- A high level of exertion
- High-fat, high-protein, low-carbohydrate diets
- A higher altitude

A related disorder, acute mountain sickness (AMS), which commonly occurs at altitudes exceeding 6,600 feet (2,000 meters), produces the following symptoms:[12, 13]

- Nausea
- Poor sleep
- Headache
- Lassitude
- Cough
- Dyspnea on exertion and at rest
- Ataxia
- Altered mental status
- Fluid retention (higher antidiuretic hormone production)

An assessment of athletes competing in the Primal Quest Expedition Adventure Race in Colorado found that 4.5 percent had altitude illness at the start of the race; 14.1 percent had altitude illness during the race that required medical treatment (of which 13.3 percent was AMS; .8 percent was pulmonary edema); and 14.3 percent withdrew from the race because of altitude-related illness.[14] This race begins at an altitude higher than 9,500 feet (2,900 meters) and rises to an altitude of more than 13,500 feet (4,100 meters). Illness occurring at high altitude should be treated by descent to a lower altitude and by administering oxygen, if available. Individuals with worsening symptoms should never delay descent because worsening symptoms may evolve to high-altitude cerebral edema (HACE) or high-altitude pulmonary edema (HAPE), both of which are life threatening.[15] Capillary leakage in the brain or lungs is the cause of this edema. Symptoms of HACE, which can progress rapidly and result in death within a matter of a few hours, include the following:[16]

- Gait ataxia (walks like someone intoxicated)
- Confusion
- Psychiatric changes of varying degree
- Disturbances of consciousness that may progress to deep coma

The cause of HAPE (fluid in the lungs) is not well understood, but it rarely occurs at altitudes below 8,000 feet (2,400 meters). A failure to treat HAPE immediately, typically by immediate descent, may result in death. Symptoms of HAPE result from a lower oxygen–carbon dioxide exchange and include the following:[17]

- Extreme fatigue
- Breathlessness at rest
- Cough, possibly with pink sputum
- Gurgling or rattling breaths
- Chest tightness, fullness, or congestion
- Blue or gray lips or fingernails

Obese individuals are more likely to suffer from acute mountain sickness (AMS) than are nonobese individuals.[18] However, people with periodic altitude exposures appear to adapt and reduce the symptoms of AMS.[19] Other strategies, including magnesium supplementation and Ginkgo biloba supplementation, have been tried for reducing AMS, but these have not been found successful.[20, 21]

The combined impact of AMS symptoms is a severe appetite depression with a concomitant reduction in foods and fluids. The high caloric requirements and fluid consumption difficulties of cold weather, combined with the anorexia of high altitude, create the two most serious problems of work at high altitude: maintenance of weight and fluid balance.

Even those who are part of well-organized mountain-climbing expeditions and regularly exposed to high altitude typically fail to consume sufficient calories, which leads to a loss of body weight. An assessment of people taking part in a Himalayan trek found that body weight was significantly reduced by the end of the trek, and energy intake was significantly lower at high altitude than at low altitude.[22] It has been found that food intakes are usually 10 to 50 percent lower at high altitude, depending on the speed of the ascent. This appears to be true even when people are not exposed to severe cold (as in a hypobaric chamber).[23] Only when there is a conscious effort to consume more food, often with forced eating, do individuals at higher altitude have energy intakes that approach physiological needs.[24]

The level of sweat loss in extremely cold environments can equal that of hot and humid environments. It has been estimated that moderate to heavy exercise in typically insulated winter clothing will result in a sweat loss of nearly 2 liters per hour.[25] Therefore, the principle strategy for ensuring adequate hydration is to have enough fluids readily available so they can be consumed frequently and in appropriate quantities. There are real problems, however, in making enough fluids available and ready to drink in cold, high-altitude environments. Fluids can freeze unless there are means of keeping them fluid . . . not an easy task in environments that are often well below freezing temperatures. In addition, fluids are heavy to transport in sufficient quantity to meet needs. One option is to acquire fluids from the local environment by melting and purifying ice and snow, but this option has been found to be extremely costly in heating fuel. It has been estimated that it could take more than 6 hours and a half gallon (2 liters) of gas to melt enough ice and snow to support the fluid needs of a single person.[26]

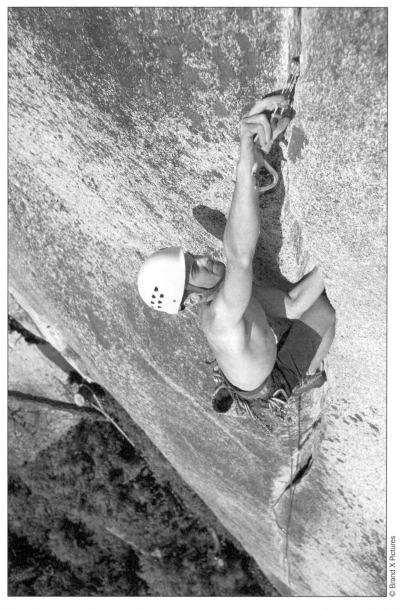

© Brand X Pictures

Because AMS depresses the appetite, mountain climbers need to make sure their level of energy intake is high.

Meeting Energy and Nutrient Needs

Energy expenditures of humans climbing Mount Everest average 2.5 to 3.0 times higher than at sea level.[27] It is easy to understand why weight loss from reduced energy intake is a common outcome of exercise in cold or high-altitude environments.[28] Athletes performing in these environments should make a conscious effort to eat at frequent intervals. They should focus on carbohydrate foods because these foods take less oxygen to metabolize than do fat or protein foods, help replace glycogen stores, and have a protein-sparing effect. In addition, inadequate carbohydrate consumption will eventually result in low blood sugar, which leads to mental confusion and disorientation. Some reports indicate that mountaineers show a preference for carbohydrates and an aversion to fat.[29] However, this finding is not consistent; other studies indicate that athletes at high altitude do not shift their food selections away from high-fat items and toward high-carbohydrate foods.[30] The same report indicates that high-altitude environments blunt the sense of taste, which may contribute to inadequate energy intake. This inadequate energy intake leads to a weight loss (including muscle weight) that negatively affects strength, endurance, and the capacity to produce heat. The goal should therefore be to consume an adequate volume of food to provide sufficient calories rather than place undo importance on the distribution of energy substrates. Athletes should have foods available to them that they know they will eat in large quantities and that make them feel good after they are consumed. To make matters even more difficult, the time to cook a meal doubles for each 5,000-feet (1,500 meter) climb in elevation. Prepackaged, high-carbohydrate snacks and foods are a good alternative for most meals, with cooked meals reserved for those times when athletes have available water and time.

The intake of vitamins and minerals is something better considered before exposure to either cold or high altitude. Iron status in particular should be excellent before attempting a high-altitude trek because oxygen-carrying capacity is stretched to its limit in this environment. Taking iron supplements while on the climb is not likely to be of much benefit because it takes a great deal of time (months) to improve a poor iron status. Oxidative stress may be higher in hot and cold environments, so consumption of foods that contain antioxidants or periodic consumption of a multivitamin and multimineral supplement should be considered.[31] A study of oxidative stress in humans at high altitude found that those receiving an antioxidant mixture had lower breath pentane (a marker of oxidative stress) compared with those receiving single antioxidant supplements. Consuming a variety of antioxidants, such as ascorbic acid, beta-carotene, selenium, and vitamin E (as would be present in a broad-spectrum supplement), is therefore likely a better strategy than focusing on a single antioxidant.[32]

Meeting Fluid Needs

Consuming sufficient fluids in cold and high-altitude environments presents unique challenges, all of which must be overcome to ensure an adequate hydration state.

These factors include providing adequate availability of drinking fluids, avoiding the freezing of drinking fluids, and overcoming voluntary dehydration.

Providing Adequate Availability of Drinking Fluids   Fluids are heavy and not easy to transport in the best of circumstances. In cold weather and treacherous high-altitude terrains, fluid availability becomes an even greater issue. The basic strategy is for each person to ensure an availability of a minimum of 2 liters of fluids and prefer-ably 4 liters of fluids per day. The 2 liters is truly a minimum because hard physical work in a cold, high-altitude environment may result in 2 liters of water loss per hour. The base-camp strategy of moving large amounts of food, water, and other living essentials to the highest possible altitude with the use of helicopters, automobiles, or animal packs is a logical strategy. Climbing to a higher altitude could then proceed from the base camp, with climbers carrying sufficient food and fluid for the amount of time away from the base camp. Using melted snow or ice as the source of fluids is not a reasonable planning option; melting snow and ice at high altitude takes a great deal of time and adds significant weight in fuel, pots, and stoves. In addition, it is possible that the available ice and snow is impure and not fit for consumption. It has been reported that Giardia lamblia, a diarrhea-causing intestinal parasite, is present in high-altitude regions.[29] Of course, in emergency situations any available fluids should be consumed, but the risk of infection is present if purification devices are not used.

Avoiding the Freezing of Drinking Fluids   Climbers should carry drinking fluids close to the body to keep them from freezing and should even consider keeping fluids with them inside their sleeping bags while sleeping. The alternative (frozen fluid) is simply too difficult to deal with. A unique strategy for keeping fluids from freezing is to add glycerol (see chapter 4), which may improve fluid retention, adds calories to fluids, and reduces the freezing point.[33] The last characteristic of glycerol is rarely considered, but for the athlete working in a cold environment, it is extremely important. The added calories are also an important benefit of glycerol because both cold-weather and high-altitude work commonly induce a hypocaloric state.

Overcoming Voluntary Dehydration   When left to their own devices, athletes typically consume less fluid while exercising than is needed to sustain an optimal hydration state. This condition, termed voluntary dehydration, may be an even greater problem when athletes exercise in the cold than when they exercise in the heat. The basis for this remains unclear, but two theories, one physiological and one practical, have been suggested as the possible cause:[34] (1) There is a possibility that cold skin or lower core body temperature modifies the thirst sensation and (2) the voluntary restriction of fluids seems to occur most often late in the day, an act that blunts the necessity for an athlete to leave a warm tent to urinate in a cold and unfriendly environment during the night. The only reasonable solution to avoid voluntary dehydration is for athletes to place themselves on a fixed drinking schedule, whether or not the sensation of thirst exists.[35] Having small sips of fluids at regular intervals also eliminates the need to consume a large volume of fluid at one time, which may stimulate the need to urinate.

11 | Gender and Age

Although this book focuses on the nutrition recommendations that will help athletes achieve at their conditioned best, there are extra considerations for female athletes and subgroups within the athlete population. Female athletes have a unique set of stressors that should be considered to sustain health and optimize performance. The female athlete triad (eating disorder, menstrual dysfunction, and low bone density) should be addressed with a series of strategies that, as much as possible, prevents its development. Child athletes and older athletes are on opposite ends of the developmental scale, a fact that alters nutrition requirements and risks. Children have fewer sweat glands that produce less sweat per gland than adults; children are also susceptible to voluntary dehydration.[1] These factors place them at increased risk of overheating unless established programs are in place where children are involved in sporting activities. Heat illness, impaired growth and development, menstrual dysfunction, eating disorders, and higher injury risk are all potential outcomes of inadequate nutrient and energy intakes in athletes.[2] Older athletes have a different set of concerns, particularly as they relate to increased heat-stress risk, normal changes in body composition, and the rate of recovery from strenuous athletic endeavors.

The Female Athlete

A quick review of the Dietary Reference Intakes (DRIs) demonstrates clearly that females have different nutrient requirements than males. Many of the requirement differences are based on body size (males being larger than females), but some are due to clear physiological differences, as is the case with iron (females require twice as much).

Energy intakes, for all athletes, are based on total weight, weight of the metabolic mass, and duration and intensity of exercise. Surveys of female athletes commonly report an underconsumption of energy, leading many to conclude that female athletes are at elevated risk of developing eating disorders regardless of the type of sport they are participating in.[3] In addition, the literature is filled with reports of the impact that intense exercise has on the female reproductive system, with amenorrhea or oligomenorrhea a common outcome. These reports suggest that increasing caloric intake to offset the high energy demand may be sufficient to reverse the menstrual dysfunction and halt the associated reduction in bone mass.[4] The reduction in bone mass caused by menstrual dysfunction is clinically relevant for female athletes because it places them at current increased risk for stress fractures and later increased risk for osteoporosis. In one study of 46 female athletes (31 with multiple stress fractures and 15 without stress fractures), nearly half of all athletes with stress fractures had menstrual irregularities, with a particularly high prevalence observed in endurance runners with high weekly training mileage.[5] Although consuming sufficient calories and calcium will not correct the biomechanical factors associated with stress fractures, including a high longitudinal foot arch and leg-length inequality, it will substantially reduce risk if this strategy helps females return to normal menstrual function.[6] (See table 11.1 for stress fracture risks.)

The energy substrate distribution is of interest to female athletes. Studies indicate that females have a higher lipid, lower glycogen (carbohydrate), and lower protein utilization than do male athletes in endurance exercise.[7] Because glycogen storage is limited, the lower rate of glycogen utilization gives female athletes what appears to be a clear advantage over men in long-duration, lower-intensity athletic events.[8] This also gives rise to the following question: Should female endurance athletes have a different energy substrate consumption pattern than male endurance athletes given the difference in the pattern of substrate utilization? No solid evidence indicates that there should be a difference in intake, and the nature of endurance and ultraendurance events still makes carbohydrate storage (glycogen) the limiting substrate in performance. Whether an endurance athlete is male or female, when glycogen is depleted the athletic performance will drop (or stop). A series of studies assessing the carbohydrate consumption pattern of female athletes involved in different sports indicated a wide range of intakes (see table 11.2). Few of the assessed female athlete groups meet the recommended carbohydrate intake of 5 to 7 grams per kilogram per day for general training and 7 to 10 grams per kilogram per day for endurance athletes.[9]

The general (nonathlete) recommendation for protein consumption in adults is .8 grams per kilogram per day. The athlete recommendation is approximately double

Table 11.1   Risks for Developing Stress Fractures

Risk factor	Nutritionally related (yes/no/possibly)
Genetics	Possibly (if related to food allergies or intolerances)
Female gender	No
White ethnicity	No
Low body weight	Possibly (if not related to genetic predisposition)
Lack of weight-bearing exercise	No
Intrinsic and extrinsic mechanical factors	No
Amenorrhea	Yes
Oligomenorrhea	Yes
Inadequate calcium intake	Yes
Inadequate caloric intake	Yes
Disordered eating	Yes

Reprinted, by permission, from A. Nattiv and T.D. Armsey Jr., 1997, "Stress injury to bone in the female athlete," *Clin Sports Med.* 16(2): 197-224.

Table 11.2   Carbohydrate Consumption Patterns in Female Athletes

Study	Amount CHO (g/kg/day)	Sport
Gabel et al., 1995[a]	18	Ultraendurance cycling (14 to 16 hours per day)
Peters & Goetzsche, 1997[b]	4	Ultraendurance
Steen et al., 1995[c]	4.9	Heavyweight collegiate rowing
Walberg-Rankin, 1995[d]	3.2 to 5.4	Anaerobic sports (gymnastics, bodybuilding)
Walberg-Rankin, 1995[e]	4.4 to 6.2	Aerobic sports (running, cycling, triathlon)

this and ranges between 1.2 and 1.8 grams per kilogram per day, depending on the degree to which the athlete is involved in endurance activity.[10] This recommended level is likely to be greater than actual needs, provided adequate total energy consumption is obtained. It should be noted that no specific protein requirement data are available for female athletes, so these values are derived from mixed-athlete or male studies. Until female-specific protein requirement data are determined, female athletes should try to consume a protein level within the currently established range.

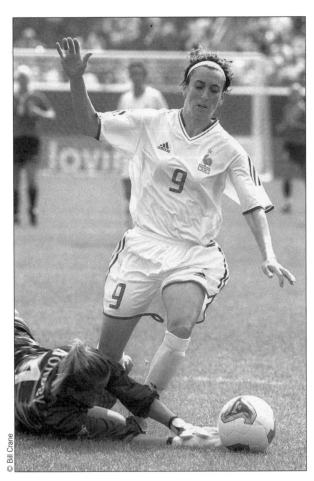

© Bill Crane

Female athletes must consciously and accurately monitor their fat, calcium, and iron intakes, assuring adequate consumption on a day-to-day basis.

Fat consumption is targeted by female athletes wishing to lower body weight, as indicated in a study showing amenorrheic athletes have a fat intake that is 6 percent lower than eumenorrheic athletes.[11] To obtain a sufficient energy intake, fat consumption should not be eliminated from the diet. Given the high energy needs of athletes, plus the fact that female athletes have an excellent system for catabolizing fat for energy, fat intakes should range in the area of 20 to 25 percent of total energy intake.

Female athletes appear to have less than adequate vitamin B_6 intake, assessed either in absolute values or in ratio to protein consumption.[12, 13] With the exception of this vitamin, female athletes who are not on energy-restrictive food intakes appear to obtain adequate vitamins to sustain health and physical activity.

There is no question that calcium and iron intakes are of concern in the diets of female athletes. Adequate calcium consumption is necessary to develop and maintain high-density bones that are resistant to fracture, and iron is necessary for oxygen delivery to working cells. For athletes concerned about dairy product consumption, calcium-fortified orange juice is an excellent alternative and, per equal volume, has the same calcium concentration as fluid milk. It should be understood that calcium intake, by itself, does not guarantee good bones. Although calcium, vitamin D, estrogen, and physical stress are all needed for bone development, ensuring an adequate calcium intake is within easy reach of every athlete.

Surveys have found low storage iron (ferritin) in female runners and other studies have found that female athletes with anemia can improve aerobic performance through a program of iron supplementation.[14, 15] Unnecessarily taking iron or other supplements in the absence of iron deficiency is not desirable. Given the very real risks that iron depletion poses, female athletes should regularly (at least yearly) have iron status assessed, with the inclusion of ferritin in the assessment protocol.

General Recommendations for Female Athletes

1. Female athletes should be made fully aware of the negative consequences associated with menstrual dysfunction and the role energy inadequacy plays in its development.[16] Put simply, female athletes should consume sufficient energy to, at the very least, eliminate the risk that menstrual dysfunction results from inadequate energy consumption.

2. A pre-participation physical examination should be a standard feature for all athletes involved in all sports. For the female athlete, the screening should include an assessment for the presence of the female athlete triad and any of its sequelae.[17]

3. Calcium and iron intakes and status should be assessed and, if inadequate, corrected through a program of altered food intake (preferred) or through a doctor-supervised supplementation program. A reasonable means of assessing calcium status is to periodically assess bone density (once every 3 years if no osteopenia or osteoporosis; more often if bone disease is present). In addition, a dietary intake analysis will determine if consumed foods are providing sufficient calcium. Iron status should be assessed yearly, with special attention paid to stored iron. In the event of iron deficiency, a supervised program of iron supplementation with follow-up blood tests should be immediately implemented.

Female athletes are at higher risk than male athletes for eating disorders, inadequate bone density attainment, and inadequate iron consumption. They also have the unique risk of dysmenorrhea. Most of these difficulties can be controlled with the intake of a nutritionally balanced diet that delivers an adequate caloric load. To achieve this, female athletes should understand that an underconsumption of calories, while lowering weight, is likely to have a greater catabolic impact on lean mass than on fat mass. This altered body composition, by forcing the athlete to consume a still lower food intake to achieve a desired body profile, will place the athlete at greater future risk of malnutrition and associated diseases.

The Young Athlete

The energy and nutrient requirements for growth and development are so high that it is difficult to imagine how growing children who are involved in regular, intense physical activity can possibly meet their nutrition needs unless extraordinary measures are taken.[18] An inadequate energy supply may result in a failure to achieve the genetically prescribed growth potential, and insufficient nutrients may result in poor development of organ systems. For instance, a poor calcium uptake during the adolescent growth spurt will result in less than optimal bone density, which has a lifetime of health implications. Careful attention to the provision of an adequate energy and nutrient intake is the essential construct for ensuring that youth sports result in healthy outcomes. In particular, athletes who achieve elite status at a young age, as is typical of female gymnasts, may fail to obtain sufficient nutriture at a time when growth and sports-related training and performance stresses are at their highest. These athletes should be frequently assessed to ensure they remain in a healthy state and have a normal growth velocity.

The adolescent growth spurt in girls begins around the age of 10 or 11 and reaches its peak by age 12; girls typically stop growing by age 15 or 16. The adolescent growth spurt in boys begins about 2 years later at age 12 or 13 and reaches a peak by age 14; boys typically stop growing by the age of 19. It is common for girls and boys to grow approximately 11.8 inches (30 centimeters) between ages 5 and 10; but boys have a greater than 3.9 inch (10 centimeter) per year growth during the adolescent growth spurt, and adolescent girls have a greater than 3.5 inch (9 centimeter) growth per year during the adolescent growth spurt. It is estimated that 25 percent of the total bone mass is acquired during the adolescent years.[19] Although the stimulation imposed on the skeleton through physical activity is important for bone development, adequate calcium, protein, and energy intakes are also critical during this period. (See table 11.3 for a summary of height and weight values of children and adolescents.)

Adolescence is the time when girls achieve menarche. Less than 10 percent of girls in the United States start to menstruate before 11 years, and 90 percent of all girls in the United States are menstruating by 13.75 years of age, with a median age of 12.43 years.[20] Athletic females typically begin menstruating 1 to 2 years later.[21]

The blood loss experienced approximately every 4 weeks by girls who are having menstrual periods is an important nutrition consideration. The iron loss in conjunc-

Table 11.3 Normal Height and Weight Values of Male and Female Children and Adolescents

Age	Height, females (in.)	Height, males (in.)	Weight, females (lb)	Weight, males (lb)
1	27 to 31	28 to 32	15 to 20	17 to 21
2	31.5 to 36	32 to 37	22 to 32	24 to 34
3	34.5 to 40	35.5 to 40.5	26 to 38	26 to 38
4	37 to 42.5	37.5 to 43	28 to 44	30 to 44
6	42 to 49	42 to 49	36 to 60	36 to 60
8	47 to 54	47 to 54	44 to 80	46 to 78
10	50 to 59	50.5 to 59	54 to 106	54 to 102
12	55 to 64	54 to 63.5	68 to 136	66 to 130
14	59 to 67.5	59 to 69.5	84 to 160	84 to 160
16	60 to 68	63 to 73	94 to 172	104 to 186
18	60 to 68.5	65 to 74	100 to 178	116 to 202

Reprinted from the CDC (Centers for Disease Control and Prevention).

tion with the periodic bleeding may predispose adolescent girls to iron deficiency or iron-deficiency anemia that, if allowed to occur, would have a significant impact on endurance capacity. Although all adolescent girls should be cognizant of the importance of obtaining an adequate iron intake, athletic girls must make a particular effort to obtain enough of this mineral. The DRI for iron is 15 milligrams per day for girls between the ages of 14 and 18. This represents nearly a 100 percent increase over the iron requirement for girls between the ages of 9 and 13, when the DRI for iron is 8 milligrams per day. Obtaining 15 milligrams of iron per day is not easy, even if the athlete is a red-meat eater. For non-meat-eating athletes, regularly obtaining 15 milligrams of iron daily becomes nearly impossible without iron supplementation.[22] (See table 11.4 for the iron content of selected foods.) If adequate iron consumption from food is not possible, the risk of iron deficiency, reduced performance, and impaired immune function associated with inadequate iron intake should motivate athletes to seek a well-tolerated strategy for consuming enough iron.[23]

Consumption of sufficient energy is critically important for ensuring normal growth and development and supporting physical activity. It appears that substrate distribution is less important for young athletes than it is for adults. The general adult recommendation for the distribution of substrates is 60 percent from carbohydrate, 15 percent from protein, and 25 percent from fat, but the energy utilization pattern of children may allow for a greater proportion of calories from fat. Studies have found that children use more fat and less carbohydrate than adults during endurance activities and more intense activities.[24, 25] Because fat is a more concentrated source of energy, a slightly higher fat intake may make it easier to satisfy the high caloric requirements of these young athletes.

Adolescent females, including adolescent female athletes, often diet to control the change in body morphology and weight associated with growth. Dieting may increase the risk of eating

Table 11.4   Iron Content of Selected Foods

Food	Iron (mg)
Apple (raw)	0.2
Beef steak (3 oz)	2.7
Bread, white (2 slices)	1.4
Broccoli (1 cup)	1.1
Burrito, bean	2.7
Chicken breast (3 oz)	1.8
Chicken filet sandwich	2.7
Cola (12 oz)	0.4
French fries (regular serving)	1.4
Grapes (raw)	0.6
Grilled cheese sandwich	1.6
Hamburger (1/4 pounder) with bun	4.5
Hot dog with bun	2.3
Milk (1 cup)	0.0
Orange juice (1 cup)	0.4
Peanut butter (1 tbsp)	0.4
Pizza, cheese (1 large slice)	0.9
Rice (1 cup)	1.9
Taco with meat	1.0

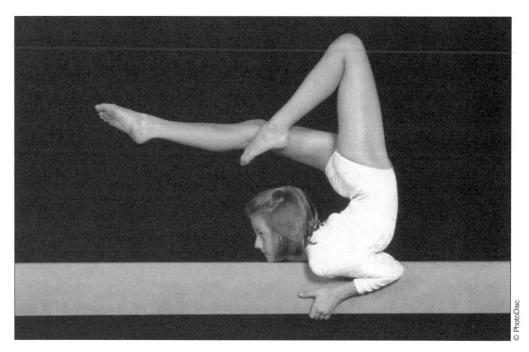

© PhotoDisc

To decrease the risks of osteoporosis and bone fractures, young athletes need to consume adequate calcium, especially in sports where appearance and size are issues, including gymnastics and diving.

disorders, particularly among adolescent female athletes involved in sports where appearance and size matter (e.g., diving and gymnastics). Compared with athletes in team sports, athletes in these sports are at greater risk of having inadequate intakes of energy, protein, and some micronutrients including calcium and iron. These are not minor issues; an inadequate calcium intake could predispose a young athlete to stress fractures and later osteoporosis, and an iron deficiency leads to poor endurance. Studies have confirmed that energy and nutrient intakes of male and female adolescent athletes, despite being better than that of nonathletes, are below recommended levels, which increases disease and injury risk and diminishes athletic performance potential.[26]

Typical school schedules that mandate a breakfast before school, a moderate lunch at midday, and a dinner that often follows sports practice create an environment that guarantees an energy imbalance. Athletic children should eat at frequent intervals to increase their total energy and nutrient exposure, to guarantee that sufficient energy is provided when it is most needed, and to reduce the chance of energy deficits that can encourage the loss of lean mass and the relative increase in fat mass.

The risk of athletes developing musculoskeletal injuries during periods of fast growth is high. This is not to say that physical activity is bad for children. On the contrary, the right amount and intensity of physical activity stimulates musculoskeletal development. However, excess physical activity that does not allow for sufficient rest and nutrient intake can result in overuse injuries, including tendinitis, Osgood-Schlatter disease, and stress fractures.[27] In addition, secondary amenorrhea often

No Logic in School Eating Patterns

When children are in elementary school, they are often provided with a midmorning and midafternoon snack of milk and a cookie, with lunch between the snacks. This is a desirable and needed strategy. However, when children move up to junior high school, just at the time they are hitting their adolescent growth spurt and in need of a huge amount of nutrients and energy, the cookie and milk snacks are removed. This makes no sense whatsoever. Junior high school teachers often complain that this is the most difficult school age to deal with but do nothing to ensure a stable blood sugar, a strategy that could have a major beneficial effect on behavior and nutrition status. Maintaining a snack in elementary, junior high, and high schools would help satisfy energy needs and, as an aside, do much to control undesirable behavior. It's not fun to be around people who are hypoglycemic.

occurs during periods of intense physical activity. To avoid overworking specific muscle groups or skeletal areas, it has been suggested that young children should participate in a variety of sports and specialize in a specific sport only after puberty. Those who follow this strategy perform better, have lower injury risk, and continue in the sport longer than those who specialize in a single sport early.[28]

Hydration issues remain a concern for young athletes because, compared with adults, they have lower sweat rates, produce more heat per unit of body weight, experience a faster rise in core body temperature, are predisposed to voluntary dehydration, and do not acclimatize as quickly to warm environments.[29] These factors dramatically increase a young athlete's risk of developing heat injury. As a result, coaches and parents should become fully aware of the mental and physical signs of dehydration and heat injuries and should pay careful attention to the ambient temperature and humidity to take appropriate measures for reducing risk. The fact that young athletes are predisposed to voluntary dehydration (i.e., they consume insufficient fluids to maintain hydration state even when they are available) should persuade adults to encourage drinking and observe drinking patterns. It is also useful to have beverages available that young athletes are more likely to consume.[30] These include beverages that have a sweet taste and include small amounts of salt to help sustain blood volume and sweat rates.

General Recommendations for Young Athletes

1. Energy intake level should be sufficient to support normal growth and development plus the added energy requirement of physical activity. As a general guide, young athletes should track normally on charts that measure height for age, weight for age, and weight for height (often used by pediatricians). A flattening of the growth percentile is a sign of inadequate energy intake.

2. To estimate the energy requirement of physical activity in young athletes it is important to remember that children use more energy per unit of body weight to do the same activity as adults. Add 20 to 25 percent to the adult energy

expenditure values for children 8 to 10 years old; add 10 to 15 percent for children 11 to 14 years old.[31]

3. The distribution of energy substrates is important, but parents and coaches should understand that total energy intake adequacy is more important than the amount of carbohydrate or fat in the diet. Slightly liberalizing the fat intake from 25 percent to 30 percent of total calories will make it easier for young athletes to obtain the calories they need. Protein intake is important but need not rise above 15 percent of total calories or 1.5 grams per kilogram of body weight provided total energy intake adequacy is satisfied.

4. Young athletes tend to underconsume fluids, predisposing them to dehydration and increasing the risk of heat illness. Athletes should be encouraged to take regular drinks by supervising adults, even when fluids are readily available. This may require fixed time-schedule drinking patterns that involve stoppage of play every 10 to 20 minutes, depending on the ambient heat and humidity.

5. Young female athletes are at risk for primary and secondary amenorrhea, both of which may be caused by excess physical activity, inadequate energy intake, and other factors. If a young female has a delayed menarche beyond age 14, she should be assessed by a pediatrician to make sure there is no underlying problem. In addition, the adequacy of nutrient and energy intake should be carefully assessed.

6. Young athletes should not diet because delayed eating and severe low-calorie intakes are counterproductive to achieving ideal body weight and body composition and negatively affect growth and development. The eating strategy should allow for frequent eating, with an opportunity to consume food approximately every 3 hours.

7. It is difficult for young female athletes to obtain sufficient iron, and surveys suggest that calcium intake is also marginal. Therefore, the parents of young athletes should consult with the family doctor to determine if iron or calcium supplements are warranted.

Young athletes have an extraordinary nutrition burden because they must satisfy the combined nutrition needs of growth plus the needs of physical activity. Young athletes should receive a minimum of six eating opportunities to ensure that nutrition needs can be met. Fluid consumption should be planned to lower dehydration risk. In addition, pediatricians should be satisfied that young athletes are maintaining normal and expected growth patterns at annual pre-participation physical examinations. Adolescent female athletes should be assessed for primary or secondary amenorrhea, with steps taken to resolve the amenorrhea as quickly as possible.

The Older Athlete

There are far too many examples of older athletes performing well to suggest that there is a definite time to put away the athletic shoes. The World Masters Athletics

Association lists many athletes who are still competing above 60 years of age in virtually every athletic discipline including steeplechase, pole vault, marathon, and the 10,000-meter run. The world-record holder for the men's outdoor 100 meters in the 100-year-old group is Philip Rabinowitz from Russia, with a time of 30.86 seconds, and Ron Taylor from Great Britain holds the record for 60-year-olds, an impressive 11.70 seconds! Older female athletes also excel. In 1994 Yekaterina Podkopayeva (Russia) won the world indoor 1,500 meters at the age of 42 with a time of 3:59:78. At the age of 80, Johanna Luther from Germany ran the 10,000 meters in an impressive time of 58:40:03. Clearly, being older does not make stopping exercise mandatory. Nevertheless, the aging process does bring with it certain undeniable changes that should be addressed to ensure that exercise remains a healthful activity. Of particular concern are the age-related changes in body composition and the impact this has on resting energy expenditure; the lowered capacity to quickly recover from intensive or long bouts of exercise; a gradually diminishing bone mass; subtle changes in GI tract function that could influence nutrient absorption; and the possibility of a progressively lower heat tolerance.[32, 33]

The issue of increased risk of heat stress in older athletes should be seriously considered because the result of heat exhaustion and heatstroke is often death. During periods of high heat and humidity, those most likely to become seriously ill or die are the elderly. Although the elderly population should not be confused with the older athlete population, even if they are in the same age group, there may be an age-related drop in the capacity to dissipate heat regardless of fitness level.[34] (See table 11.5.)

An important factor in sweat production and cooling capacity is the ability to increase blood flow to the skin. Blood flow to the skin in older, fit athletes is lower than in younger athletes.[35, 36] In addition, the lower blood flow associated with increasing age appears to be independent of hydration state. It also appears that, although sweat-gland recruitment is similar to that of younger athletes, older athletes produce less sweat per gland.[37] There is a wide genetically based variability in sweat production, but these studies suggest that older athletes should be vigilant about following a regular fluid-consumption schedule while exercising to optimize

Table 11.5   Factors That Change With Age That Could Affect Heat Tolerance, Regardless of Chronological Age

1. Lower aerobic capacity and associated variables
2. Sedentary lifestyle
3. Lower lean body mass; higher relative fat mass
4. Chronic hypohydration from lower fluid intake or higher fluid excretion by the kidneys, or both
5. Higher prevalence of chronic diseases, including hypertension, diabetes, and heart disease
6. Higher use of medications, including diuretics, adrenergic blockers, vasodilators, and anticholinergics

Reprinted, by permission, from W.L. Kenney, 1993, "The older athlete: Exercise in hot environments," *GSSI Sports Science Exchange*, #44, 6(3).

their capacity to produce sweat. Older athletes and their exercise partners should be cognizant of the symptoms of heat exhaustion and heatstroke. They should also be aware that most heat exhaustion occurs before heat acclimatization. Therefore, normal exercise intensities and durations should be reduced for the first few days in a new environment until the athlete has adapted.

Bone density becomes progressively lower with age, and females experience a faster drop in bone density after menopause when they lose the bone-protective action of estrogen. This is one of the primary reasons why it is so important to achieve a high bone density by young adulthood so that, even with a progressive loss of density later on, there will be sufficient density to avoid reaching the fracture threshold in older age.

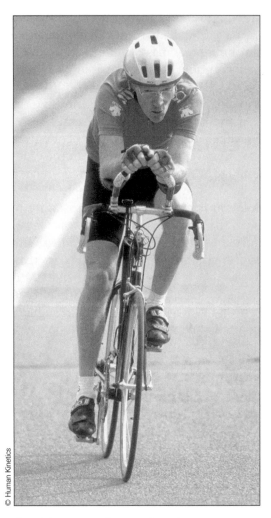

© Human Kinetics

As athletes age, they produce less sweat per gland. A systematic hydration schedule enables older athletes to compensate for less sweat production.

The rate of change in bone density can be altered through an adequate intake of calcium, periodic and regular exposure to the sun for vitamin D, and regular stress on the skeleton through weight-bearing exercise. In addition, women may choose to take, through the advice of their doctors, estrogen replacement therapy (ERT). ERT may be particularly useful when there is a family history of osteoporosis or a woman has been diagnosed with low bone density. Certain cortisone-based drugs taken for the control of pain or osteoarthritis appear to be catabolic to bone, so regular use of these drugs would place the older athlete at increased risk of low bone density. The fact that older athletes continually stress the skeleton through regular physical activity is a major protective factor in keeping bone density elevated.

It would be expected that older athletes experience some degree of progressive GI dysfunction and changes in nutrient requirements, although no athlete-specific studies confirm that this, indeed, occurs. The typical effects of age on the GI tract include reduced motility; decreased absorption of dietary calcium, vitamin B_6, and vitamin B_{12}; and greater requirement for fluid and fiber to counteract reduced GI motility. The absorption of iron and zinc may also be a concern.[38] Energy expenditure decreases approximately 10 calories each year for men and 7 calories each year for women after the age of 20. However, fit individuals who maintain their lean body (muscle) mass are typically able to sustain energy metabolism. It is unclear, therefore, how or if the typical reduction in energy metabolism affects older athletes.

Changes in immune function should also be considered, but regular long-term exercise appears to attenuate the changes in the immune system that are typically associated with aging.[39] Vitamin and mineral supplementation is common among older athletes, often in an attempt to boost the immune system. There is little evidence that this is a useful strategy, but if the supplements target nutrients that aren't well absorbed, they may be warranted. Rather than guess, however, older athletes should consult with their doctors to determine the best strategy for delivering needed nutrients. In some cases, as in the case of vitamin B_{12}, a periodic injection may be the only strategy that reduces the risk of pernicious anemia. Taking oral supplements of vitamin B_{12} simply does not work. Good protein status is an important component of a stable immune function, but there is no evidence that protein intake should in any way be increased beyond the normal values established for athletes (~ 1.5 grams per kilogram per day). On the contrary, aging often brings with it a reduction in kidney function, so reducing the amount of nitrogenous waste by lowering protein intake may be warranted. A good strategy would be to consume less protein but of higher quality to reduce the amount of nitrogenous waste produced.

General Recommendations for Older Athletes

1. Older athletes should take steps to reduce the risk of dehydration. Developing a fixed drinking schedule and being aware of the signs of heat stress are important because older athletes are likely to have lower sweat rates than younger athletes involved in the same activity.

2. GI function may require additional vitamin and mineral intake, perhaps through supplements. Older athletes should regularly consult with doctors to determine the biological need for specific supplements and take them only in reasonable, prescribed doses. Vitamins and minerals of particular concern are calcium, iron, zinc, vitamin B_6, and vitamin B_{12}.

3. Reduced gut motility requires a slight increase in fiber consumption, but this should always take place in conjunction with additional fluid intake. Focusing on fresh fruits and vegetables as well as whole grain products is an excellent means of obtaining additional fiber, plus these foods provide needed carbohydrate energy.

4. Frequent illness may be a sign that immune function is depressed. There is no perfect weapon for combating a reduction in immune function, but exercising reasonably, eating well, and resting well are useful strategies. Older athletes with frequent eating patterns should consult with their doctors.

5. It takes longer for older athletes to adapt to new environments, so reducing exercise intensity and frequency for several days after travel is a logical and useful step to avoid overheating and illness.

Older athletes can expect some slowing of the metabolic rate, which makes it more difficult to sustain a desirable body composition and weight without making the appropriate reduction in energy consumption. At the same time, nutrient requirement mandates the consumption of a diet with a high-nutrient density (i.e., a higher nutrient-to-calorie ratio). The avoidance of overtraining is important for injury reduction and sustaining immune function. This is particularly important because healing time for both injury and disease is longer with increasing age. Finally, adequate fluid intake is critically important to avoid dehydration and to sustain gut motility because the frequency of urination associated with advanced age may inhibit fluid consumption.

Body Composition and Weight

12

The strength-to-weight ratio is a critical factor in overcoming resistance (drag) associated with sport, and in many sports the marker of success is related to the athlete's appearance (e.g., diving, rhythmic gymnastics, artistic gymnastics). Common strategies athletes use for weight loss are counterproductive, however; they may temporarily lower weight, but at the cost of an undesirable change in body composition. Ideally, the athlete should understand the best strategies for overcoming sport-specific resistance while enhancing the capacity to sustain power output during practice and competition. This requires an understanding by athletes of how to achieve ideal weight without losing muscle and power and without increasing body fat percentage in the process. In addition, athletes and their coaches must understand the risks associated with the cyclic weight-loss patterns often experienced by many female and some male athletes. These risks include the development of eating disorders and the associated bone-density problems. The bone-density problems lead to stress fractures, which ultimately may take the athlete out of the sport. At the very least, poorly achieved weight loss nearly always reduces muscle mass and increases fat mass, making it more difficult for the athlete to steadily attain top performance.

This chapter helps athletes understand weight loss and body composition issues so they can apply the appropriate strategies to achieve the optimal strength-to-weight ratio for their sports. In addition, the chapter provides an up-to-date review of the methods commonly used for assessing body composition, with the aim of helping athletes better understand what the values derived from these methods really mean. Finally, this chapter discusses eating disorders and how they can develop from the cyclic weight-control strategies so often followed by athletes.

Weight Loss and Body Composition

The body is made up of different components (water, muscle, fat, bone, nerve tissue, tendons, and so on), and each has a different density. From a functional standpoint, tissues are grouped together into those that are mainly fat (fat mass), which is mainly anhydrous (has little water associated with it), and those that have little fat (fat-free mass), which is hydrous (has a great deal of water associated with it). The fat-free mass is also commonly referred to as lean mass, although this is viewed by many to be an inaccurate description because the fat-free mass includes a great deal of water (greater than 65 percent). Because techniques for estimating body composition are widely available, bone mass is now also included as a third commonly assessed component of body composition. In this book the components of body composition are referred to as fat mass (the body tissue that is mainly fat) and fat-free mass (the body tissue that is mainly free of fat, including muscle and bone).

Fat mass is composed of essential fat and storage fat. The essential fat is a required component of the brain, nerves, bone marrow, heart tissue, and cell walls that we cannot live without. Approximately 12 to 15 percent of total body weight in adult females is essential fat, the majority of which is associated with reproductive function and includes the additional fat associated with breast tissue. Because males do not have this reproductive function, their essential-fat levels are considerably lower. Storage fat, on the other hand, is an energy reserve that builds up in adipose tissue underneath the skin (subcutaneous fat) and around the organs (interabdominal fat). It is common for healthy men and women to have a storage-fat level that contributes 11 to 15 percent to total body weight. Combining the essential-fat and storage-fat components, normal body fat percentage for males is approximately 15 percent (3 percent essential; 12 percent storage), while normal body fat percentage for females is 26 percent (15 percent essential; 11 percent storage).[1]

Women with extremely low body fat percentages are at risk of developing reproductive system difficulties, commonly manifested as irregular menstrual periods (see table 12.1). Oligomenorrhea and amenorrhea are associated with increased fracture risk and low estrogen production, which increases the risk of osteoporosis (a bone disease associated with low bone density). It appears that a body fat percentage of 17 to 22 percent is needed to maintain a normal menstrual cycle in most women.[2]

Women who develop an excessively low body fat percentage typically exercise excessively for the amount of energy they consume, or they have an eating disorder. The female athlete triad, a condition prevalent in many female athletes, includes

Table 12.1   Common Terms Related to the Menstrual Cycle

Term	Definition
Amenorrhea	Absence of the menstrual period for 6 months or absence of the menstrual cycle for 3 cycles
Dysmenorrhea	Painful menstrual periods
Eumenorrhea	Normal menstrual frequency; no abnormalities of flow, timing, or pain
Oligomenorrhea	Infrequent menstrual frequency; fewer than 8 periods a year or periods at intervals greater than 35 days
Background	The hypothalamus (an organ in the brain) detects a lowered amount of estrogen and progesterone in the bloodstream during a period and secretes *gonadotropin releasing hormone* (GnRH), which stimulates the pituitary gland to secrete *follicular stimulating hormone* (FSH), which stimulates the ovaries to make estrogen to build up tissue in the uterus and to mature an egg within a follicle that holds it until ovulation; and *luteinizing hormone* (LH), which stimulates the release of that egg (ovulation). After ovulation, the remaining emptied follicle makes progesterone, which matures the built-up tissue in the uterus in preparation for implantation (pregnancy). Without implantation, the hormone levels fall, and the built-up uterine lining cannot hold together. The sloughing away of the uterine lining is referred to as the *menstrual period.*

the interrelated presence of an eating disorder; amenorrhea; and low bone density, osteopenia, or osteoporosis (figure 12.1).

Fat-free mass is mainly water and protein but also includes small levels of minerals and stored carbohydrate (glycogen). The main constituents of fat-free mass include skeletal muscle, the heart, and other organs. Although total body weight is approximately 60 percent water, the water content of the fat-free mass is 70 percent. This can be compared with the water content of the fat mass, which is below 10 percent.[3] Athletes typically have a higher fat-free mass and a lower fat mass than do nonathletes.

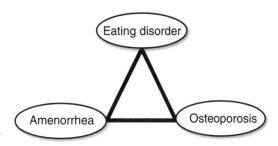

Figure 12.1   The female athlete triad.

Weight

The measurement of weight (pounds) or mass (kilograms) by itself does not discriminate between fat mass and fat-free mass so is not a measure of body composition.

Therefore, the statement "My weight is increasing, so I must be getting fat" is common but not necessarily correct. It is possible for an athlete to increase fat-free mass (i.e., muscle) without increasing fat mass. The result would be an increase in weight but not an increase in fat weight. It is also possible for an athlete to maintain weight but experience changes in fat or fat-free mass. This could be either desirable or undesirable depending on which element is increasing. All athletes, regardless of sport, find it desirable to achieve a high strength-to-weight ratio, which is associated with a relative increase in the ratio of fat-free mass to fat mass. This can be achieved by maintaining the fat-free mass while fat mass is decreased (lower total weight); increasing the fat-free mass while fat mass is maintained (higher total weight); increasing the fat-free mass while fat mass is decreased (lower total weight); or increasing the fat-free mass more than the increasing fat mass (higher total weight). As you can see, monitoring a change in weight alone is an inadequate means of understanding what really matters: the components of weight change. Although tracking weight is an appropriate measure for understanding the athlete's energy balance, it does nothing to explain whether the components of the weight are changing in a desirable direction. It is for this reason that body composition evaluation should be a standard component of the athlete assessment protocol.

Ideal Weight

There are several common means of predicting ideal body weight, but they should all be considered of limited value when used with athletes. The most common formulas for predicting ideal body weight are those of BJ Devine (1974), JD Robinson (1983), and DR Miller (1983):

Devine Formula

Males: ideal body weight (in kilograms) =
50 kilograms + 2.3 kilograms per inch over 5 feet

Females: ideal body weight (in kilograms) =
45.5 kilograms + 2.3 kilograms per inch over 5 feet

Robinson Formula

Men: ideal body weight (in kilograms) =
52 kilograms + 1.9 kilograms for each inch over 5 feet

Women: ideal body weight (in kilograms) =
49 kilograms + 1.7 kilograms for each inch over 5 feet

Miller Formula

Men: ideal body weight (in kilograms) =
56.2 kilograms + 1.41 kilograms for each inch over 5 feet

Women: ideal body weight (in kilograms) =
53.1 kilograms + 1.36 kilograms for each inch over 5 feet

Body Mass Index

Body mass index (BMI) is a useful tool for categorizing weight. However, it is not likely to be useful for athletes because athletes have more muscle than do nonathletes, which increases the weight-to-height ratio. BMI considers weight in relation to height using one of the following formulas:

BMI = weight in kilograms divided by height in meters squared
BMI = kg/m^2
BMI = weight in pounds divided by weight in inches squared multiplied by 703
BMI = ([lb/in^2] × 703)

Table 12.2 gives BMI values and their corresponding classifications.

Weight Issues

There is no question that total body weight is an important issue for athletes because it influences how easily they can perform their skills. A study assessing the relationships between body composition and fundamental movement skills among children and adolescents found that unhealthy weight gain reduced movement skill.[1] However, looking at weight by itself may provide athletes with a misleading picture of what is good or bad about their body composition. In a number of sports, athletes will increase the time or intensity of a training regimen to improve performance, but then they inappropriately use changes in weight as a marker of success or failure. Imagine a football player who comes to training camp at a weight much higher than the coach is accustomed to seeing in this player. It may well be that the football player worked hard during the off-season to increase muscle mass, and the increase in weight is a result of more muscle. Wouldn't the coach be wrong in telling that player that he has to lose weight? Gymnasts often reach their competitive peak during adolescence, a time when fast growth is the normal biological expectation. Despite this, gymnasts and other athletes are often weighed weekly or more often to make certain they are maintaining their weight. Shouldn't all the training they're doing increase their muscle mass and therefore their weight? Shouldn't they be growing and thus increasing their weight? These are examples of how weight is often used arbitrarily and incorrectly. Tracking the constituents of weight makes much more sense and provides valuable information on the nature of body changes that are occurring.

The principle of energy thermodynamics is always with us. Consumption of more calories than the body burns leads to a weight gain; consumption of fewer calories than the body burns leads to a weight loss; and consumption of exactly the same number of calories that the body burns leads to weight stability. But making a change in body weight is not as straightforward as the principle of energy thermodynamics may make it appear to be.

The most common belief is that low-calorie dieting is an effective but unpleasant means of weight and fat loss. It seems logical that a 25 percent reduction in energy intake will lead to a 25 percent reduction in weight. The reality, however, is that energy expenditure after weight loss is less than would be expected by the amount

Table 12.2   BMI Classification

Classification	BMI value
Underweight	<18.5
Normal	18.5 to 24.9
Overweight	25.0 to 29.9
Obese	≥30

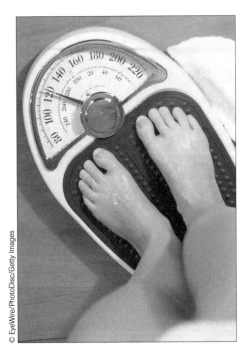

EyeWire/PhotoDisc/Getty Images

Training should naturally increase not decrease weight.

of weight that was lost.[4] This means that the adjustment in energy expenditure to inadequate intake is greater than the mathematical expectation and leads to a return to the original weight, even with a lower energy intake (i.e., the less you eat, the less you can eat to maintain weight). A close look at the reason for this lower metabolic rate is clear. With an inadequate caloric intake, the body catabolizes the metabolic (lean) mass so it can survive on less energy.

Logic also suggests that a 25 percent increase in energy intake will lead to a 25 percent increase in weight. In fact, although weight gain does occur, it doesn't appear to increase as much as the increase in energy intake suggests it should, but it's close. When people are purposefully overfed to gain weight, the amount of weight gain is proportionate to the amount of overfeeding.[5-8] These studies strongly suggest that we have homeostatic mechanisms during periods of energy deficit that help us maintain our weight. This may be a "survival of the species" mechanism that helps humans survive periods of famine. We also appear able to store energy effectively (as fat) during periods of excess. This may be another survival mechanism that enables us to store energy when we are lucky enough to have excess food available.

Since major energy surpluses and deficits appear to activate homeostatic mechanisms, a possible means of making a desired change in weight and body composition is to avoid major energy-balance shifts. Exercise should be at the core of any desired body composition change (i.e., an increase in lean mass and a decrease in fat mass, coupled with a small decrease in weight). But such a change might be easier to achieve if the energy deficit and energy surplus created are never too large during the day. See figure 12.2 for an example of what can happen to body composition with three different eating patterns. Energy surpluses and deficits are represented, respectively, by variations above and below the perfect energy-balance line (zero). In the figure, when the line moves above zero, the athlete has consumed more energy than was expended. When the line moves below zero, the athlete has expended more energy than was consumed. Eating pattern 1 represents an athlete eating small meals frequently; there are no energy surpluses or deficits that exceed 400 calories. Eating pattern 2 represents infrequent eating, with excess calories (high surplus energy peaks) consumed at each meal. Eating pattern 3 represents an athlete who spends the majority of the day in an energy-deficit state from not eating enough when the energy is needed, a condition that stimulates the breakdown of muscle tissue for energy. At the end of the day, a very large meal brings the athlete into energy balance, but much of this meal will be stored as fat. Within any given day, energy balance is important for both performance and body composition.

Weight is the best indicator of the adequacy of caloric intake, and body composition helps determine if the calories are being consumed in the proper amounts and at the correct intervals. See figures 12.2 and 12.3 for illustrations of how to optimally fuel your activity, and see chapters 16 to 18 for sample diet plans.

Since the standard three-meal-a-day schedule forces athletes to consume a large amount of energy at each meal to obtain the necessary energy, staying in energy balance is easier on a six-meal pattern. Frequent consumption of small meals to maintain a steady energy flow can be an important strategy in making the desired changes. Chapter 6 discusses the importance of meal timing.

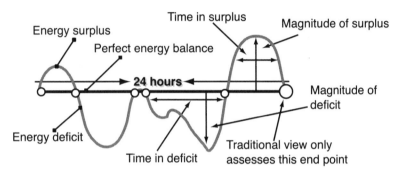

Figure 12.2   Sharp deviations in energy balance during the course of a day can affect body composition.

Adapted, by permission, from D.R. Lamb, 1995, "Basic principles for improving sport performance," *GSSI Sport Science Exchange*, #55, 8(2).

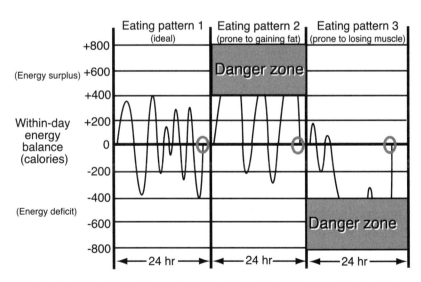

Figure 12.3   An individual's eating pattern has the potential to greatly affect body composition.

Body Composition

The purpose of body composition assessment is to determine an athlete's distribution of fat-free mass and fat mass. A high ratio of fat-free mass to fat mass is typically synonymous with a high strength-to-weight ratio, which is typically associated with athletic success. However, there is no single ideal body composition for all athletes in all sports. Each sport has a range of lean mass and fat mass associated with it, and each athlete in a sport has an individual range that is ideal for him or her. Athletes trying to achieve an arbitrary body composition that is not right for them are likely to place themselves at health risk and will not achieve the performance benefits they seek. In fact, athletes nearly always perform less well when they try to achieve a weight or body composition that is inconsistent with their history and genetic makeup. Therefore, the key to body composition assessment is the establishment of an acceptable range of fat-free mass and fat mass for the individual athlete. It is important to regularly monitor the fat-free mass and fat mass to ensure the stability or growth of the fat-free mass and a proportional maintenance or reduction of the fat mass. Just as much attention should be given to changes in fat-free mass (both in weight of lean mass and proportion of lean mass) as the attention traditionally given to body fat percentage.

The "fat mass and fat-free mass" model of body composition assumes that the combined weight of fat mass and fat-free mass equals total body weight. The assessment of body composition typically results in the prediction of body fat percentage, or the proportion of total weight that is composed of fat. As an example, assuming an athlete weighs 150 pounds (68 kilograms) and has a body fat percentage of 20 percent, the athlete has 30 pounds ($150 \times .20 = 30$) (13.6 kilograms) of fat weight and 120 pounds (54.4 kilograms) of fat-free weight. If this same athlete were to experience a reduction in body fat percentage to 15 percent while maintaining weight, this translates into 22.5 pounds ($150 \times .15 = 22.5$) (10.2 kilograms) of fat weight and 127.5 pounds (57.8 kilograms) of fat-free weight. This increase of 7.5 pounds (3.4 kilograms) in fat-free weight and reduction in fat weight means the athlete is now smaller (pound for pound, lean mass takes up less space than fat mass because it has a higher density), which means he or she should be able to move more quickly and more efficiently (less drag) than before, despite being the same weight. However, if this 150-pound athlete were to maintain weight but increase fat mass while reducing lean mass, potential speed and efficiency of movement would be reduced. Weight, in the absence of knowledge of its components, is a poor measure for predicting athletic success and should not be used by itself for this purpose.

Body Composition and Performance

Athletic performance is, to a large degree, dependent on the athlete's ability to sustain power (both anaerobically and aerobically) and to overcome resistance, or drag. Both of these factors are interrelated with the athlete's body composition. Coupled with the common perception of many athletes who compete in sports where appearance is a concern for both the athlete and the common perception of these athletes (swimming, diving, gymnastics, figure skating), attainment of an "ideal" body composition often becomes a central theme of training. Besides the aesthetic and performance reasons for wanting to achieve an optimal body composition, there may also be safety reasons.

In the minds of athletes, there is an inherent conflict between overcoming the resistance, or drag, associated with sport and having enough energy to sustain power output over the entire course of a competition or training session (see figure 12.4). Athletes view weight reduction (i.e., being smaller) as an effective means of overcoming resistance (imagine the position and profile of a cyclist or speedskater to reduce drag), and the common way to achieve weight reduction is to reduce caloric intake. However, having the capacity to sustain power output requires eating to at least a state of energy balance. It appears that many athletes believe this latter point (i.e., sustaining power output) is not as important as reducing drag, so the athletes consume inadequate calories.

An athlete who is carrying excess weight may be more prone to injury when performing difficult skills than the athlete with a more optimal body composition. However, when athletes attempt to achieve an optimal body composition, their methods are often counterproductive. Diets and excessive training often result in such a severe energy deficit that, although total weight may be reduced, the constituents of weight also change, commonly with a lower muscle mass and a relatively higher fat mass. The resulting higher body fat percentage and lower muscle mass inevitably result in a performance reduction that motivates the athlete to follow regimens that produce

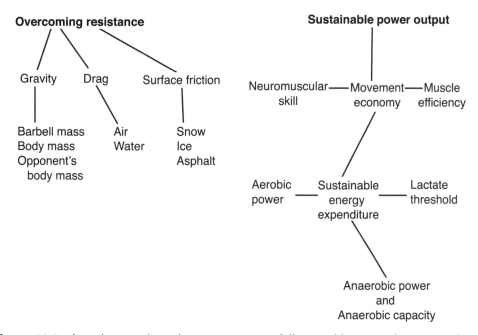

Figure 12.4 In order to train and compete successfully, an athlete must have enough energy to sustain the necessary power to overcome drag.

Adapted, by permission, from D.R. Lamb, 1995, "Basic principles for improving sport performance," *GSSI Sport Science Exchange*, #55, 8(2).

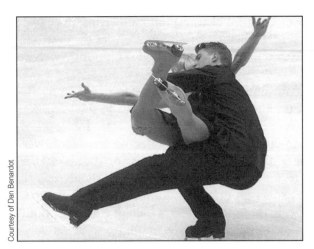

Courtesy of Dan Benardot

At times, wrongly, achieving ideal body composition becomes the focus of training instead of sustaining power and overcoming drag, a line that blurs in sports like swimming, diving, gymnastics, and figure skating.

even greater energy deficits. This downward energy intake spiral may be the precursor of eating disorders that place the athlete at serious health risk. Therefore, although achieving an optimal body composition is useful for high-level athletic performance, the processes athletes often use to attain an optimal body composition may reduce athletic performance, place athletes at a higher injury risk, increase health risks, and predispose them to eating disorders.

Many people have the unhealthy mind-set that food, regardless of the amount and type, is "fat producing." A much healthier (and from the point of view of an athlete, more appropriate) mind-set is that food is the provider of the fuel and nutrients associated with muscle energy.

Body fat percentage should be thought of as having an approximate range for different sports, and it's OK for athletes to fall anywhere on that sport-specific range. Within some reasonable bounds, having a relatively low body fat percentage may aid athletic performance by improving the strength-to-weight ratio: For a given weight, more of it is represented by lean mass that is power producing and less of it by fat mass that represents stored fuel. It also helps by lowering the resistance, or drag, an athlete has as he or she moves through the air, swims in water, or skates on ice; the smaller the body profile, the less resistance the body is likely to produce.

Less resistance is so important for some sports (typically the faster you go, the greater the importance of drag reduction) that performance techniques are based on reducing drag. After their initial strides off the starting line, for instance, speed-skaters spend the entire race bent over to reduce wind resistance. Cyclists wear special streamlined helmets and clothing, position their bodies on the bicycle to reduce drag, and even strategize about the best time to sprint ahead of the cyclist in front of them. Going too soon can lead to premature exhaustion because it takes a great deal more energy (12 to 17 percent more) for the cyclist in the lead facing the air resistance to go the same speed. A gymnast who weighs 110 pounds (50 kilograms) and is 5 feet (152 centimeters) tall with a body fat percentage of 15 percent will have a lower air resistance (i.e., less drag) tumbling through the air than a gymnast with the same weight and height but with a body fat percentage of 20 percent. Figure skaters are increasingly required to perform jumps with more in-air revolutions to stay competitive. The greater the number of revolutions, the more difficult it is for a larger figure skater to complete the jump. For some sports, however, this may make little or no difference. It's hard to imagine how a lineman on a football team is concerned about air resistance. Nevertheless, even for this athlete, having a high strength-to-weight ratio makes a difference because the lineman who can move his mass more quickly and powerfully will knock over the lineman who moves more slowly. Even a powerlifter gains an advantage if, in meeting a weight category, more of the lifter's weight is composed of muscle and less is composed of fat. In sports where being aerodynamic helps, body composition makes a difference because, pound for pound, fat takes up more space than lean tissue does because it is less dense. Table 12.3 compares common body composition values found in different sports.

Table 12.3 Body Fat Percentage Ranges for Male and Female Athletes in Different Sports

Sport	Body fat percentage (range of average)	
	Males	Females
Baseball (age 20–28)	12–16	
Basketball (age 25–27)	7–11	20–27
Cycling	8–9	13–15
Figure skating	9–10	12–13
Football, defensive backs (age 19.3–20.3)		13–14
Football, offensive backs (age 17–24.5)		10–12
Football, linebackers (age 17–24.7)	9–12	
Football, quarterbacks (age 24.1)	13–14	
Hockey (age 22.5–26.3)	13–15	
Rowing (age 25.6)	5–7	
Racquetball (age 21–25)	8–9	13–14
Speedskating (age 21)	9–11	
Skiing, alpine (age 16.5–21.8)	9–11	20–21
Skiing, cross-country (age 20.2–25.6)	7–13	15–22
Skiing, Nordic (age 21.7)	8–9	
Soccer, U.S. junior (age 17.5)	9–10	
Soccer, U.S. Olympic (age 20.6)	9–10	
Soccer, U.S. collegiate (age 20)	9–11	
Soccer, U.S. national (age 22.5)	9–10	
Swimming, all strokes, distances (age 15.1–21.8)	5–11	26–27
Swimming, sprints		14–15
Swimming, middle distance		24–25
Swimming, distance		17–18
Synchronized swimming (age 20.1)		23–24

(continued)

Table 12.3 *(continued)*

Sport	Body fat percentage (range of average)	
	Males	**Females**
Track and field, distance running (age 20–26)	5–7	15–19
Track and field, middle distance (age 20–25)	6–13	
Track and field, sprint (age 20–47)	5–17	19–20
Track and field, cross country (age 15.6)		15–16
Track and field, race walking (age 26.7)	7–8	
Track and field, discus (age 21–28)	16–17	24–26
Track and field, hurdles (age 20.3)		20–21
Track and field, shot put (age 21.5–27)	16–20	27–29
Triathlon	7–8	12–13
Volleyball (age 19–26)	11–13	17–22
Weightlifting, power (age 24.9–26.3)	9–20	
Weightlifting, Olympic (age 25.3)	12–13	
Weightlifting, bodybuilding (age 25.6–29)	8–14	13–14
Wrestling (age 11.3–27)	4–15	

Note: The values presented are estimates from limited numbers of athletes assessed in different settings using skinfolds or hydrodensitometry and should *not* be considered ideals. The values in this table can be used to compare common body composition values found in different sports.

Adapted from *Training for sport and activity: The physiological basis of the conditioning process*, 3rd ed., 1988, edited by J. Wilmore and D. Costill, with permission of The McGraw-Hill Companies.

Body Composition Estimation

It is extremely difficult to determine body composition, with accuracy, by weighing a person or by looking at him or her. There are many "thin" people who have lost so much lean mass that they actually have a relatively high body fat percentage, and there are also many "large" people who are actually relatively lean. Even with modern equipment and sophisticated equations it is extremely difficult to accurately measure body fat percentage and to consistently repeat that measure. We have no direct means of assessing body composition (the subject wouldn't survive if we tried), so all the techniques available to us are attempting to accurately estimate the fat mass or the fat-free mass. Each technique uses a different means of making this estimate, so cross-comparisons between techniques should not be made. As an example, athletes who have had body fat percentage estimated via skinfolds should not compare the values from that method with values obtained by bioelectrical impedance analysis. The values obtained from these techniques are likely to be sufficiently different that, at the very least, the athlete will be confused. The common methods for assessing body composition include

- hydrostatic weighing (underwater weighing),
- skinfold measurements applied to prediction equations,

- bioelectrical impedance analysis (BIA), and
- dual-energy X-ray absorptiometry (DEXA).

Hydrostatic Weighing (Hydrodensitometry)

Hydrostatic weighing is the classic means of determining body composition. It uses what is known as Archimedes' principle,[9] which states that for an equal weight, lower-density objects have a larger surface area and displace more water than higher-density objects. From a body composition standpoint, this principle is applied in the following way:

- The subject is weighed on a standard scale to get a "land weight."
- Using specialized equipment, the subject's lung volume is estimated (the subject blows into a tube).
- The subject sits on a chair that is attached to a weight scale.
- The chair and weight scale are positioned over water, and the chair is slowly lowered into the water.
- When the subject is lowered into the water just below the chin, he is asked to fully exhale and completely lower his head into the water to be completely immersed.
- While immersed, "underwater weight" is read off the scale that is attached to the chair the subject is sitting on.

Subjects weigh less in water than out of water because body fat (regardless of the amount present) makes the subject more buoyant. The greater the difference between in-water weight and out-of-water weight is a function of how much body fat the subject has. A very obese subject with a high level of body fat appears lighter in water relative to land weight. Lung volume is measured before taking the "water weight," and there is an adjustment for the buoyancy that can be attributed to the air in the lungs. To minimize the lung–air effect, the subject is asked to exhale before full submersion, but there is always some remaining air in the lungs, referred to as residual volume.

Although there is some potential for error with hydrodensitometry related to a person's hydration status and residual volume, this technique is useful for determining the change in body composition over time if the technicians performing the measurements are good at precisely replicating the measurement procedure. It is also a useful means of determining the body composition of a population because the errors associated with the technique are likely to average themselves out over many measurements. However, individuals within that population would never be sure if their personal body composition results were accurate. Good laboratories that do research in body composition have invested a great deal for the equipment needed to accurately do hydrostatic weighing. Further, they also invest in making sure they have highly qualified people to take the measurements.

Skinfolds

Skinfold calipers, which vary in cost from free to $500, are used to measure a double thickness of the fat layer under the skin. This fat layer (called subcutaneous fat) is hypothesized to represent approximately 50 percent of a person's total body fat. Therefore, if you can get a good estimate of the subcutaneous fat layer, you should be able to predict the total body fat level. The prediction equations commonly used to determine body composition from skinfolds are based on the body composition determinations derived from hydrodensitometry. It works something like this: You measure a group of people using hydrodensitometry to determine their body fat percentages. Then you measure these same people with a series of skinfolds, which are used in statistics to predict the body fat percentage obtained from hydrodensitometry. If the skinfolds, when applied to the newly created equation, can successfully predict the hydrodensitometry value, then you have a skinfold equation for predicting body fat percentage.

A number of different equations are available for the general population, and several equations have been developed specifically for athletes. In general, using an equation that is more specific to the person you're measuring yields more accurate results. Also, equations that use more skinfold measurements are generally more accurate. For instance, one equation may require height, weight, age, triceps skinfold, and abdomen skinfold. Another equation may require height, weight, age, and skinfolds at the triceps, subscapular, midaxillary, suprailiac, abdomen, and midthigh sites.

It's important to say a word about the values that are derived from skinfold equations and used to predict body fat percentage. Many of the equations used for athletes are actually meant for the general (i.e., nonathlete) population. Since many athletes are considerably leaner than the average nonathlete, the results derived from skinfold equations are unrealistically low. Many athletes come to the lab saying they have a body fat percentage of 2 or 3 percent, and I know immediately that these are estimates from equations that have not been normalized on athletes. It's simply not possible to have such a low body fat percentage. When these athletes are given the true value from a more realistic assessment (using either better, more population-specific equations or a more accurate technique), they don't usually respond positively when they receive the new number (usually somewhere between 8 and 18 percent). It's important for you to remember that when skinfold equations are used, the single number you get is not going to be perfectly accurate. However, that number can be used as a baseline to determine change over time if the same technique and same equation are used to get the second value. It is completely inappropriate to compare the first value with one that was obtained using a different set of skinfolds and a different equation.

Bioelectrical Impedance Analysis (BIA)

For those of you who know what to do if you're in a swimming pool and begin to hear thunder nearby, you already know the principle behind bioelectrical impedance analysis (BIA). Water is a good conductor of electricity, and most body water is found in the lean mass. Fat, which has almost no water in it, is such a poor conductor of electricity that it actually impedes the electrical flow. BIA equipment comes in two basic forms. In one form, the subject lies down and the right wrist and right ankle are fitted with electrodes, which produce an electrical current that runs from the wrist to the ankle. In another form, the subject stands on a platform with bare feet, and an electrical current runs from the right foot, up the right leg, down the left leg, and out the left foot. Regardless of the BIA equipment used, the principle behind the technique is the same. If you know the beginning level of energy (electricity) that enters the system and you can measure the level of energy that exits the system, you know how much of the energy has been impeded in the system. Since muscle is an efficient conductor of electricity (because of the water and electrolytes it contains) and fat is an efficient insulator of electricity, the greater the impedance, the greater the level of fat. If you start with 100 units of electricity going into your system, and 80 units of electricity come out of the system, you have more water and muscle than someone who has 100 units going in and 60 units coming out.

Of course, a number of adjustments to the prediction are necessary. The electrical current would run a longer distance in a taller person, so a taller person would automatically have a greater level of impedance. The ratio of weight to height is also important because it helps predict the distance the current is running and the composition of the tissues it is running through. Since body composition commonly changes with age (people become less lean and more fat as they get older), age is also an important predictor of body composition. At the initiation of the adolescent growth spurt, males and females begin to differentiate themselves on body composition, with women having relatively more fat than men do. So gender is also an important consideration in this prediction. Therefore, when performing a BIA, the variables age, height, weight, and gender are included in the equation that predicts body fat percentage.

Although BIA has an excellent theoretical basis for making good body composition predictions, several important protocols must be followed for the results to be accurate and repeatable. Since the technique is dependent on electrical conductivity through the lean mass, the hydration state of the subject can alter the results. If someone having a BIA test is not well hydrated, the electrical current will not be conducted through the lean mass as well, so the subject will appear to have more fat mass than they actually do. Therefore, it is critically important that the person being measured be in a well-hydrated state. It is generally believed that drinking alcohol, exercising, consuming large amounts of coffee, and spending time outside in hot and humid weather within 24 hours of a BIA test lead to sufficient dehydration that the results will not be accurate. Since serious athletes exercise most days, this technique may provide results that indicate more body fat than they really have. Therefore, athletes who are measured with this technique should wait until after a day of rest and should make certain they are well hydrated. An easy hydration check is to see if the urine is clear. The more clear it is, the better hydrated you are.

Dual-Energy X-Ray Absorptiometry (DEXA)

Dual-energy X-ray absorptiometry (DEXA) is the latest, most accurate, and most expensive means of determining body composition, and it is generally considered the current gold standard for this purpose. The information you can derive from a full-body scan on an athlete is invaluable, including bone density; body fat percentage; lean body mass; fat mass; and the distribution of fat and lean tissue in the arms, trunk, and legs. DEXA output even provides the differences in lean mass and fat mass between the left and right sides. This information can be particularly important for athletes who wish to develop symmetrical bodies or who, because of the nature of the sport, need to produce the same muscular power in each leg or in each arm.

DEXA works by passing two X-ray beams through the subject and measuring the amount of X ray absorbed by the tissue it has passed through. One beam is high intensity and one is low intensity, so the relative absorbance of each beam is an indication of the density of the tissue it has passed through. The higher the tissue density, the greater the reduction in X-ray intensity. Don't be frightened by all this talk of X-ray beams passing through your body. In fact, the amount of radiation energy that is used with DEXA is extremely small. You would need to have approximately 800 full-body DEXA scans before being exposed to the same amount of radiation received from one standard chest X ray. In fact, the level of radiation is so low that DEXA is approved by the FDA as a screening device to predict body composition. Usually, X-ray devices are reserved as diagnostic instruments because of the amount of radiation they impart, but not so for DEXA.

The procedure for DEXA, which was originally developed to determine the density of bone, couldn't be easier. The subject lies on the DEXA table for approximately 20 minutes, and the pencil-beam X rays pass through the subject and are interpreted by a mechanical arm above the subject. Because metal has such a high density, the subject is asked to remove all jewelry and must wear clothing that contains no metal. The resultant value is translated into a density value for bone, lean, and fat tissue. Because the density values are derived from a direct assessment of tissue density, this is as close as we can get to directly assessing tissue density (short of surgery). If you can find a lab with DEXA, the usual cost for a full-body scan is somewhere between $100 and $250.

Changes in Body Composition

Body composition changes. We can influence that change by taking charge of what we eat and how we exercise. The general rule for lean mass (including bone mass) is "use it or lose it." We're wonderfully adaptive creatures, and we quickly adapt to our environments and our activities. We know, for instance, that the bones of astronauts quickly demineralize because the gravity-free environment of outer space eliminates the need for a strong skeleton. We would do quite well in that environment looking like a jellyfish, and the bones quickly adapt by releasing lots of calcium. The effect of this environment is so strong that astronauts must spend a significant amount of time doing exercise that places stress on the skeleton. Again, we're adaptive creatures, so placing this artificial stress on the bones helps keep them strong, even in a gravity-free environment. The same thing happens when people are bedridden because of an injury. Both bone and muscle masses are rapidly reduced because they simply aren't needed when you're lying in bed. The important thing to remember about our tissues is that they are alive and will do what's needed to adapt to their current situation. Even bone, which to the casual observer might appear to be a hard, rocklike, nonadaptive structure, is actually very much alive and changing itself all the time. Minerals move in and minerals move out, and this process leads to a constant remodeling of bone.

When you consider the influences on body composition, they boil down to the following:

- **Genetic predisposition.** This is everyone's bottom line, and no matter how hard you try, you can't change it. People have different inherited body types, and each type has a different predisposition toward accumulating more or less fat. Endomorphs (large trunk, short fingers, shorter legs) have a predisposition toward higher body fat percentages, and ectomorphs (long legs, long fingers, shorter trunk) have a predisposition toward a slender build with less body fat. What you're born with can't change, so all you can hope to do is optimize what you've been given.

- **Age.** People generally develop a lower lean mass and higher fat mass after the age of 30. However, although this age-related change in body composition is normal, it isn't inevitable. It has been clearly shown that a good diet and regular activity can keep you lean. Since energy metabolism drops about 2 percent for each decade after age 30, it gets progressively more difficult to maintain a desirable weight and body composition. To maintain what you've got, you would have to make either a 2 percent increase in energy expenditure or a 2 percent decrease in energy intake each decade after 30 to match the drop in energy metabolism. Although this 2 percent difference seems small, it could make a major difference in your body composition. Consider that the average person consumes about 2,500 calories per day. If you need 2 percent less than this and don't make an adjustment, that represents a 50-calorie error of excess each day. Multiply that over 365 days and it represents 18,250 excess calories per year. Since an excess of 3,500 calories represents a 1-pound weight gain, in the course of 1 year this small 50-calorie error would manifest itself as a weight gain of more than 5 pounds (2.3 kilograms). In 5 years, that's a weight gain of 25 pounds (11.5 kilograms), and in 10 years, that's a weight gain of a whopping 50 pounds (23.0 kilograms).

- **Gender.** All other things being equal, women have a higher body fat percentage than do men. Nothing can be done to alter this, and there is certainly nothing wrong with it. The gender difference is just a manifestation of the different biological expectations of men and women. However, there are many women who have a lower body fat percentage than some men because they exercise more and eat better. Therefore, despite this baseline difference, doing the right things can help you (regardless of your gender) optimize your body composition for your sport.

- **Type of activity.** Different types of activities place different stresses on the system, and as you would expect, the body responds differently to these stresses. Aerobic exercise is the standard for reducing body fat percentage. However, there is good evidence that any type of activity (including anaerobic activity) will reduce body fat percentage. High-intensity activity (such as performed by sprinters and weightlifters) may increase lean body mass and reduce body fat percentage, so the impact on weight may be minimal. Nevertheless, this shift in body composition is still likely to make the person appear slightly smaller, since pound for pound, fat weight takes up more space than lean-mass weight. Low-intensity activity, on the other hand, appears to reduce body fat percentage with minimal impact on lean body mass, so weight is reduced. When energy expenditure (calories burned) is equivalent, both anaerobic and aerobic activity appear to lower body fat to the same extent.

- **Amount of activity.** Clearly, the more a person exercises, the greater the potential benefits in desirably altering body composition. However, activity must be supported by an adequate intake of energy. Increasing the time of activity without also increasing the amount of energy intake causes a breakdown of muscle mass to support energy needs. There is no question that this would be an undesirable change in body composition for an athlete. In addition, overtraining, although it will not necessarily lead to a reduction in lean body mass, causes an increase in muscle soreness and reduces muscular power and endurance. Therefore, the amount of activity should be carefully balanced with adequate energy intake and with adequate rest to ensure maintenance of muscle mass and athletic performance.

- **Nutrition.** Eating too much or too little can both negatively affect body composition. Eating too much, either over the course of a day or at one time, is likely to increase fat storage; eating too little will lower both lean (muscle) mass and fat mass. In addition, certain nutrients are important for metabolic processes. A failure to consume an adequate level of these nutrients (B vitamins, zinc, iron, and so on) may reduce your ability to properly burn fuel, thereby limiting your ability to burn fat through exercise.

Body Composition Assessment Issues

Body composition has become an important part of athlete assessment. The amount of muscle and fat an athlete has can be predictive of performance, and bone mass assessment is important for understanding if developmental problems exist or if the athlete will face current or future risk for fracture. A periodic assessment of body composition also helps the athlete understand if the training regimen is causing the kinds of physical changes that are being sought. However, there are some important things to keep in mind when assessing body composition.

You can alter body composition by changing your diet and exercise, but these two should be considered together when making changes. Making dramatic changes in either direction is likely to cause unpredictable problems in your body composition. If you increase your training regimen, it is necessary to increase your energy intake to support the increase in energy expenditure. Putting yourself in a severe energy-deficit state by increasing exercise and maintaining or lowering energy intake is likely to lower metabolic rate, increase fat storage, and cause a breakdown of muscle to support energy needs. Eating too much is also likely to increase fat storage. It's best to maintain energy intake throughout the day, so athletes should be careful to consume enough energy to support exercise rather than make up for an energy deficit at the end of the day.

Athletes often compare body composition values with other athletes, but this comparison is not meaningful and may drive an athlete to change body composition in a way that negatively affects both performance and health. Health professionals involved in obtaining body composition data should be sensitive to the confidentiality of this information. They should also explain to each athlete that differences in height, age, and gender are likely to result in differences in body composition, without necessarily any differences in performance. Strategies for achieving privacy and helping the athlete put the information in the proper context include the following:

- Assess only one athlete at a time to limit the chance that the data will be shared.
- Give athletes information on body composition using phrases such as "within the desirable range" rather than a raw value, such as saying, "Your body fat level is 18 percent."
- Provide athletes with information on how they have changed between assessments rather than offering the current value.
- Increase the focus on muscle mass, and decrease the focus on body fat.
- Use body composition values as a means of explaining changes in objectively measured performance outcomes.

Different methods for assessing body composition produce different standard results. Therefore, it is inappropriate to compare the results from one method with the results of another. If athletes are being evaluated to determine body composition change over time (an appropriate use of body composition assessment), this comparison should be made only if the same method has been used for the entire assessment period. For instance, the difference in two DEXA scans taken several months apart provides valuable information on how body composition has changed in an individual, as does the difference in two skinfold assessments. However, the difference between body composition values from a DEXA scan and a skinfold equation is not useful in determining change. Even within methods, the same prediction equations should be used to determine if an athlete's body composition has changed between measurements.

Most athletes would like their body fat level to be as low as possible. However, athletes often try to seek a body fat level that is arbitrarily low (so low that it has nothing to do with the norms in the sport or their own body fat predisposition), and this can increase the frequency of illness, increase the risk of injury, lengthen the time the athlete needs before returning to training after an injury, reduce performance, and increase the risk of an eating disorder. Body composition values should be thought of as numbers on a continuum that are usual for a sport. If an athlete falls anywhere on that continuum, it is likely that factors other than body composition (e.g., training, skills acquisition) will be the major predictors of performance success.

Seeking arbitrarily low body fat levels or weight is an issue in sports where making weight is a common expectation. Wrestlers in particular make dangerous efforts—sometimes leading to death—to lower body fat levels and weight to be more competitive. Read more about this subject in the section on wrestling in chapter 13 (p. 259).

Athletes who are assessed frequently (weight or skinfold measurements recorded regularly) are fearful of the outcome because the results are often (and inappropriately) used punitively. Real changes in body composition occur slowly, so there is little need to assess athletes every week, every two weeks, or even every month. Assessing body composition two to four times each year is an appropriate frequency to determine and monitor body composition change. In some isolated circumstances when an athlete has been injured or is suffering from a disease, such as malabsorption, fever, diarrhea, or anorexia, it is reasonable for a doctor to recommend a more frequent assessment rate to control for changes in lean mass. Coaches who have traditionally obtained weight or body composition values much more frequently (e.g., weekly, monthly) should shift their focus to a more frequent assessment of objective performance-related measures.

Pathologic Weight Control in Athletes: Eating Disorders

It is unclear whether athletes in general are at greater risk of developing eating disorders than are the nonathlete population. In a study of both athletes and non-athletes it was found that the risk for developing eating disorders was not related to whether or not the subjects were athletes.[2] A similar finding was observed in ethnically diverse urban female adolescent athletes and nonathletes; the athletes were not at higher risk for disordered eating.[3] This study also found that Hispanic and Caucasian urban adolescent females were at higher risk for eating disorders than were African-American urban adolescent females. However, athletes involved in sports that emphasize appearance or that have a weight requirement are clearly at a higher risk of developing an eating disorder, and the risk is higher in female athletes than in male athletes.[11]

There are clear differences in pubertal development in male and female artistic gymnasts, differences that are associated with adequacy of energy intake. Although female gymnasts display delayed menarche and delayed pubertal development, the male gymnasts' developmental patterns appear normal.[12] But there are exceptions to the occurrence of developmental delays in female athletes. A study of British female synchronized swimmers (a subjectively scored sport where appearance is important) found that this group is relatively free of menstrual disturbances associated with eating disorders. None of the 23 national-team members who were assessed had amenorrhea, and only 3 of the 23 had oligomenorrhea.[13]

The traditional view of eating disorders (see figure 12.5) is that a combination of genetic, social, and psychological factors create the basis for their development. In athletes, however, there may be yet another important factor in the development of eating disorders involving a desire to perform well athletically. Because attainment of an ideal weight and body composition is critical for high-level sports performance,

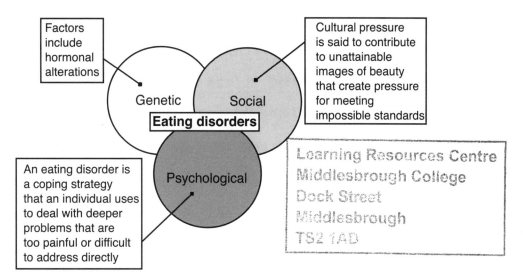

Figure 12.5 The various causes traditionally believed to contribute to an eating disorder.

many athletes are predisposed to placing themselves on restrictive intakes. Restrictive intakes in athletes, particularly female athletes, are common. In a study of male and female collegiate athletes, 23 percent of the males and 62 percent of the females had inadequate energy intakes because they wanted to lose weight.[14] However, because restrictive intakes lower the metabolic mass, this makes it more difficult for athletes to eat normally without gaining weight, so they are forced into lower and lower caloric intakes that, ultimately, cause them to develop eating disorders.

The most common eating disorders among these athletes are anorexia nervosa, bulimia, and anorexia athletica; in female athletes, these conditions often manifest themselves with low bone density and amenorrhea, referred to as the female athlete triad. Athletes and coaches should be sensitive to the warning signs of eating disorders, which include the following:[15]

- Preoccupation with food
- Preoccupation with weight
- Frequently stated concerns about being fat
- Frequent criticism about the eating patterns of teammates
- Going to the bathroom during or after meals
- Complaints about feeling cold
- Use of laxatives
- Frequently eating alone
- Additional exercise outside the normal training regimen

Anorexia Nervosa and Anorexia Athletica

Anorexia nervosa and anorexia athletica are typified by restrained eating from a fear of becoming fat, with a resultant loss of weight that places these athletes at serious health risk. Individuals with anorexia athletica may have abnormal exercise patterns, including the desire to exercise while injured and compulsive exercise beyond the normal training regimens (see table 12.4).

The restrictive caloric intakes of anorexia are associated with lower bone density, a failure to reach a desirable peak bone density in adolescence, and an increased risk of stress fractures.[16] Although these conditions are serious in and of themselves, it should also be remembered that mortality rates from anorexia nervosa have been reported as high as 18 percent, usually attributable to fluid and electrolyte abnormalities or suicide (see figure 12.6 for possible relationships between energy deficits and disordered eating).[17, 18] Hormone replacement therapy (i.e., estrogen replacement) is a strategy for dealing with the sequelae of amenorrhea, but it seems logical to either decrease the intensity and duration of exercise or increase the caloric intake, or both, to return athletes diagnosed with this condition to an energy-balanced state. To successfully achieve this, athletes must understand that proper eating can better optimize athletic performance and appearance by encouraging muscle mass development while discouraging fat mass development.[19] It is important that athletes understand the difference between wanting to be "thin" and needing to be "lean."

Table 12.4   Criteria for Anorexia Athletica

Weight loss > 5% of expected body weight	Excessive fear of becoming obese
Delayed puberty (no menses by age 16— primary amenorrhea)	Restriction of caloric intake (diets < 1,200 calories)
Menstrual dysfunction (amenorrhea or oligomenorrhea)	Use of purging methods (vomiting, laxatives, and diuretics)
GI complaints	Binge eating
No medical illness explaining disorder	Compulsive exercising
Disturbance in body image	

Adapted, by permission, from J. Snudgot-Borgen, 1994, "Risk factors for the development of eating disorders in female elite athletes," *Med Sci Sport Exerc* 26(4): 414-419.

Bulimia Nervosa

Bulimia nervosa is characterized by compulsive eating binges, during which individuals consume enormous quantities of foods, followed by purging episodes through vomiting or laxative intake to rid themselves of the consumed foods. The bingeing–purging cycles of bulimia nervosa are often referred to as "gorge–purge syndrome." These athletes are often normal or near normal weight and, for this reason, may be more difficult to identify than those with anorexia nervosa. Symptoms include corrosion of teeth and gums (from frequent gastric acid exposure due to vomiting),

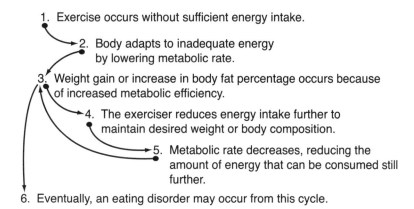

1. Exercise occurs without sufficient energy intake.

2. Body adapts to inadequate energy by lowering metabolic rate.

3. Weight gain or increase in body fat percentage occurs because of increased metabolic efficiency.

4. The exerciser reduces energy intake further to maintain desired weight or body composition.

5. Metabolic rate decreases, reducing the amount of energy that can be consumed still further.

6. Eventually, an eating disorder may occur from this cycle.

Figure 12.6   As this figure illustrates, there is a possible relationship between energy deficits and eating disorders.

Reprinted, by permission, from D. Benardot and W.R. Thompson, 1999, "Energy: The importance of getting enough and getting it on time." *ACSM's Health and Fitness Journal* 3(4): 14-18.

edema, electrolyte abnormalities, dehydration, depression, and excessive bathroom visits.[11]

Eating Disorders and Sports Performance

Although many athletes initially experience an improvement in sports performance with weight loss, this improvement is generally short lived if it was due to a drastic reduction in food intake. A major decrease in food consumption depletes energy and can be indicative of an eating disorder. Lower plasma volume, impaired thermoregulation, and lower glycogen storage are all associated with eating disorders and can lower the levels of anaerobic and aerobic endurance.[20, 21]

In addition, lowered food intake also predisposes athletes to multiple micronutrient deficiencies that can lower athletic performance and increase the risk of injury. This is evidenced when examining the abnormal menstrual patterns that often accompany eating disorders. Females who have stopped menstruating have lower levels of calcium in their bones, increasing their risk for stress fractures. The menstrual abnormalities correlate to a negative balance of energy and are also associated with a lower resting-energy expenditure, which is typically the result of a decreased metabolic rate and lean mass.[22]

Body composition can be a useful tool in helping the athlete and coach understand the changes that are occurring as a result of training and nutrition factors. Health professionals involved in obtaining body composition data should focus on using the same technique with the same prediction equations to derive valid comparative data over time. Care should be taken that body composition values are used constructively as part of the athlete's total training plan. Ideally, the emphasis should be on a periodic (semiannually or quarterly) monitoring of the athlete's body composition to determine change of both the lean and fat mass. Many athletes are sensitive about body fat, so care should be taken to use body composition values in a way that enables their constructive use in an athlete's general training plan. Athletes suspected of having an eating disorder should be quickly assessed and treated if necessary. It is likely that helping young athletes understand appropriate nutrition strategies for attaining a desirable body profile, weight, strength, and endurance will help reduce future eating disorder risk.

Part IV

Nutritional Strategies for Specific Energy Systems

13 Anaerobic Metabolism for High-Intensity Bursts and Power

Athletes in power events such as weightlifting, hammer throw, and shot put must maximize their potential for success by improving muscular strength, speed, and power. Power development is a function of the maximum amount of energy that a muscle can produce quickly and is largely dependent on the distribution and trained state of type IIa and type IIb muscle fiber. These muscle types can quickly produce power by simultaneously recruiting more fibers than type I fibers are able to recruit; type I fibers are more associated with endurance sports. Since athletes in power sports follow training regimens that increase their muscle mass, they have unique nutrition requirements for supporting or enlarging this mass. These athletes must consume enough energy so the nutrients, including protein, needed to support this larger mass are available for anabolic use and are not catabolized to meet energy requirements. In addition, eating strategies must be carefully planned so the consumed energy is available for muscular use at the time the muscles are in greatest need. Some power sports require "making weight," while others place a premium on gaining weight. However, the resultant weight loss or weight gain should always value the maintenance or increase of muscle mass. This chapter presents the full spectrum of nutrition tactics power athletes can employ to meet the specific needs of their sports, whether it is to increase mass to be a more competitive lineman on a football team, or to make weight for a wrestling competition.

Nutrition Tactics for Power Athletes

Different activities place special metabolic requirements on muscle systems, and these differences alter the nutrition requirements among athletes involved in various types of sports. Sports that require a high level of power and speed over short distances have a high anaerobic component. Athletes in these sports are not interested in their ability to move efficiently over long distances for long periods of time; they want to be there first in short distances. When a baseball player steals a base, there is virtually nothing about that 4- to 5-second experience that requires aerobic efficiency. The sprint to the next base is entirely dependent on anaerobic metabolism, which is almost entirely dependent on phosphocreatine and glycogen as fuels. Bodybuilders need explosive power to train but almost never place continuous stress on the muscles for longer than 1.5 minutes, which is the approximate time limit for anaerobic activities.

There has been an evolution in the way athletes eat to support top athletic performance. Around AD 200, Diogenes Laertius wrote that the training diet of Greek athletes of the time consisted of dried figs, moist cheeses, and wheat products.[1] American Olympians at the Berlin Games of 1936 had a daily intake that included beefsteak, lots of butter, three eggs, custard, 1.5 liters of milk, and as much as they could consume of white bread, dinner rolls, fresh vegetables, and salads. With each successive Olympic Games, athletes have consumed certain foods and avoided other foods depending on the state of nutrition knowledge. Since the 1960s, however, there has been a purposeful scientific effort to learn what athletes need and why they need it. This scientific endeavor has led to a much-improved understanding of how muscles work for power and how they work for speed. The science of sports nutrition has also helped us understand the different nutrition demands associated with different types of activities. A failure to consider the nutrition implications of the activity will most certainly lead to problems in training and to performance outcomes that are below the capabilities of the athlete.

Our current knowledge of nutrition requirements for anaerobic activity is substantial, with the clear understanding of what it is that muscles use in this type of activity: phosphocreatine and glycogen. Of course, there is also a question of how to obtain and sustain the larger muscle mass typically needed by athletes involved in anaerobic activity, and the answer to this question is also known: more calories. However, despite the well-established nature of these facts, anaerobic athletes place an unyielding focus on protein intake to satisfy the phosphocreatine, glycogen, and muscle requirements of their activities.

Anaerobic Metabolic Pathways

Athletes have the capacity to obtain a limited amount of energy quickly without oxygen. Events that are predominantly anaerobic (i.e., they require maximal power and energy over a limited period of time) rarely last longer than 90 seconds because the anaerobic energy supply would be exhausted. In some anaerobic events, such as boxing, each round is followed by a period of rest to allow the cells to prepare for the next bout of intense work. What follows is a description of the anaerobic metabolic pathways.

Phosphocreatine (Phosphagen) System

Anaerobic metabolic processes supply ATP from phosphocreatine (PCr) and glycolysis without oxygen. The in-muscle concentration of preformed ATP is 25 to 33 percent of the concentration of PCr. The enzyme creatine kinase can break apart PCr into inorganic phosphate and creatine, with a resultant release of energy. The free inorganic phosphate is united with ADP to reform ATP. The breakdown of PCr is not reversible until energy is obtained from other sources (mainly through oxidative metabolic processes). The volume of energy that can be supplied by the breakdown of PCr is vast, and it can be produced instantaneously. However, the length of time that this high volume of energy can be supplied is never greater than 10 seconds because of the limited amount of PCr stored in tissue. The formation of energy from PCr breakdown is directly linked to the intensity of exercise: The higher the exercise intensity, the greater the reliance on PCr breakdown as a source of energy. Athletes performing maximal exercise for 8 to 10 seconds (sprint, vault, jumps) must take a break of 2 to 4 minutes to allow for the regeneration of PCr before undertaking another maximal bout of exercise.

Creatine monohydrate supplementation is popular because athletes want to increase the storage of PCr, with the hope of increasing both capacity and power.

Glycolysis (Glycolytic System)

Glycolysis refers to the anaerobic breakdown of glucose or glycogen for energy. As indicated in table 13.1, there is a delay of 5 to 10 seconds after the initiation of activity before the glycolytic system can supply energy to working tissues. The six-carbon glucose molecule is phosphorylated and broken into two three-carbon molecules (glyceraldehydes-3-phosphate, or G3P). Each molecule of G3P is converted into pyruvate with the formation of ATP. The glycolytic reaction creates two molecules of ATP for each molecule of glucose; it creates three molecules of ATP for each molecule of glucose if glycogen is the initial substrate. The pyruvate may be converted to acetyl-CoA for later storage as fat or conversion to lactate. In either case, the fat or lactate created from pyruvate can be oxidative sources of energy. As indicated in table 13.1, glycolysis has half the power to create energy as the PCr system but has three times the capacity. The combination of PCr and glycolysis can support

Table 13.1   Capacity and Power of Anaerobic Systems for Producing ATP

System	Capacity (mmol ATP/kg)	Power (mmol ATP/kg)	Delay time
Phosphocreatine system	55-95	9.0	Instant
Glycolytic system	190-300	4.5	5–10 sec
Combined	250-370	11.0	–

Adapted, by permission, from M. Gleeson, 2000, Biochemistry of exercise. In *Nutrition in sport*, edited by R.J. Maughan (London, England: Blackwell Science), 22-23.

predominantly anaerobic maximal work for approximately 90 seconds, often referred to as the anaerobic maximum.

A Sampling of Sports Relying on Anerobic Metabolism

Anaerobic sports require maximal effort over relatively short periods of time. Imagine a baseball player swinging the bat or running to first base; imagine a gymnast sprinting down the runway to perform a vault. In both of these cases the athlete is using mainly existing energy stores that are both limited and easily depleted. You could never imagine a baseball player running to first base, back to home, and back to first base over and over again for 30 minutes with the same power and speed shown while running to first base a single time because it is physiologically impossible to do so. Nor could you ever ask a gymnast to repeatedly perform the floor routine over and over again without a break because it would be impossible to do. What follows is a sampling of sports that have these special characteristics: They involve extreme intensity performed with breaks between each bout of intense effort.

Baseball

Baseball is a wonderful sport that requires an almost equal combination of teamwork and individual effort. It's also a highly mental game, requiring that the athlete stay constantly alert to make split-second judgments for the right play. It's safe to say that physically tired baseball players are also likely to be mentally tired (glucose is the fuel for both the brain and muscles) and prone to bad judgment and poor physical performance. David Halberstam, in his book *Summer of '49* (New York: William Morrow, 1989), describes the 1949 pennant race between the Red Sox and Yankees. A central theme of this book is how players get worn out during the long baseball season, with the outcome of the pennant race determined, to a degree, by the number of players who remain relatively fresh by the end of the year. Clearly, many factors contribute to wear players down during a long season, including frequent travel, hard-fought games, and constant time-zone changes.[2] Nutrition factors also come into play: The foods and fluids consumed over the long summer and fall season do make a difference in the outcome. When steak and beer are constantly on the menu, as was common for many baseball players in the past, it is predictable that physical and mental fatigue will eventually take its toll. Alcohol interferes with B-vitamin metabolism (and therefore energy metabolism) and also increases dehydration risk. Red meat is a useful means of supplying good-quality protein, iron, and zinc, but it should not be the focus of a baseball player's diet. What baseball players really need is plenty of bread, cereal, fruits, and vegetables to constantly replace the glycogen used up in the quick and powerful actions of the game, as well as enough calories to support their muscle mass. Keeping this in mind, baseball players must consider the following nutritionally relevant factors for their sport.

As a primarily summer sport, baseball is often played in a hot and humid environment. Optimally hydrated muscles are composed of more than 70 percent water, and it should be the athlete's goal to maintain this optimal hydration state. A failure to do so will lead to a progressive reduction in total body water with a concomitant reduction in athletic performance. Evidence suggests that poor hydration makes an athlete more prone to injury by reducing mental function (poor hydration is associated with higher core temperatures that can reduce coordination) and by making muscles less resilient (thus increasing the risk of muscle tears and pulls).

Baseball players (particularly pitchers) are known to experience a reduction in peak torque arm strength between pre- and postseason measurements, with some of this

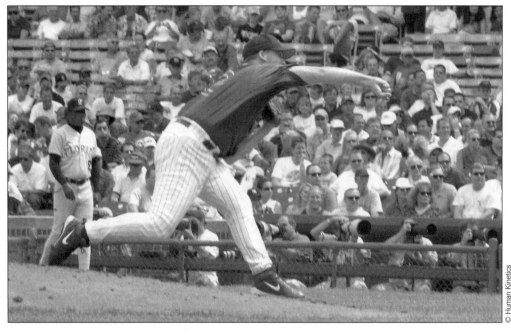

© Human Kinetics

Baseball players, especially pitchers, need to continually replenish their glycogen storage as continued play drains mental and physical ability, resulting in poor play.

power reduction caused by overuse injury to the pitching arm.[3] Reduced throwing power could also be due to reduced leg strength, which could negatively alter the throwing motion and exacerbate the risk of injury.[4] It seems likely that the degree to which the progressive reduction in power occurs could be reduced with a regular program of optimized hydration and energy intake.[5]

A study of baseball players strongly suggests that conditioning plays an important role in the ability of the athletes to maintain an optimal hydration state. At fixed exercise intensities, the better-conditioned baseball players were able to maintain body temperature with a lower sweat rate than that of players who were less fit.[6] Another study found that blood flow to the pitching arm (in pitchers) increased up to 40 pitches but steadily declined after that. By the 100th pitch, blood flow to the pitching arm was 30 percent below baseline.[7] The decrease in blood flow to the pitching arm matches a decrease in the general hydration state of the pitchers. Since it is established that blood volume is a key factor in the maintenance of athletic performance, the performance of pitchers may be strongly influenced by their ability to stay hydrated.

Given the possibility of frequent exposure to hot and humid environments, baseball players should consider the following strategy for maintaining their hydration state:

1. During the preseason, weigh yourself before and after each game and practice to learn how much weight has been lost. Then determine how much fluid should be consumed during a typical game (1 pint of fluid equals 1 pound of body weight). The goal should be to drink enough fluids to maintain body weight (±1 pound) during the game. Different people have different sweat rates, so your drinking schedule is likely to be different from those of your teammates.

2. Drink plenty of fluids before each game (a minimum of 16 ounces 1 hour before the game, followed by a constant sipping of fluids).

3. Use each opportunity between innings to consume fluids. Since baseball involves multiple bouts of high-intensity movements, the drain on stored glycogen is high. Therefore, fluids consumed should be carbohydrate containing. Fluids containing a 6 to 7 percent carbohydrate solution are best both for replacing carbohydrate and for encouraging a fast fluid absorption.

4. Immediately after the game, eat and drink enough carbohydrate to reconstitute your glycogen stores and body water.

5. Avoid or limit the consumption of alcohol and caffeinated beverages. With sufficient intake, both alcohol and caffeine have a diuretic effect that could place an athlete in a negative water balance.

Baseball requires a combination of power and speed, both of which place a high reliance on phosphocreatine and carbohydrate (primarily glycogen) for muscular fuel. Phosphocreatine is synthesized from three amino acids (from protein), so an adequate intake of protein is necessary to ensure that sufficient phosphocreatine can be manufactured. However, the protein consumption must be in the context of an adequate total intake of energy (calories). It is easier for fully grown baseball players to obtain sufficient energy (baseball players reach their peak at around age 28).[8] However, younger players must supply enough energy to support the activity plus enough energy to support growth. Inadequate energy intake causes the consumed protein to be burned as a fuel, making it unavailable for use as a substrate for the manufacture of other substances, such as creatine. With sufficient energy, even a modest protein intake of between 1.2 and 1.7 grams per kilogram is sufficient to support the synthesis of creatine and support a stable or growing muscle mass. In the context of an adequate energy intake, baseball players should consume a diet that derives 60 to 65 percent of its energy from carbohydrate, 20 to 25 percent of its energy from fat, and 15 percent of its energy from protein.

Many games are played during the season, with several games played each week. This frequency of games and practices can easily lead to overtraining, with the associated problems of fatigue, weakness, and increased risk of illness. A key to limiting the impact of overtraining is adequate rest and the consumption of a high-carbohydrate diet to maintain muscle glycogen levels. It has been shown that daily practices or competitions will lead to a progressive reduction in muscle glycogen storage, with a related reduction in endurance and performance. Since baseball players are highly dependent on muscle glycogen as a fuel, a reduction in glycogen from inadequate carbohydrate intake would lead to a discernable lowering of performance with time.

Games typically last 2 to 3 hours. Normal blood glucose flux is approximately 3 hours. That is, from the time you finish eating a meal, blood glucose stays in the normal range for about 3 hours. After this, blood glucose falls below the normal range (80 to 120 milligrams per deciliter), a physiological event normally associated with hunger. In the exercising person, blood glucose is likely to fall below the normal range more quickly. Because blood glucose is an important factor in maintaining normal mental function, and is also important for delivering fuel to muscles that have exhausted stored carbohydrate, baseball players should take steps to maintain blood glucose during the entire game by consuming a carbohydrate-rich beverage at every opportunity.

Pitchers work harder when they're pitching than other players on the team, which is why they are able to pitch effectively only every three to five games. Pitchers are better able to maintain muscular power (both in the legs and arms) by maximizing glycogen storage and hydration state before and during each game. The principle of glycogen loading (a general tapering of activity coupled with a high carbohydrate and fluid intake—refer to chapter 6 for more detailed information) can be followed with starting pitchers because they typically have several days between starts.

The weight and insulating effect of the equipment worn by catchers adds to their energy and fluid requirements. Catchers are constantly in motion, working with the pitcher, and since they tend to play on a more frequent rotation than starting pitchers, it's safe to say that, pound for pound, catchers have the highest energy and fluid requirements of any of the baseball positions.

Bodybuilding

Bodybuilders strive for a physique that is the extreme of high muscle mass and low body fat. The low body fat is a necessary adjunct to performance, which requires a high level of muscular definition to achieve a high score. A high body fat level would mask the underlying muscle formation because approximately 50 percent of all body fat expresses itself subcutaneously. To achieve this high level of muscle mass, body-builders must place a high level of repetitive stress (typically via free weights and muscle-resistance equipment) on each muscle group. This is never done aerobically (i.e., low-level muscular force over long time periods). Instead, bodybuilders rely on high-intensity repetitions that rarely last longer than 30 seconds per muscle group and never last longer than 1.5 minutes. In preparation for competition, bodybuilders couple this hard muscle training with the consumption of extra energy to support an enlargement of the muscle mass or reduction of the fat mass.[9] Diets of bodybuilders are often high in protein and protein-related supplements and creatine.[10]

Once the muscle mass is enlarged, bodybuilders go into a second training phase that involves a reduction in energy coupled with a small aerobic component in the training.[11] This second phase is aimed at reducing body fat levels (particularly subcutaneous fat) to allow for a greater visual muscle definition. During the week before competition, bodybuilders typically decrease total energy intake and increase carbohydrate intake to glycogen load the muscles. There is also a great deal of fluid and sodium manipulation to aid in muscle definition. During this week, both fluids and sodium are typically restricted. There is evidence that fluid restriction is dangerous, particularly in younger bodybuilders, where both low blood potassium and phosphorus have been observed.[12] There is also evidence that the energy restriction common during the period immediately before the competition causes a loss of lean body (muscle) mass, suggesting that the energy restriction is counterproductive.[13]

Perhaps no sport is as prone to nutrition misinformation as bodybuilding. In a study evaluating advertisements in bodybuilding magazines, no scientific evidence was offered for 42 percent of the products for which beneficial nutrition claims were made. Only 21 percent of the advertised products had appropriate documentation to support their claims, and 32 percent of the products that had some scientific documentation were marketed in a misleading manner.[14] A study of male and female bodybuilders found widespread multidrug abuse (up to

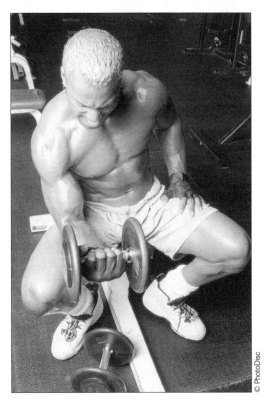

© PhotoDisc

For bodybuilders, extra energy must be consumed to support their larger muscle mass, but contradictory to the belief of many bodybuilders, consumed energy should be balanced between carbohydrate, fat, and protein—not just excess protein.

40 percent of the subjects), and a majority of bodybuilders reported following regimens that led to severe dehydration.[15] In this same study, the female bodybuilders had extremely low calcium intakes and nutrition practices that placed them, as a group, at high risk for poor health. Keeping this in mind, bodybuilders must consider the following nutritionally relevant factors for their sport.

Bodybuilders strive for a high level of muscle mass, a goal that mandates a higher need for energy. Although the total amount of protein needed to maintain this larger mass is slightly greater than what athletes with a stable muscle mass require, the proportion of protein provided by typically consumed foods is likely to satisfy need. Ideally, bodybuilders should consume between 1.5 and 1.7 grams of protein per kilogram of body weight, but this should be consumed in the context of adequate total energy consumption where most of the energy is derived from carbohydrates.

Studies of bodybuilders strongly suggest that protein consumption is usually much higher than the body's capacity to use it anabolically (i.e., to use it to build tissue). Therefore, the excess protein is simply burned as a fuel or, in the case of excess total energy consumption, stored as fat. This has been confirmed by the findings in one study, which determined that bodybuilders had significantly higher protein intakes than did lean control subjects, and they also relied more heavily on protein as a fuel to meet the energy requirements of the muscles.[16] The belief that the excess protein is a requirement for building muscle is pervasive among bodybuilders, but in truth, this extra protein is merely a source of needed calories that would be more efficiently provided through the non-nitrogenous energy substrates. The key to building muscle mass is to consume enough energy to support the larger mass. A bodybuilder now weighing 180 pounds (82 kilograms) who wishes to weigh 190 pounds (86 kilograms) should eat enough energy to support the larger mass. In doing so, the increase in calories should not come solely from protein but rather a proportionate increase in protein, carbohydrate, and fat where carbohydrates remain the major source of energy. Data from successful bodybuilders suggest that the ideal composition of diets should emphasize carbohydrates (55 to 60 percent of intake) and be relatively low in fat (15 to 20 percent of intake), with the remainder from protein (25 to 30 percent of intake).[17]

Bodybuilders strive for an extremely low level of fat mass. Body fat percentage is, to a great degree, determined by a person's genetic makeup but can also be influenced by dietary and exercise habits. From a dietary standpoint, it is most important to consume only enough energy to meet physiological need because excess energy intake will manifest itself as stored fat. Dietary fat is the most concentrated source of energy, so consumption of excess fat may most easily create an excess total energy intake, and it is easily converted to stored fat. Carbohydrates are more efficiently burned as a fuel for high-intensity muscular work and are not as efficiently converted to fat for storage. For these reasons, fat intake should be kept relatively low (15 to 25 percent of total calories). This level of intake is slightly below the general population recommendation that no more than 30 percent of total calories be provided from fat. The consumption of small and frequent meals is also a useful strategy because it helps suppress the manufacture of fat by lowering the insulin response to food. If you eat 1,500 calories in a single meal, the normal processing of so much energy at one time will inevitably lead to an important percentage of this intake being stored as fat. Were this 1,500-calorie meal to be consumed in two meals that are 3 hours apart (750 calories per meal), the energy could be more effectively processed without storing a significant proportion of it as fat. Therefore, eating the right amount of calories to maintain an energy-balanced state (something that is easier on a moderately low-fat diet) and eating small but frequent meals are both important strategies for obtaining a low body fat percentage.

Bodybuilders commonly go through repetitive patterns of weight gain and weight loss in an attempt to build muscle and then reduce body fat levels. The average reported weight loss experienced during the competitive season is 15 pounds (6.8 kilograms), and the average reported weight gain is 14 pounds (6.3 kilograms). This cyclic dieting leaves bodybuilders with a food preoccupation that leads to binge eating after competitions, as well as psychological stress.[18] A much more logical approach to building muscle safely is to consume a moderate excess in calories (300 to 500 calories beyond current needs) from complex carbohydrate to support a larger muscle mass, coupled with activities that sufficiently stress the muscles to encourage their enlargement.

Bodybuilders appear to be excessively dependent on nutritional and quasi-nutritional products and ergogenic aids to achieve the desired body composition. Self-experimentation with ergogenic aids and nutritional products is common in many sports. However, bodybuilders are especially targeted by marketing efforts for these products. To make matters more complex, the placebo effect in nutrition is very real. That is, if an athlete believes a product will help him or her meet specific goals, then it probably will have some benefit even if there is no physiological or biological basis for this improvement. Ideally, athletes should consume products and foods that have a physiological and biological basis for achieving their goals. If the athletes also believe these products and foods work, they may realize an even greater benefit (i.e., the placebo effect).

It is common for bodybuilders to rely on strategies that increase body water loss to achieve the desired cut appearance. Dehydration is dangerous (numerous deaths occur yearly from dehydration, among both athletes and nonathletes) and diminishes athletic performance. With bodybuilders, even though it is important to have a "cut" appearance, achieving this through dehydration is an unacceptable strategy because it can lead to organ failure and death. Bodybuilders should achieve their desired appearance through hard work and the development of a relatively low level of body fat using the strategies discussed already.

Nutrient intake appears to be inadequate for many in this population. The focus on nutritional products (protein powders and shakes, amino acid supplements, creatine monohydrate supplements, and so on) rather than nutrient-rich foods may place bodybuilders at nutrition risk. Consumption of low-fat, high-carbohydrate, moderate-protein foods that provide adequate energy (calories) will ensure a good nutrient intake. An excessive reliance on supplements appears to provide an unnecessarily high protein intake and may not satisfy the nutrients most lacking in the diets of these athletes. Blindly consuming individual vitamin and mineral supplements is also not a useful strategy because athletes rarely know what specific nutrients are most needed. Consumption of a wide spectrum of foods that exposes these athletes to all the nutrients is the best strategy, with supplements playing a role only where the adequate intake of energy substrates or nutrients is impossible.

Football (American)

Football is the epitome of an anaerobic sport, with the length of plays almost never exceeding 15 seconds, followed by a rest period between each play. However, when the ball is in play, the players are giving maximal muscular effort to move, or stop the movement of, the ball. Football players also carry the extra burden of heavy equipment, which adds to the energy requirement. The fuels most used in this type of activity are phosphocreatine and muscle glycogen, making the traditional "steak and potato" pregame meal less than ideal for ensuring an optimal storage of muscle glycogen because there is a relative overemphasis of protein (steak) and a relative underemphasis of carbohydrate (potato). Football players are in need of nutrition education, particularly on the use of dietary supplements.[19] A study of college football players found that supplementing with creatine monohydrate had a performance-enhancing effect by improving lifting volume and repeated sprint performance.[20] Another study of football players found that creatine supplementation was useful for enhancing peak force and maximal strength.[21] However, findings from this and other studies should be reviewed carefully before embarking on a path of ergogenic-aid supplementation because the total energy intake adequacy of the subjects in this study was not evaluated. It is unclear, therefore, if the apparent benefit of creatine monohydrate supplementation would be sustained if the total energy intake of the football players was adequate. In one of the few studies assessing the safety of long-term creatine supplementation, creatine monohydrate showed no long-term detrimental effects on kidney or liver function in the absence of other supplements.[22]

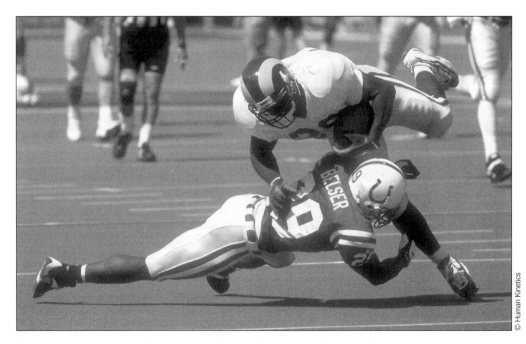

© Human Kinetics

The stop-and-go anaerobic nature of football increases the need for strictly monitoring fluid intake and fluid loss on, and off, the football field.

In another study evaluating nutrient supplementation on athletic performance, football players who consumed chromium picolinate supplements for 9 weeks experienced no improvement in either body composition or strength when compared with a group of football players who did not supplement.[23]

The stop-and-go nature of football, which vacillates between bouts of maximal effort and rest during a game, is also associated with a high level of body water loss. This loss of body fluid negatively affects cooling ability, athletic performance, and concentration.[24] A study of the consumption of carbohydrate-containing beverages among football players showed that these beverages were better able to maintain plasma volume than water alone.[25] Since maintenance of plasma volume is strongly associated with athletic performance, football players should consider consuming a well-designed sports beverage to maintain endurance and performance. Adequate fluid consumption before, during, and after games and practices should be an important part of the training regimen.

Football players at every level have recently been getting bigger and stronger each year and have a relatively positive body image when compared with other male athletes.[26] In a survey of high school all-American football teams from 1963 to 1971 and from 1972 to 1989, significant increases were found in the ratio of weight to height (body mass index) in the 1970s and 1980s that did not exist earlier.[27] In other words, football players are getting heavier (relative to their heights) at a rate much higher than existed before 1963.

Increased weight by itself may not be a good thing for football players. One study found that football linemen with higher body fat percentages and higher body mass indexes had higher rates of lower-extremity injuries.[28] In another study, football players with higher body fat levels had a 2.5 times higher relative risk of injury than those with lower body fat levels.[29] In addition, an unexpectedly high rate of obesity was found among adolescent football players. Since body image is inversely related to body fat percentage in male athletes (i.e., higher body fats are associated with poor body image), it is important to help athletes understand how to increase weight properly if higher weight is desirable.[30] Taken together, these findings strongly suggest that increasing lean (muscle) mass rather than simply increasing weight should be a priority for football players.

Many have questioned whether the recent increases in player size are due to improved preselection in a sport that attracts larger individuals, improved nutrition, or an increased reliance on anabolic steroid hormones. It is possible, of course, for all or any combination of these factors to contribute to the recent increases seen in the body mass index. Football players appear to be eating better than their non-football-playing counterparts. In a study of junior high school and high school football players, it was found that, in general, their nutrient and energy intakes were better than those seen in the U.S. population of same-age boys.[31] Energy intakes, which are often below recommended levels in other sports, appear to meet close to 94 percent of the requirement in the assessed football players. One nutrient found to be low in this study was zinc. In another study of football players, low zinc levels negatively affected maximal workloads. Since zinc is most easily obtained through the consumption of red meat, football players should consider a regular consumption of meat. However, meat consumption should not interfere with or replace the consumption of carbohydrates, which are essential for maintaining performance in stop-and-go activities. Vegetarians may be at higher risk for inadequate zinc intake, so they should be assessed by a qualified medical professional to determine if zinc supplements are warranted.

Weight loss is often an issue for lightweight football players. These players, who must maintain weight below a given threshold to be eligible to play, often display eating patterns that are unhealthy. In one study, 20 percent believed their weight-control practices frequently interfered with their thinking and other activities, and 42 percent had a pattern of dysfunctional eating. Almost 10 percent of those surveyed were practicing binge–purge (bulimic) eating behaviors.[32]

As with athletes in other professional sports, time-zone changes make a difference in performance outcomes. It has been found, for instance, that when games are played at night, west coast teams have a clear advantage over eastern and central time-zone teams.[33] The west coast teams feel as if they're playing earlier in the day relative to the other teams, so they do not suffer from end-of-day fatigue to the degree that other teams do. West coast teams have a 75 percent and 68 percent winning percentage when playing central and east coast teams, respectively, and still maintain a high winning percentage even when playing in away games (approximately 68 percent). These data strongly suggest that football players who travel across time zones to play should do whatever it takes to return to normal circadian rhythms. Among the positive actions that players can take are eating small amounts of foods frequently and consuming plenty of fluids during travel. Keeping this in mind, football players must consider the following nutritionally relevant factors for their sport.

Football requires a high level of strength and speed of short duration but high frequency. Football players are involved in activities that require repeated bouts of high effort interspersed with periods of rest. This type of activity requires a high level of carbohydrate to properly fuel the muscles. Therefore, football players should enter the game with their muscle glycogen levels full. However, even with muscle glycogen storage at its peak, a player cannot play an entire game without depleting muscle glycogen in specific muscle groups. Therefore, football players should take every opportunity to consume a carbohydrate-containing beverage during breaks in the game.

Linemen require a high mass. Although high mass affords linemen a clear advantage, the ability to move the mass quickly is equally important. Therefore, linemen should strive for a high level of muscle mass rather than just higher weight. To achieve this, consumption of a diet that meets the energy requirements plus 300 to 500 calories for the higher mass is needed, along with a relatively low intake of fat (less than 25 percent of total calories) and a moderate intake of protein (12 to 15 percent of total calories or about 1.5 grams of protein per kilogram of body weight). This type of diet, coupled with exercise that places stress on the muscles, helps enlarge the muscle mass. Increasing total energy intake through the consumption of a high level of fatty foods greatly enables an increase in fat storage (and therefore mass), but fat does not contribute to strength. Thus, fatty foods negatively alter the strength-to-weight ratio and make it more difficult for a lineman to move quickly and powerfully off the line.

Backfield defensive positions and pass receivers require high agility, speed, and quick reaction time. High speed and agility require a relatively low level of body fat. Therefore, these football players should have an eating pattern that limits fat storage (i.e., a high-carbohydrate, low-fat intake with the consumption of small, frequent meals). Since multiple 40-yard sprints down the field to catch (or defend against) long passes will quickly deplete muscle glycogen storage, consumption of carbohydrate-containing beverages at natural breaks during the game is desirable. During hot and humid days, consuming these beverages will also enhance the ability to maintain a desirable hydration state.

Repeated high-intensity activity while carrying equipment (e.g., pads, helmet) translates into high sweat losses. The fluid in sweat must be replaced to maintain optimal performance. To do this, consumption of sports beverages that contain a 6 to 7 percent carbohydrate solution are useful for maintaining the body's water level and replenishing carbohydrate fuel. When assessed, athletes typically place themselves in a state of voluntary underhydration, so there is every reason to set up a strategy that makes football players consciously consume fluids during every possible break in the game.

Gymnastics

The number of young gymnastics competitors continues to increase, so it is especially important that growth, weight, bone health, eating behavior, and other developmentally important factors be carefully monitored. In gymnastics, small athletes have become the norm, and gymnasts themselves commonly view this small body image as ideal. Weight is a prevailing theme in gymnastics, regardless of the gymnastics discipline. Even in men's gymnastics, it is suggested that controlling energy intake to achieve lower weight is an appropriate and desired approach if a gymnast is to achieve success.[34] However, growth in children is expected, so there should be a concomitant expectation of increasing weight. Not recognizing this fact, many young gymnasts may try to achieve a low weight through unhealthy means. There is evidence that the delayed puberty and growth found in female gymnasts are most probably associated with an inadequate caloric intake.[35, 36] Of course, inadequate caloric intake is associated with nutrient intake, and female gymnasts are at a particularly high risk of nonanemic iron deficiency, which could diminish health and performance.[37] Although it is true that lowering excess body fat will reduce body mass and, perhaps, lower the risk of traumatic injuries to joints, trying to achieve this through inappropriate means may also place the gymnast at risk.[38]

Elite-level gymnastics has four separate disciplines, including men's artistic gymnastics, women's artistic gymnastics, women's rhythmic gymnastics, and women's rhythmic group gymnastics. Although the total time spent in gymnastics practice is high for elite gymnasts (up to 30 hours of practice each week), the actual time spent in conditioning and skills training is considerably less. Gymnasts begin practice with a series of stretches and then initiate a series of basic skills on the floor mat as part of the warm-up routine. After warm-up, each gymnast takes a turn practicing one of the events. The time performing a skill in practice never exceeds that of the

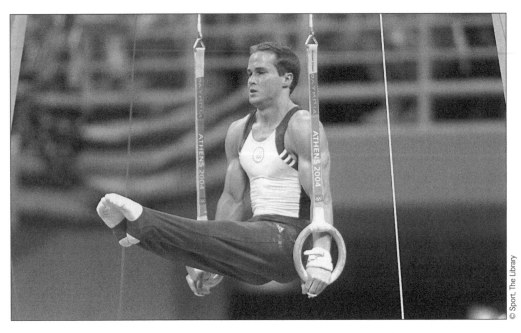

Male gymnasts, along with their female teammates, also run the risk of consuming inadequate amounts of energy, iron, and calcium when training to achieve a strong and lean build.

competition maximum and is usually a small fraction of it. Because practice involves repeated bouts of highly intense, short-duration activities, gymnasts rest between each practice bout to regenerate strength (i.e., regenerate phosphocreatine). With the exception of the group competition in rhythmic gymnastics, none of the events within each of these disciplines lasts longer than 90 seconds. This maximal effort and short duration categorizes gymnastics as a high-intensity, anaerobic sport.

As anaerobes, gymnasts rely heavily on type IIb (pure fast twitch) and type IIa (intermediate fast twitch) muscle fibers.[39] These fibers, while capable of producing a great deal of power, are generally regarded as incapable of functioning at maximal intensity for longer than 90 seconds. Type II fibers have a low oxidative capacity, which limits fat usage as an energy substrate during gymnastics activity, and a poor capillary supply, which deprives these fibers of nutrient, oxygen, and carbon dioxide exchange during intensive work. Because of these factors, gymnastics activity is heavily dependent on creatine phosphate and carbohydrate (both glucose and glycogen) as fuels for activity.

A number of studies evaluating the nutrient intake of elite gymnasts have found inadequate intakes of energy, iron, and calcium.[40-42] Heavy gymnastics training and inadequate nutrient intake are implicated as causative factors in the primary amenorrhea experienced by many young gymnasts and may also contribute to the secondary amenorrhea experienced by older gymnasts.

Although inadequate calcium intake is associated with poor bone development and increased risk of stress fractures, inadequate iron intake is associated with anemia, a risk factor in the development of amenorrhea (see table 13.2).[43]

Table 13.2 **Amenorrhea Definitions**

Primary amenorrhea	A woman 18 years of age and older who has never had a period (delayed menses) is considered to have primary amenorrhea.
Secondary amenorrhea	A woman who has experienced menses in the past but is not currently experiencing periods over a span of time (several months or even years) is considered to have secondary amenorrhea.

Keeping this in mind, gymnasts must consider the following nutritionally relevant factors for their sport.

Gymnasts are required to perform difficult tumbling and acrobatic skills that are easier for smaller people to do. Artistic gymnasts are commonly small (30th percentile for height-to-age ratio) but extremely muscular (90th percentile for arm muscle circumference).[40] This tendency for small stature may be due to a self-selection in the sport (i.e., only those who are naturally small remain in the sport competitively because they tend to be more successful) or because of an inadequate nutrient intake. Both of these factors are possible, either together or separately. Gymnasts and gymnastics coaches know that the top gymnasts tend to be small, so many try to achieve this small size by reducing food intake. There are numerous problems with this strategy, not the least of which is the possibility of delayed growth, with resultant poor skeletal development. In the relatively few cases where this occurs because of an overzealous coach or a gymnast who has made severe cuts in food intake, the outcome may be grim, leading to life-threatening eating disorders. Luckily, however, the vast majority of gymnasts do very well in this sport, have a high self-esteem as a result of participating in this sport, thrive as adults, and have healthy families.

Unhealthy athletes do not remain competitive, so it's in everyone's interest to eat enough to sustain health and growth. Toward that end, gymnasts should think more about optimizing body composition rather than achieving an arbitrarily low weight. A difficulty arising from low-calorie dieting is that weight goes down more from a loss of muscle than from a loss of fat. At some point the muscle loss will inhibit the capacity of gymnasts to perform the required skills, and the downward spiral in the muscle-to-fat ratio may cause gymnasts to further reduce food intake. The progressive reduction in food intake can eventually lead to an eating disorder, with all the dangerous implications that this involves.

Gymnasts are sensitive to the strength-to-weight ratio both from appearance and performance standpoints. It is impossible to avoid the reality that appearance is a factor in how highly a skill is scored. High strength enables gymnasts to more easily accomplish the required skill, and the appearance of effortlessness is a factor in the score (i.e., it enables an artistic gymnast to look more artistic). Gymnasts are constantly being reminded to smile while in competition, emphasizing that the performed skills are easily accomplished. The key is to be sufficiently conditioned and strong, factors requiring a stable muscle mass, so the skills can be completed with ease.

In a number of countries there is concern that gymnasts start learning skills too early, when they should be focusing on conditioning. A well-conditioned athlete can learn a skill more quickly and with a lower risk of injury. However, there are tremendous pressures on coaches to demonstrate that the gymnasts are making progress, and the best way to do that is to put them in junior competitions. A more balanced approach that focuses mainly on conditioning early in the gymnast's career while delaying the introduction of specific gymnastics skills may improve the skills acquisition learning curve later on.

To improve conditioning, gymnasts must consume sufficient energy and nutrients to meet the combined demands of growth, maintenance, and improvement in musculature. The focus of gymnastics training should be on getting strong, with a relatively low body fat percentage, rather than on staying (or getting) small, and this can only be accomplished through a training program that satisfies nutrition needs.

Gymnasts and many other female athletes have delayed menarche, which may play a role in bone health. Gymnasts failing to achieve menses by age 16 should see a doctor to determine the cause and, if needed, to seek a remedy. There are many possible causes for a delay or cessation of menses:

- Low body fat
- Poor iron status
- High physical stress
- High psychological stress
- High cortisol level (cortisol is a hormone produced by the body to counteract the soreness created from activity; it is commonly high in athletes and interferes with estrogen production)
- Low energy intake

It is conceivable that gymnasts may have all of these factors. Regardless of the cause(s), a delay in menstrual onset may negatively affect bone health and increase the later risk of early osteoporosis development. To reduce the risk of delayed menstrual onset, gymnasts should periodically assess both iron status and body composition to ensure a maintenance or enlargement of the muscle mass with age.

The competitive peak for female gymnasts is commonly reached at about age 16 to 18. With the exception of figure skating and diving, it is difficult to conceive of athletes who achieve this level of accomplishment at such a young age. For this to occur, a tremendous amount of time must be spent in conditioning and skills acquisition while the athlete is in the adolescent growth spurt. The combination of training and growth during these years places a tremendously high nutrition burden on the athlete that cannot be properly met without careful planning. However, with appropriate nutrition planning, it is possible to meet the combined needs of growth, physical activity, and tissue maintenance. Gymnasts who follow a sound nutrition program look better, perform better, enjoy the sport more, and stay in the sport longer.

Hockey

Regardless of whether it's played by men or women, hockey is a no-holds-barred, high-intensity, full-effort sport. If you watch hockey closely, you'll notice that the athletes play in shifts, staying on the ice for roughly 1.5 minutes before the next shift takes the ice. This system allows hockey players to play at full tilt for the entire time they're on the ice, while the bench time allows for the regeneration of phosphocreatine so the players are capable of more quick-burst activity when they return to the ice. This intense effort is highly anaerobic and, therefore, highly reliant on phosphocreatine and glycogen stores. It is possible to make positive changes in the diets of hockey players that can help them maintain weight during the off-season and improve anaerobic endurance during the season.[44]

Findings from a study of elite Swedish hockey players found that the distance skated, the number of shifts skated, the amount of time skated within shifts, and the skating speed all improved with carbohydrate loading.[45] Another study reached a similar conclusion, suggesting that hockey performance would be enhanced by carbohydrate ingestion.[46] It was concluded that individual performance differences among hockey players are directly related to muscle glycogen metabolism, a finding confirmed in a study of seven professional hockey players. In this study, 60 percent of the muscle glycogen in the quadriceps muscles was burned during a single game.[47] Since hockey players frequently skate in practice or play on successive days, it is possible for muscle glycogen to become depleted on an inadequate carbohydrate intake. Data from this study reveal that most players consume a diet high in protein and low in carbohydrate, a diet that is guaranteed to cause fuel-supply problems in muscles working anaerobically.

Shifting away from a high-fat, high-protein intake toward one that is higher in carbohydrate is not easy, however, and may result in inadequate energy consumption because of the lower caloric density of carbohydrate compared with fat. A study in which hockey players were placed on a special reduced-fat, reduced-protein, higher-carbohydrate intake resulted in an inadequate total energy intake.[48] Therefore, if a switch is made from a higher-fat diet to one that is lower in fat and higher in carbohydrate, care must be taken that the total energy intake is sufficient to meet the athlete's needs.

Keeping this in mind, hockey players must consider the following nutritionally relevant factors for their sport.

Frequent games place a high demand on muscle glycogen, which requires the consumption of foods high in carbohydrate (60 to 65 percent of total energy) for glycogen replenishment. The strategies for optimizing glycogen storage must also be considered. The pregame meal should consist almost entirely of carbohydrates that are mainly starch based, such as pasta, potatoes, rice, breads, and cereals. Fruits, vegetables, and high-bran (i.e., high crude fiber) foods may increase gas production in the gut so should be avoided or consumed sparingly in the pregame meal. Every opportunity should be taken during games to provide carbohydrate-containing beverages during breaks in play and between periods. Postgame carbohydrate consumption during the first hour after the game is critical to capitalize on the circulating glycogen synthetase.[49] The

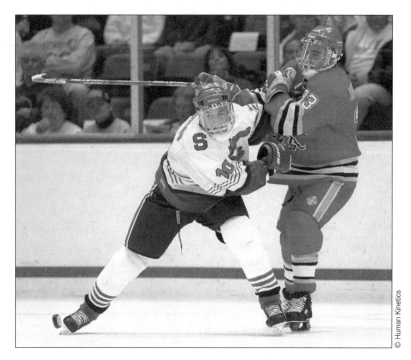

© Human Kinetics

Although hockey is a sport of speed and strength, the high-protein diets of hockey players need to be tailored to include more carbohydrate to compensate for glycogen loss during games.

typical food intake not associated with games or training should focus on starch-based complex carbohydrates, but the during-game and immediately postgame carbohydrates should be more sugar-based simple carbohydrates.

Changing food intake to provide more carbohydrates may result in inadequate energy consumption. Surveys of hockey players strongly suggest that usual energy intakes tend to be high in fat, high in protein, and low in carbohydrate, an energy substrate distribution that does not adequately support the type of energy metabolic processes associated with hockey. However, because of the higher energy concentration of fats, it is easier for hockey players to obtain the total amount of energy they need. For the same weight of food, fats provide more than twice the caloric content of carbohydrates (9 calories per gram versus 4 calories per gram). Therefore, making a switch to foods that are lower in fat and higher in carbohydrate while maintaining the same eating frequency may create a negative energy balance that could also be detrimental to performance.[50] Inadequate energy intake in physically active people guarantees a catabolism of muscle, an outcome that reduces athletic performance in a power sport. A possible solution to this undesirable outcome is to make certain that hockey players increase their eating frequency to six times per day (breakfast, midmorning snack, lunch, midafternoon snack, dinner, evening snack) to create more eating opportunities while fat is being reduced and carbohydrate intake is being increased.

High-intensity activity causes body temperature to rise quickly, with a concomitant rise in sweat rate. This fact, plus the amount of equipment worn by hockey players, places them at high risk of dehydration. Following a good hydration plan is critical, therefore, for success. Hockey players should consume plenty of fluids before the game and take every opportunity to consume fluids during and after the game. Given the need for carbohydrates and the need for fluids, a good strategy is to consume a carbohydrate-containing beverage whenever possible. (See chapter 3 for additional information on hydration protocols.)

Track and Field (Sprints, Jumps, and Throws)

Track and field competition includes a number of events of short duration that rely on power through anaerobic energy. Sprints and hurdle events include races up to and including 400 meters, while field events include jumps and throws of short duration and maximal effort. There is evidence that male and female sprinters, jumpers, and throwers have less than optimal nutrition habits, with a majority having below-standard intakes of at least one vitamin or mineral.[51] There is also evidence that stress fracture risk, considered an outcome of inadequate energy and calcium intake, is high in track and field athletes.[52]

It is hard to imagine an overweight sprinter, strongly suggesting that aerobic activity is not necessary for lowering body fat. A study assessing the fat-lowering impact of high-intensity versus low-intensity activity found that they were equally effective in lowering body fat.[53] Sprinting has been recommended as a normal component of interval training in many sports. Regardless of whether it's done for training or it represents the sport itself (as in the 100-meter dash), sprinting has specific energy requirements that must be accounted for and satisfied to perform optimally. Sprints, which by their very nature rarely last longer than 10 seconds, primarily use the fuels phosphocreatine and glycogen. Muscles with an adequate storage of phosphocreatine can support high-intensity exercise for 8 to 10 seconds, making it likely that most athletes use primarily phosphocreatine for the entire duration of the sprint. A study assessing creatine monohydrate supplementation found that it increased the muscular storage of phosphocreatine, promoted gains in fat-free (i.e., muscle) mass, and improved sprint performance.[54] This is consistent with a number of studies in other sports that produced similar findings.[55] Carbohydrate intake also makes a difference in sprint performance. In a study evaluating the impact of high-, moderate-, and low-carbohydrate intakes, the high-carbohydrate intakes produced better initial sprint performance than did lower carbohydrate intakes.[56]

In some sports, the "sprint" may be the difference between winning or losing even when the majority of time is spent on lower-intensity activities. For instance, 10K runners and marathoners run almost the entire distance at the highest pace at which they are capable of sustaining aerobic metabolic processes. At the end of these races, however, the athlete goes into a sprint pace (referred to as the "kick") that exceeds his or her oxidative capacity. A study emulating this high-pace aerobic running followed by an anaerobic kick found that a higher carbohydrate intake aided performance.

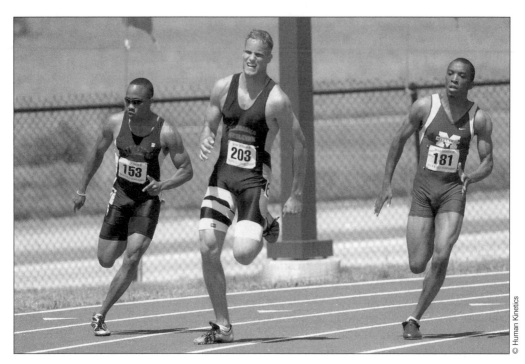

© Human Kinetics

Sprinters need to consume a diet high in carbohydrate but should not participate in any carbohydrate loading, as the body stores extra water with the extra glycogen, and the water weight may leave the sprinter feeling too heavy.

Over 4 consecutive days, a high carbohydrate intake, when compared with a moderate carbohydrate intake, was more capable of maintaining muscle glycogen in athletes working at a high intensity of aerobic capacity (~75 percent of $\dot{V}O_2$max) followed by five 1-minute sprints.[57]

Keeping this in mind, track and field athletes must consider the following nutritionally relevant factors for their sport.

Sprinting demands a large amount of phosphocreatine and carbohydrate fuels. By its very definition, a sprint requires the fastest possible movement over a short prescribed distance. Metabolic limitations control the maximum distance humans can sprint, and sprints never last longer than 1.5 minutes. During short sprints, there is a primary dependence on phosphocreatine as a fuel. It has been hypothesized that the ingestion of extra creatine, typically as a supplement in the form of creatine monohydrate, may improve phosphocreatine storage. (Refer to chapter 4 for more detailed information.) This increased storage of phosphocreatine could increase the number of short all-out sprints an athlete is capable of performing and might also improve the maximal time muscles can rely mainly on phosphocreatine as a fuel. There is evidence that supplementing with creatine monohydrate does, in fact, improve both sprint frequency and sprint distance. However, inherent design weaknesses are present in some of these studies, so athletes should refrain from jumping on the creatine supplement bandwagon. For instance, these studies did not evaluate the energy intake adequacy of the athletes, so the inherent limits of synthesizing creatine without adequate energy may have been inhibiting performance, a problem that could be more easily and cheaply resolved through a greater energy intake, preferably from carbohydrate. Also, the issue of the safety of frequent and long-term creatine monohydrate ingestion has not yet been adequately addressed.

Creatine is a normal constituent of the diet and is plentiful in meats (beef, pork, poultry, fish). Therefore, in the context of a high-carbohydrate diet, it seems useful for sprinters to consider consuming small amounts of lean meats regularly. For nonmeat eaters, care should be taken to consume sufficient protein and calories so the synthesis of creatine can occur in the body. However, even more important than protein intake is satisfying total energy requirements so the athlete is capable of synthesizing all the creatine needed to sustain optimal performance.

Pure sprinters may be inhibited by carbohydrate supercompensation, while endurance athletes may require carbohydrate supercompensation to support the end-of-race "kick." Pure sprinters must move their mass quickly over a relatively short distance, and the amount of mass that must be moved is a factor in how quickly it can be moved. Sprinters with high strength-to-weight ratios have advantages over those with lower strength-to-weight ratios. One of the effects of carbohydrate loading (or supercompensation) is to force more carbohydrate (glycogen) into the muscles so it is available for muscular work. Glycogen is stored with water in a 1 to 3 ratio. That is, for each gram of glycogen stored, the body stores 3 grams of water. At times, athletes who undergo a carbohydrate-loading regimen mention that they feel stiff and heavy. Clearly, this is not the way a sprinter should feel at the beginning of a race, but it is a perfectly acceptable feeling for long-distance runners. Therefore, pure sprinters should regularly consume a high-carbohydrate intake that provides sufficient total calories but should avoid any carbohydrate-loading regimen that might force additional glycogen and water into the muscles.

Swimming (100 to 400 Meters)

Perhaps there is no other sport where so much time must be spent practicing to gain such incrementally small levels of improvement. Swimmers spend a considerable amount of time in the water to perfect techniques that will better overcome drag and to improve their capacity to sustain both aerobic and anaerobic energy production. In the shorter (sprint) distances where races are typically less than 2 minutes in length, the majority of energy is predominantly derived anaerobically from phosphocreatine and glycogen (see table 13.3). Although these sprint races are short in duration, the amount of energy needed to sustain a high level of power output is tremendously high, and the majority of this energy (more than 55 percent) must come from glycogen and phosphocreatine.

The time spent training has a high energy and nutrient cost that must be considered when developing a training plan. A study of national developmental-training-camp swimmers found that the average energy (5,221 calories for males; 3,573 calories for females) and nutrient intakes were adequate, but there was a large between-swimmer

Table 13.3 **Relative Contribution of Aerobic and Anaerobic Energy Sources During Exercise of Different Lengths**

Time	Anaerobic %	Aerobic %
0-30 seconds	80	20
30-60 seconds	60	40
60-90 seconds	42	58
90-120 seconds	36	64
120-180 seconds	30	70
Expressed Cumulatively		
0-60 seconds	70	30
0-90 seconds	61	39
0-120 seconds	55	45
0-180 seconds	45	55

Note: As the exercise time increases, power production decreases and a greater proportion of energy is derived aerobically. Aerobic metabolism is less reliant on glycogen and phosphocreatine because of an ability to metabolize fat for energy.

Adapted, by permission, from D.R. Lamb, 1995, "Basic principles for improving sport performance," *GSSI Sport Science Exchange*, #55, 8(2).

variation in intake.[58] This variation, coupled with a tendency for these swimmers to consume excessive amounts of fat and insufficient amounts of carbohydrate, suggests that a large proportion of swimmers may have dietary habits that do not optimally support training and competition needs. In addition, there is evidence of poor iron status among female collegiate swimmers, which could compromise training and exercise performance.[59] The desire for higher-fat foods from meats and dairy products has been tested in male swimmers, and it was found that they tend to like the sensory appeal of fat-containing animal products, even when undergoing a high level of exercise.[60]

High-level swimmers, often high school students and college-age adults, must spend a great deal of time in the pool to gain a speed improvement, which commonly translates into multiple training sessions each day. Swimmers typically practice in the early morning and late afternoon (before and after school), and they generally accept that they must get an hour or two of laps in before classes begin (often at 5 A.M.) to have a chance of improving. The problem, therefore, is ensuring that swimmers consume enough energy at the right time and in the right form to make it supportive of the training plan. Ideally, swimmers should make the time between and during practices an opportunity to consume a significant amount of high-carbohydrate foods. However, swimmers must do this in a way that ensures the stomach is empty before getting into the water. This means that the focus, during practice and swim competitions, should be on carbohydrate-containing sports beverages. Having large amounts of solid foods shortly before getting into the water causes a fluid shift away from the muscles and into the GI tract and may cause cramping.

Keeping this in mind, swimmers must consider the following nutritionally relevant factors for their sport.

Swimmers train for many hours and have an intensive training protocol. Competitive swimmers work hard and long at getting better, and all that work translates into a tremendously high caloric need. Since swimmers often have an early-morning practice, it is important that they consume some carbohydrates immediately upon awakening to give the food or beverage enough time to leave the stomach before practice. A failure to consume at least 100 to 200 calories of carbohydrate before practice may limit the benefits the athlete could derive from practice.

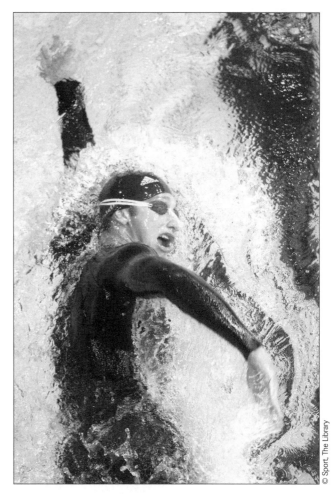

Elite male swimmers need to take in over 5,000 calories per day to adequately fuel their training and racing energy requirements.

Fluids (apple or grape juice or a sports beverage) are good to sip on during the trip to the pool. After the morning practice, swimmers should consume some high-carbohydrate breakfast foods (cereal, toast, bagel) that should be immediately available. This will help replenish the energy consumed during practice and begin the process of storing more energy for the afternoon practice. Also, because so much energy is needed, high school swimmers should seek approval from school administrators to consume a midmorning snack of 200 to 400 calories. Swimmers who practice sprinting in the pool should be aware that phosphocreatine (a major fuel for sprints) is likely to become depleted in muscle cells, and it takes time to regenerate the phosphocreatine to get the cells ready for the next sprint. When total sprinting time meets or exceeds 2 minutes, there should be a recovery period of up to 4 minutes to allow cells time to replenish the depleted phosphocreatine. A failure to allow for this recovery period will force the swimmer to work at a lower intensity and for shorter periods on subsequent sprints. If that happens, the swimmer will be learning to sprint in a way that could adversely affect competitive times.[61]

Some swimmers believe body weight reduction may be necessary to improve bathing suit appearance and reduce drag. The paper-thin material used for racing suits makes it impossible for swimmers to hide their physiques. Since everyone wants to look good, swimmers may be motivated to reduce body weight. However, many swimmers could easily experience a reduction in performance if weight loss results in a loss of muscle with a secondary loss of power. If weight were lost in a way that reduces drag, there could be a performance benefit, but most weight-loss strategies backfire and hinder performance. Therefore, swimmers wishing to lose weight to either look better or go faster (or both) should do so only under the direct supervision of a qualified health professional. Also, the focus should be on fat reduction and muscle maintenance rather than weight reduction per se.

Swimmers rely heavily on glycogen and phosphocreatine, and sprinting performance is highly dependent on carbohydrate (to make stored glycogen) and phosphocreatine. With sufficient total energy intake that focuses on carbohydrates (at least 30 calories of carbohydrate per kilogram of body weight) and the inclusion of an adequate amount of protein (about 1.5 to 2.0 grams per kilogram of body weight), there is every reason to believe that athletes can store enough glycogen and make enough phosphocreatine to properly fuel their muscles. However, there is tremendous motivation for athletes to consume creatine monohydrate supplements (a precursor to phosphocreatine) to gain a competitive edge. Although creatine monohydrate supplements may improve the number of high-intensity sprints a swimmer is able to do, swimmers should be aware that regular creatine consumption is associated with an increase in weight. Since this weight increase is likely to be from water, it could reduce buoyancy and increase drag. It is likely that a greater benefit could be achieved by creating opportunities to eat so as to ensure an optimal total energy intake.

Swimmers need to consume fluid. It is difficult to imagine that, with so much water around, swimmers could be at risk for dehydration. The fact that swimmers work in a hypothermic environment (water is usually colder than air temperature) makes it easier for the excess heat generated from muscular work to be dissipated. However, there are other good reasons for swimmers to consider whether their hydration state is adequate. A poorly hydrated athlete may develop a lower blood volume that causes the heart to work harder to bring oxygen and nutrients to cells, and there is less volume in which to place metabolic by-products. Also, many competitions take place outside, where swimmers spend a great deal of time waiting for their events, and where they can easily become overheated. Excess water storage could clearly cause a problem for swimmers by increasing weight and drag, but insufficient body water can influence performance and concentration. Therefore, a good rule of thumb is to constantly sip small amounts of water or sports beverage while avoiding strategies that could force an excess water storage (e.g., glycogen loading, glycerol, creatine).

Wrestling

Wrestling has been around as a sport for thousands of years. Early sculpted artifacts and paintings from France, Egypt, and ancient Babylon show wrestlers involved in holds that are essentially the same as those used today. In the early Olympic Games in Greece, the wrestling competition was the premier event.[62] The basic strategy in all this time has not changed: Wrestlers attempt to force the shoulders of the opponent onto the mat to win the match. If neither wrestler is able to score such a fall, the winner is determined by officials, who use a point system involving the provision of points for near falls, holding an opponent close to his back, and controlling the opponent.

In 1997, news coverage of the tragic deaths of three collegiate wrestlers initiated a needed discussion about the techniques used by wrestlers to "make weight." Jeff Reese, a University of Michigan junior, died of kidney and heart failure while working out in a rubber suit in a 92 degree Fahrenheit (33 degree Celsius) room so he could qualify for a lower weight class. Billy Saylor (19 years old and three-time Florida State champion) of Campbell University and Joseph LaRosa (22 years old) of the University of Wisconsin also died while trying to lose a large amount of weight to qualify for a lower weight class. The outrage resulting from these deaths has finally led to serious examination of the rules that encourage the manipulation of normal weight and the techniques used (supplements, dehydration, fasting) to achieve a weight well below the athlete's natural weight to permit qualification in a lower weight class. An important outcome of this discussion should be an improvement in the information wrestling coaches have about weight loss, sports nutrition, training diets, dehydration, and body composition. In surveys of wrestling coaches that evaluate knowledge in these areas, a high proportion

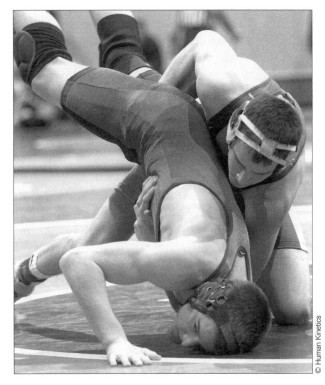

In light of major concerns about the hazards of "making weight" in the wrestling world, coaches and wrestlers need to be properly educated about healthy weight-loss strategies.

© Human Kinetics

of the coaches have a less-than-adequate knowledge level to provide appropriate guidance to young athletes.[63] The American College of Sports Medicine's position on weight loss in wrestlers states:[64]

> Despite a growing body of evidence admonishing the behavior, weight cutting (rapid weight reduction) remains prevalent among wrestlers. Weight cutting has significant adverse consequences that may affect competitive performance, physical health, and normal growth and development. To enhance the education experience and reduce the health risks for the participants, the ACSM recommends measures to educate coaches and wrestlers toward sound nutrition and weight control behaviors, to curtail "weight cutting," and to enact rules that limit weight loss.

The general goal of this weight-loss strategy (cutting) is to qualify for a weight class during a weigh-in on the night before a match and to gain as much weight as possible between the weigh-in and the match the next day. A survey assessing weight-loss practices of college wrestlers determined that 40 percent were following the new NCAA rules and curbing their risky weight-loss practices.[65] Although this is a positive outcome, the majority of wrestlers have maintained risky weight-loss behaviors. Sadly, there is evidence that wrestling at a weight below the predicted minimum wrestling weight appears to be associated with greater wrestling success.[66] But there is also evidence that successful weight gain during this short period is important for success. In one study evaluating the relative weight gains of wrestlers, the heavier wrestler was successful 57 percent of the time.[67]

There is concern on many levels about the weight-loss techniques commonly practiced by wrestlers. Some evidence suggests that undernutrition may lead to altered growth hormone production in wrestlers that, if present over several seasons, could lead to permanent growth impairment.[68] Another study determined that dietary restriction reduced protein nutrition and muscular performance.[69] These data are confirmed by findings indicating that weight loss by energy restriction significantly reduced anaerobic performance of wrestlers. Those on a high-carbohydrate refeeding diet tended to recover their performance, while those with lower intakes of carbohydrate did not.[70] Besides the obvious physiological changes that occur from rapid weight loss, there is good evidence that rapid weight loss in collegiate wrestlers causes an impairment of short-term memory, a fact that could affect scholastic achievement in these student athletes.[71]

Keeping this in mind, wrestlers must consider the following nutritionally relevant factors for their sport.

"Making weight" is a hazard to both performance and health. Ample evidence suggests that the weight cycling associated with making weight (i.e., weight loss to make weight followed by weight recovery for performance) is dangerous and can lead to glycogen depletion, a lower muscle mass, a lower resting energy expenditure, and an increase in body fat.[72] Should this occur with frequency, it is likely that the reduction in resting energy expenditure could make it more difficult for the athlete to achieve the desired

weight through dietary restriction, leading the wrestler to take more draconian (and more dangerous) measures to achieve the desired weight outcome. Wrestlers and coaches should follow a reasonable model for achieving desired weight, such as that offered by the Wisconsin Interscholastic Athletic Association, to avoid health and performance difficulties.[73] This program develops reasonable goals for weight and provides nutrition education information to help wrestlers achieve desired weight reasonably and to understand the implications of improper weight-loss methods. In these weight-achievement guidelines, a cap is placed on the maximum amount of weight change that can occur during the course of a season, and a monitoring system has been added to ensure that sudden and dramatic weight change does not occur at any point in the season.

The anaerobic nature of wrestling implies a high need for carbohydrate. Although there is an aerobic component to Olympic wrestling (matches may continue for 5 minutes without a break), high school wrestling is primarily an anaerobic sport (three 2-minute periods). The demand for carbohydrate in this type of activity is extremely high, and there is evidence that wrestlers perform better on high carbohydrate intakes. It is also of great concern that wrestlers commonly resort to dehydration as a means of achieving desired weight. Nothing could be more dangerous or more performance reducing than competing in a dehydrated state. Wrestlers should resist inducing dehydration because of the clear dangers (including organ failure, heatstroke, and death) associated with this strategy and should understand that well-hydrated athletes perform better than dehydrated ones.

Wrestlers and coaches should become better educated on the potential hazards of improper nutrition. Trying to achieve an arbitrarily low weight in growing athletes is disease inducing rather than health enhancing (the ultimate goal of sport). It is not acceptable to place a young athlete in harm's way to achieve a falsely low weight goal, especially since the achieved weight has nothing to do with the weight at which the wrestler actually competes. Everyone involved in the sport should endorse the development of widely accepted weight-to-height norms that can be applied reasonably to wrestlers. Further, weight should be taken immediately before the competition rather than at a time that permits drastic and dangerous shifts in eating behaviors. Until the rules change, wrestlers and coaches should all be made aware of the hazards associated with the current "making weight" procedures.

Athletes in sports involving maximal power and speed should focus on the provision of an adequate total energy intake, primarily from carbohydrates, so that sufficient glycogen can be synthesized and stored for muscular work. Since phosphocreatine and glycogen are the primary fuels for high-intensity activities, protein intake should also be sufficient (about 1.5 to 2.0 grams per kilogram of body weight) to ensure that creatine can be synthesized. There is increasing evidence that creatine supplementation can significantly improve performance in short-duration, high-intensity activity.[74] However, research design issues of many of these studies fail to clarify how athletes might perform with an adequate caloric consumption and if this might encourage a greater internal synthesis of creatine. Many athletes across a wide-ranging spectrum of sports have unsatisfactory nutrition habits that should be corrected before embarking on a strategy of supplementation.[75] Fluid intake is also important because it helps maintain blood volume, a critically important factor in athletic performance, and inadequate fluid intake limits glycogen storage and also makes it difficult to maintain body temperature. Coaches tend to overvalue proteins, are excessive in recommending low-fat diets, and often use food myths rather than facts in making dietary recommendations to athletes.[76] Athletes should always adapt their carbohydrate and fluid needs to their sports, but in the case of high-intensity, short-duration activities, the needs are almost always high.[77]

14 Aerobic Metabolism for Endurance

For endurance athletes, optimizing carbohydrate storage before competition, sustaining carbohydrate delivery during competition, and maintaining an optimal hydration state before and during competition are critical factors for achieving optimal performance. Surveys of endurance athletes indicate, on average, an inadequate consumption of calories, an overreliance on protein and fat, and an underreliance on carbohydrate needed for optimal performance. In addition, endurance athletes are only beginning to consider nutrition factors that will enhance muscle recovery after daily training sessions. Endurance athletes often train in ways that do not mimic competition (e.g., they rarely consume beverages every 5 kilometers during training, although this is a standard protocol in long endurance runs), making it difficult for them to fully adapt to the competition environment. This chapter presents strategies for optimizing carbohydrate storage in preparation for training and competition, as well as hydration strategies that can sustain blood volume and sweat rates. In addition, the chapter provides a review of commonly available hydration and energy products to help endurance athletes recognize the best products in a variety of different training and competition environments.

Nutrition Tactics

Endurance events such as road cycling, long-distance swimming, marathon, triathlon, and 10K run all require a high level of endurance and place a relatively low premium on anaerobic power. These events force competitors to perform at the margin of their maximal aerobic capabilities over long distances. As training, nutrition, and selection of athletes in endurance sports improve, records continue to fall. This suggests that doing the right things can and will result in moving the known envelope of speed in endurance events. The winner of the marathon at the Atlanta Olympic Games in 1996 won with an average running pace of slightly under a 5-minute mile, a feat that is not commonly achieved. Despite this incredible speed, the athlete had to maintain this pace at a level that allowed a sufficient oxygen uptake to sustain, primarily, aerobic muscular metabolism. That is, the majority of all muscular work took place with fuel being burned in the presence of oxygen. This is an efficient means of obtaining energy, allowing the athlete to sustain muscular work for long periods of time.

Aerobic training does some wonderful things to the athlete's ability to use oxygen. The intermediary (type IIa) fibers, which tend to behave more like fast-twitch (power) fibers than slow-twitch (endurance) fibers, dramatically increase in mitochondrial content and the in enzymes involved in oxidative metabolism. The training impact on oxygen usage is well known. In studies looking at blood lactate concentration, trained athletes are far more capable of tolerating high levels of blood lactate than are untrained subjects doing the same intensity of work. The conversion of the behavior of the intermediary fibers results in an improvement in the athlete's aerobic endurance. The increased ability to use oxygen results in an improvement in the ability to burn fat as a primary fuel, reducing the reliance on carbohydrates. As you can see in table 14.1, athletes in aerobic sports have a far better ability to use oxygen than do athletes in power sports.

Since even the leanest athletes have a great deal of energy stored as fat, this increased ability to

Table 14.1 Oxygen Uptake in Olympic-Level Athletes in Selected Sports

Sport	Maximal oxygen uptake (ml/kg/min)
Cross-country skiing (male)	84
Cross-country skiing (female)	65
Runners (male)	80
Runners (female)	58
Speedskaters (male)	77
Speedskaters (female)	54
Cyclists (male)	73
Rowers (male)	62
Weightlifters (male)	55
Sedentary (male)	43
Sedentary (female)	40

Adapted, by permission, from F.I. Katch, V.L. Katch and W. McArdle, 1993, *Introduction to nutrition, exercise, and health*, 4th ed. (Philadelphia, PA: Lea & Febiger), 179.

burn fat dramatically improves endurance. However, since carbohydrate is needed for the complete combustion of fat, carbohydrate is still the limiting energy source for endurance work because athletes have relatively low carbohydrate stores. This is clearly demonstrated by findings that athletes consuming a high-fat diet have a maximal endurance time of 57 minutes; on a normal mixed diet their endurance rises to 114 minutes; and on a high-carbohydrate diet, their maximal endurance rises to 167 minutes.[1]

Aerobic Metabolic Pathways

Aerobic metabolic pathways are the means we have for obtaining energy from fuels (carbohydrate, protein, and fat) in the presence of oxygen. The controlled release of energy during aerobic metabolism allows for a large amount of the energy in glucose to be stored as energy in ATP. The chemical reaction for the full oxidation of glucose produces energy, carbon dioxide, and water:

$$\text{Glucose} + 6 \text{ O2} + 38 \text{ ADP} + 39 \text{ Phosphate} = >6 \text{ CO2} + 6 \text{ H2O} + 38 \text{ ATP}$$
$$[\text{Glucose} = \text{C6H12O6}]$$

In anaerobic metabolism, pyruvate is converted to lactate. However, in the presence of sufficient oxygen, pyruvate can be oxidized for energy in the mitochondria (often referred to as the energy factories of the cells). Glucose, a six-carbon molecule, is converted to two molecules of pyruvate, a three-carbon molecule. When pyruvate enters the mitochondria, it undergoes further conversion to a two-carbon molecule to form acetyl-coenzyme A (commonly abbreviated to acetyl-CoA).[2] Acetyl-CoA can also be created from the beta-oxidation of fatty acids that reside in the mitochondria. During beta-oxidation, carbon is cleaved from the long carbon chains of fatty acids in two-carbon units. These two-carbon molecules form acetyl-CoA. The newly created acetyl-CoA from pyruvate or beta-oxidation of fats can be oxidized to carbon dioxide (CO2) in the tricarboxylic acid cycle (TCA).[3] The critical aspect of the TCA cycle is producing hydrogen atoms for transport to the electron transport chain. It is in the electron transport chain that oxidative phosphorylation occurs to create ATP from ADP. With sufficient hydrogen to feed into the electron transport chain and enough oxygen for oxidative phosphorylation, the electron transport chain can continuously produce energy in the form of ATP.

If there is excess production of acetyl-CoA (i.e., inadequate oxidative enzymes to process the acetyl-CoA for energy or inadequate oxygen delivery), the excess can be converted to either fat for storage or to the amino acid alanine. Alanine can be converted by the liver to glucose or can be made part of larger protein structures (see figure 14.1).

Anaerobic metabolic processes have the capacity to provide ATP energy immediately but only for a short duration, while aerobic metabolic processes begin providing ATP energy more slowly but for long durations, provided there is sufficient substrate and oxygen available to the cells. We have large stores of energy that we can call upon to create ATP energy for muscular work (see table 14.2).

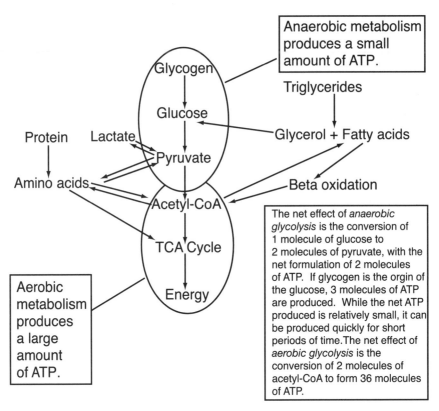

Figure 14.1 Substrate usage in energy pathways.

Table 14.2 Theoretical Average Energy Stores

	Mass (kg)	Energy (kcal)	Exercise time (min)
Liver glycogen	.08	306	16
Muscle glycogen	.40	1,529	80
Blood glucose	.01	38	2
Fat[a]	10.5	92,787	4,856
Protein	12.0	48,722	2,550

Note: There is increasing evidence that muscle triglyceride is an important energy source for endurance activity. However, it appears to increase under conditions that compete with glycogen storage. Should an effective means be found for increasing both muscle triglyceride and glycogen, this would have positive implications for endurance performance.[4]

Adapted, by permission, from M. Gleeson, 2000, Biochemistry of exercise. In *Nutrition in sport*, edited by R.J. Maughan (London, England: Blackwell Science), 29.

Of the energy stores available to us, fat is the most efficiently stored and provides the greatest mass from which we can derive ATP energy. Glycogen requires approximately 3 grams of water for storage, while fat storage is essentially anhydrous, making fat a more efficient form of energy storage. Muscle and liver glycogen stores represent a small fraction of the energy in fat stores but have the advantage of being able to be metabolized either anaerobically or aerobically, while fat can only be metabolized aerobically. Protein stores are from functional tissues that, under ideal conditions, would never be catabolized as a source of energy. Nevertheless, a small amount of protein (approximately 5 percent of total energy needs) does appear to be metabolized to meet energy requirements in most activities. In the absence of carbohydrate, protein stores are catabolized at a faster rate to provide a source of glucose (the amino acid alanine can be converted to glucose by the liver) and a source of acetyl-CoA and oxidative metabolism. However, this protein catabolism is not desirable and can be avoided with a regular supply of carbohydrates and adequate total energy consumption.

At the initiation of exercise, the majority of ATP is derived anaerobically. For highly intense, maximal-effort activities, the requirement for a high volume of energy mandates a continuous dependence on anaerobic processes. However, for lower-intensity activities the majority of ATP is initially provided anaerobically, but then the activity switches to aerobic metabolism to meet most ATP needs. Anaerobic and aerobic metabolic processes should be thought of as proceeding simultaneously, with the intensity of the activity determining the predominant metabolic pathway for the supply of ATP. High-intensity, maximal-effort activities rely more on anaerobic metabolism, while lower-intensity activities rely more on aerobic metabolism. Because far more energy is available to us aerobically (fat can only be metabolized aerobically), the high energy needs of endurance athletes force them to train muscles to be more aerobically competent. Cells of well-trained aerobic athletes have more mitochondria and more aerobic enzymes in the mitochondria, resulting in a higher capacity to derive energy aerobically.

Considerations for Endurance Sports

Endurance sports are those in which the predominant form of energy metabolism is oxidative (it occurs in the presence of oxygen). Aerobic athletes must be capable of acquiring and delivering enough oxygen to the working muscles to support the physical work that is being done. Endurance work occurs at intensities below a person's maximal work capacity. By definition, working at a higher or maximal capacity exceeds the athlete's capacity to meet oxygen needs. Sprinters, who are working at maximal capacity, can run very fast but only for relatively short distances. Endurance athletes can't run as fast as sprinters but can go much longer distances because they are metabolizing energy using a much more clean-burning and energy-efficient oxidative system. To maintain the efficiency of their systems, endurance athletes should consider factors that can influence their aerobic capacity, including overtraining, overuse injuries, and dietary adequacy.

Overtraining

A world-class runner wrote the following in an e-mail communication:

> I've just come off three weeks of particularly intense training. I went "hard" four days a week. I have plateaued and am now resting to allow my body to absorb all the good work I did but am still feeling a little bit lethargic. I sleep well but don't feel rested. My coach is concerned that I may have become anemic. As you know, my nutrition analysis has always come up good. Should I get some blood tests? Take iron? Take something else? I'm worried.

These signs are typical of an "overtrained" athlete who is suffering the consequences. Overtraining has some well-established warning signs, including increased muscle soreness, delay of muscular recovery, inability to perform at the previous training load, poor-quality sleep, decreased vigor, swelling of lymph nodes, high illness frequency, and loss of appetite. Many of these signs are a result of working at a level harder than the body's capacity to adequately recover. Overtraining rarely leads to an improvement in performance and, in fact, commonly reduces performance because it ultimately increases the likelihood that the athlete will become sick or injured.

A 26-year-old athlete who transferred to a more competitive team increased his training volume by 200 percent and after 2 months experienced continuous fatigue, tinnitus, palpitations, and insomnia. Nevertheless, he continued to play for 3 months but then became totally unfit, with sleepless nights and severe mental depression.[5] This is precisely what should never happen.

Overtraining is a problem for many athletes (10 to 20 percent of those who train intensively) and appears to be relatively common in endurance athletes. Among other factors that may increase the risk of developing this condition, a poor intake of carbohydrates and fluids is known to be a problem.[6] Overtraining syndrome is an untreated excessive training overload with inadequate rest, resulting in chronic decreases in performance and in the ability to train. Other problems may result and may require medical attention. Factors associated with the development of overtraining syndrome include

- frequent competition, particularly if it involves quality efforts;
- monotonous training with insufficient rest;
- preexisting medical conditions (e.g., colds or allergies);
- poor diet, particularly inadequate intake of carbohydrates, or dehydration;
- environmental stress (e.g., altitude, high temperatures, and humidity); and
- psychosocial stressors (e.g., work or school conflicts).

According to the American College of Sports Medicine, overtraining syndrome can be effectively eliminated through a logical training program that allows for adequate rest and recovery with proper nutrition and hydration.[7] Studies of marathon runners suggest that even athletes who consume a high-carbohydrate diet require 7 days after a marathon to return muscle glycogen to prerace levels.[8] A continuation of regular training before full muscle glycogen resynthesis will inevitably lead to performance degradation. Athletes must therefore understand that rest is a useful and necessary part of training, particularly after a hard and intensive training session. Athletes fearing that a reduction in training may diminish competitiveness may resist getting enough rest. Therefore, everyone in the athlete's training circle (family, coach, athletic trainer, and so on) should support the concept that overtraining is associated with reduced performance. Put simply, rest and recovery should be an integral part of the training plan.

Overuse Injuries

Overuse injuries occur when an athlete chronically repeats the same physical task; they may be particularly problematic in adolescent athletes experiencing rapid growth.[9] In its simplest and most benign form, a heel blister caused by the rubbing of an ill-fitting running shoe is an overuse injury. A more serious form would be, for instance, the constant pounding of legs on hard pavement that causes sufficient vibrational bone stress to induce a stress fracture. This is analogous to taking a wire clothes hanger and bending it repeatedly in the same place. After a while, the hanger develops a crack and eventually breaks. Because endurance athletes spend so many hours training, overuse injuries are a real concern.

A study of triathletes found that some developed skeletal injury early in the competition, which became worse as the competition progressed. These injuries to muscles may alter the use of energy substrates as the triathlon progresses and as the body heals after the competition.[10] Although protein breakdown and muscular damage occur during a race, well-trained athletes should experience no alteration in fitness provided nutrition status is maintained.[11] Adequately nourished athletes have a better capacity to heal the minor tissue damage that occurs during training and competition. Additionally, athletes who can maintain carbohydrate and fluid levels during exercise are likely to have better brain function, which translates into a smoother running style that is less prone to injury development. Loss of mental capacity, which can easily occur with either a carbohydrate or fluid storage deficit, causes a breakdown in coordination that can increase structural stresses that lead to injury.

Dietary Adequacy

Low glycogen stores reduce the time an athlete is capable of exercising, a fact that mandates the regular consumption of carbohydrates to maintain or replace limited glycogen stores.[12] This requires, ideally, a carbohydrate intake of between 7 and 10 grams per kilogram of body weight per day. As indicated in table 14.3, even for 100-pound (45 kilogram) athletes, this represents a substantial amount of calories from carbohydrate.

The timing of carbohydrate ingestion is also important and may influence glycogen storage and resynthesis. A study of highly trained male cross country runners found that food intake was generally adequate and well timed except for the period

Table 14.3 Energy Intake for Endurance Athletes

	Grams per pound of body weight per day	Calories per day for 100-pound athlete	Calories per day for 200-pound athlete
Carbohydrate	3.2-4.5	1,280-1,800	2,560-3,600
Protein	0.7-0.9	280-360	560-720
Fat[a]	0.35-0.6	315-540	630-1080
Total calories per day	2,808-3,888	1,875-2,700	3,750-5,400

Note: Fat values based on 20 percent of total caloric intake.

after competition. Although it is recommended that endurance athletes consume carbohydrates immediately after competition to encourage restoration of glycogen stores, these athletes delayed eating carbohydrate foods until, on average, 2.5 hours after competition.[13] A delay of this magnitude leads to poor glycogen replacement, and subsequent days of exercise showed the negative effect of reduced endurance. A study of marathon runners found that a significant proportion of total energy intake occurs after 4:00 P.M. rather than earlier in the day when it's needed the most.[14] Delayed eating represents a missed opportunity for trained endurance athletes to maximize muscle glycogen storage after exercise.[15, 16]

There is no substitute for consuming sufficient energy and carbohydrates for endurance events. Supplements and ergogenic aids appear to be ineffective. The only strategy that works effectively is to eat enough and to eat at a time that is most useful for delivering energy to needy muscles or for maximizing glycogen storage. There is also evidence that endurance athletes must focus on glycogen storage activities about 1 week before a major competition.[17] A failure to do so can have a negative effect on the athlete's endurance capacity.

Endurance athletes, because of the time spent training and competing, may need to develop their own strategies for obtaining energy and fluids during the activity. This is not easy because consuming the wrong foods or fluids or consuming them at the wrong time will have a performance-decreasing effect. The "nervous stomach" many athletes experience just before a race makes the consumption of the right energy or fluid package even more difficult. Athletes should undergo a purposeful experimentation to discover what sports beverages, carbohydrate gels, and other sources of energy and nutrients are well tolerated so they can use this information to optimize training sessions and achieve peak performances during competitions. The reliance on recommendations for the general athlete population may be a good starting point, but it is not enough to generate winning performances in tough competitive fields.

Each type of race alters slightly the proportion of carbohydrate and fat that is burned as fuel (more intensity equals proportionately more carbohydrate; lower intensity equals proportionately more fat), but it's the carbohydrate level that ultimately determines if the athlete will "hit the wall." That is, when the glycogen stores are depleted, the athlete will no longer be capable of maintaining a sufficiently strong pace. Since endurance events are long, every available opportunity must be capitalized on to ensure that the athlete has enough food energy to continue the race and to store enough energy (glycogen) to do well during the next day of racing.

Athletes should do whatever is necessary to take in sufficient energy and nutrients (bringing baggies filled with food to meetings, eating while walking to class, snacking while going to the car), or the benefits derived from training will be wasted. Athletes who do not eat effectively become more easily fatigued and injured and are more likely to try unproven products touted as having ergogenic properties. There is no doubt whatsoever that much of the attention given to ergogenic aids and nutrient supplements by athletes, whether they're cyclists, runners, or swimmers, is to overcome a failure in planning to eat enough and to eat on time.

Maintaining hydration status is important for operating at optimal physiological levels of efficiency. Endurance athletes should practice consuming fluids frequently, even in the absence of thirst, to reduce the chance of dehydration. Consumption of a carbohydrate-containing beverage with small amounts of sodium is useful for fluid absorption and for maintaining the drive to drink.

Nutrient Supplementation

Athletes who fail to consume sufficient carbohydrate or enough total energy are likely to be at increased risk of inadequate vitamin C, thiamin, riboflavin, niacin, calcium, magnesium, and iron intakes.[18] A study of marathon runners found that supplement usage (especially vitamins C and E, calcium, and zinc) was common. Forty-eight percent of the runners questioned reported using at least one supplement within the 3-day period surrounding the Los Angeles Marathon.[19] Other studies confirm that nonsupplemented marathon runners, soccer players, wrestlers, and basketball players have adequate serum concentrations of vitamin C and vitamin B_6, so supplementation of these vitamins does not appear to be warranted.[20, 21] In a study evaluating the effectiveness of magnesium supplementation on marathon runners, the supplementation did not improve resistance to muscle damage during the race, did not enhance muscle recovery after the race, and did not improve running performance.[22]

Male marathon runners were evaluated to determine if the consumption of a commercial ergogenic aid supplement containing vitamins, minerals, amino acids, and unsaturated fatty acids was useful in improving performance. Results indicate that the ergogenic aid had no effect on oxygen consumption or any other important metabolic or physiological parameter that might be useful to endurance athletes.[23]

Nutritional Concerns for Female Endurance Athletes

Female endurance athletes must consume sufficient energy and nutrients to avoid amenorrhea (cessation of regular menstrual periods). Amenorrhea occurs for many reasons, including high physical stress, high psychological stress, inadequate energy intake, poor iron status, high cortisol levels, and low body fat levels. It is conceivable that female endurance athletes have all of these factors working against them.

Although some of these factors are clearly out of a woman's control, food intake is not one of those. Female athletes should do whatever is within their means to consume sufficient total energy with a balanced nutrient intake to support good health. Amenorrhea is strongly associated with a loss in bone density and an increase in stress fracture risk. Additionally, low bone density during the running years places the athlete at higher osteoporosis risk later in life.

A Sampling of Sports Relying on Aerobic Metabolism

Aerobic sports involve submaximal effort over long periods of time. The aerobic nature of these activities results in a steady creation of ATP energy in working muscles, allowing athletes to continue working for as long as there is sufficient fuel and for as long as the body does not become overheated (hydration state is important). Athletes who can rely more efficiently on fats and less on carbohydrate (glycogen) typically have better endurance because they have more fat fuel than glycogen fuel, which has limited stores. Because fats require a high amount of oxygen for efficient metabolism, the endurance athlete with the best oxygen system (e.g., most oxidative enzymes, best ability to carry oxygen to working cells) has the best endurance. What follows is a sample of endurance sports and their special nutrition considerations.

Distance Running

Distance running is commonly thought of as any distance 10,000 meters (6.2 miles) or longer. To go these distances, runners place a premium on relying primarily on aerobic metabolic pathways during the majority of the run. Runners who are capable of doing this rely mainly on fat for the majority of fuel, enabling them to limit the usage of carbohydrate. Carbohydrate storage is finite, but fat storage is, from a practical standpoint, limitless. The higher reliance on fat enables long-distance runners to run very long distances. It also enables them to preserve carbohydrate for moments during the race when they require fast acceleration (e.g., at the end of the race or while passing another runner). According to one study, only 2 to 7 percent of the total energy burned in aerobic activity is derived anaerobically.[24] A small amount of carbohydrate is used even when maintaining aerobic activity, so distance runners must develop strategies for delivering carbohydrate during the run. A failure to do so will result in either low blood sugar or low muscle glycogen, both of which impair endurance by leading to premature muscle fatigue.

Keeping this in mind, distance runners must consider the following nutritionally relevant factors for their sport.

Long-distance runners are at risk of amenorrhea, low bone density, and stress fractures. The distances that these athletes run weekly to train may predispose them to stress fractures, despite the potential stimulating impact of running on skeletal mass.[25] Although stress fractures occur more frequently in women runners than in men, all runners should ensure that their calcium intake is adequate to reduce the risk of fracture. Female runners are at higher risk of stress fractures because hard endurance training is often associated with cessation of the menstrual cycle. The reduced estrogen associated with amenorrhea is linked to lower bone density. Therefore, runners who experience either primary or secondary amenorrhea should seek appropriate medical advice to determine if reasonable steps can be taken to return to normal menstrual status.[26]

Female runners should take the following steps to reduce the risk of osteoporosis:

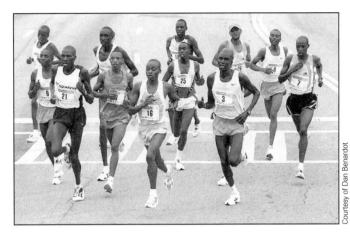

Elite runners depend heavily on both fat and carbohydrate for fuel to accelerate and vary speed over the course of a long-distance race.

- Consume calcium (1,500 milligrams per day) from food or a combination of food and supplements.
- Avoid overconsumption of protein because excess protein is associated with higher urinary calcium losses.
- Control the production of stress hormones (particularly cortisol) by maintaining hydration and blood sugar during exercise.
- Avoid overtraining, which is associated with amenorrhea.

Inadequate energy intake is a red flag that the intake of vitamins and minerals may also be low. A study comparing the nutrient intakes of trained female runners who were amenorrheic, oligomenorrheic, or menstruating normally found clear nutrition differences between these groups, despite being matched on height, weight, training distance, and body fat percentage.[27] The runners who were not menstruating had zinc intakes well below the recommended level of intake and lower than those found in the runners who had normal menses. In addition, the runners who had normal menses had higher intakes of fat and a more adequate total energy consumption. This suggests that high-carbohydrate diets, which are preferred for optimal performance, make it more difficult to consume the needed level of energy because carbohydrates have a lower caloric density than high-fat foods. Therefore, athletes should concentrate on consuming more food when carbohydrates constitute the main energy source. A failure to menstruate normally is a strong risk factor in the development of weaker bones and resulting stress fractures. Female runners have good cause to be fully aware of the adequacy of their energy and nutrient intakes because almost no injury is more frustrating or potentially career ending than the development of frequent stress fractures. Endurance runs require enormous amounts of energy (a marathon requires about 2,900 calories); they cannot be adequately trained for or run without an adequate total energy consumption. Food intake strategies, including eating snacks between meals and consuming snacks or sports beverages before, during, and after exercise, are important for ensuring that fuel consumption matches need.

Surveys of distance runners confirm that total energy and carbohydrate intakes are below the recommended levels, suggesting that runners must make a concerted effort to consume the recommended amounts before, during, and after exercise.[28, 29] In a case study assessing the nutrient intake of an ultraendurance runner during a race, it was found that if the pre-event and during-event guidelines for food and beverage are followed, then athletes will have sufficient energy and fluids to successfully complete the event.[30]

Tapering activity before a competition improves competition performance.[31] It does so by increasing glycogen stores, but it also makes the runner calmer, which gives the athlete an improved economy of running motion that enhances endurance. The importance of tapering exercise and of carbohydrate loading before an important event cannot be overemphasized.

Fluids are crucial. Fluid consumption should be on a fixed time schedule (every 10 to 15 minutes) to avoid underhydration and thirst. Perhaps no single factor is more important for ensuring a long-distance runner's success than maintaining an optimal hydration state. Athletes should drink now, drink again in 10 to 15 minutes, and when they believe they've had enough, they should drink more. Of course, the type of beverage consumed is also important. (See chapter 3 for more information of fluids and electrolytes.)

A great deal of body heat is generated over the course of an endurance run, and this heat is liberated through sweat evaporation. Studies strongly suggest that a 6 to 7 percent carbohydrate solution with electrolytes is most effective in maintaining exercise endurance.[31] It has been firmly concluded that acute heat exposure is detrimental to muscular endurance.[32] Therefore, long-distance runners should develop the habit of frequent fluid consumption to maintain body water status, whether they are thirsty or not. A fluid intake of .5 to 1 liter per hour is sufficient to prevent significant dehydration in most athletes in mild environmental conditions, but a greater intake of fluids is needed for athletes running at higher intensities or in more severe environmental conditions in order to avoid heat stress.[33]

Distance runners typically have relatively low body fat levels. Successful long-distance runners are commonly thin, and this body profile may be advantageous to them in dissipating heat during long runs.[34] However, since very low body fat levels are associated with amenorrhea, female athletes should seek a balance between low body fat levels and normal hormone function.

A critical factor in the performance of all endurance athletes is iron status, and evidence exists that endurance runners have reduced hemoglobin, hematocrit, and red blood cell counts when compared with strength and mixed-trained athletes.[35] Iron status is sufficiently important that one of the more common illegal ergogenic aids used by endurance runners is erythropoietin (EPO),[36] which stimulates the production of red blood cells, thereby enhancing oxygen-carrying capacity.[37] Iron is an essential oxygen-carrying component of hemoglobin (red blood cell iron), myoglobin (muscle cell iron), and ferrochromes (oxygen-carrying enzymes essential for making ATP) in the mitochondria. It appears that hemoglobin status is of highest priority, so iron from other cells is cannibalized to support a normal hemoglobin production when iron stores (ferritin) and intake are inadequate. Therefore, a standard blood test measuring hemoglobin may appear normal while other iron-containing cells are depleted. For this reason, it is important that blood tests in endurance athletes always include a measure of ferritin, which should be at the level of a minimum of 20 nanograms per deciliter. Besides having an inadequate dietary intake, which is most common in runners who do not eat red meat or who are vegetarian, there are several other common causes of low iron status in runners:[38-40]

- Excess iron loss in sweat
- Excess loss of blood through the GI tract
- Excess loss of blood in the urine (hematuria)
- Excess menstrual blood loss in female runners
- Poor absorption of iron
- Intravascular hemolysis

The issue of blood donations should also be considered because iron is so crucial to running success. According to Noakes (1991), runners wishing to donate blood should first assess iron status. Normal hemoglobins and ferritins above 60 nanograms per milliliter after 5 days of hard training are the margin point for safely donating blood.[41] In addition, runners who do donate blood should not exercise with normal intensity for 3 to 6 weeks after the donation to allow for sufficient time to return blood volumes and iron status back to normal levels.

Triathlon

Muscular balance in the upper and lower body is important to successful triathletes because the three events each have a different muscular focus. Since all the major muscles are put to the test in triathlons, these athletes must consume enough total energy to ensure that the fuel capacity for each working muscle starts out full. Swimmers, for instance, have a much higher upper-body strength requirement than cyclists, while triathletes require balanced strength in all the muscles.[42] Perhaps this use of all the muscles is what makes the triathlon a sport with no preference for body type or shape, making it accessible to anyone who is willing to train hard in all three disciplines.[43]

Triathlons have different lengths, depending on the location and sponsor. An Olympic-distance triathlon consists of a 1.5-kilometer swim, a 40-kilometer cycle, and a 10-kilometer run. The most well-known Ironman competition in Hawaii includes a 2.4-mile swim; a 112-mile bike race; and a 26-mile, 385-yard run. A survey of non-elite triathletes indicated that even they have training loads that most people would find impossible to follow. This survey revealed that the average swimming distance per week for these triathletes was 8.8 kilometers, the cycling distance was 270 kilometers, and the running distance was 58.2 kilometers.[44] Still, it is important for triathletes

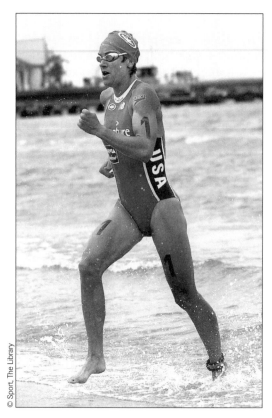

© Sport, The Library

Following the swim, the next two legs of a triathlon race put a lot of stress on the athlete's skeleton, creating a greater need for calcium intake during the training stages of the season.

to taper training before a competition. One study showed a statistically significant improvement in performance when triathletes reduced the total time spent training before an event.[45] Once again, rest before competition proves to be an effective adjunct to training.

Different sports induce athletes to consume different foods and, therefore, take in different levels of nutrients. Calcium intake was found to be lower in triathletes than in athletes participating in team sports such as volleyball and basketball. Of the athletes surveyed in a large French study with 10,373 subjects, calcium intakes were below the recommended level for the triathletes, and females had lower calcium intakes than did males.[46] This is bad news for athletes who place so much repetitive stress on the skeleton, which places them at increased risk for stress fractures.

Keeping this in mind, triathletes must consider the following nutritionally relevant factors for their sport.

Maintenance of normal hydration is difficult. Perhaps the most important performance-related factor for triathletes is creating a strategy for maintaining hydration state during this grueling event. Triathletes should find a well-tolerated sports beverage and develop a drinking schedule that results in the smallest possible weight loss by the end of the competition. Developing a workable drinking strategy of a carbohydrate–electrolyte beverage (typically between .25 to .5 liter every 15 minutes) may be the single most important ergogenic act a triathlete can do.

There is concern that triathletes who wear wet suits during the swimming phase of the triathlon (if the water temperature is warm) may predispose themselves to heat stress during the cycling and running portions of the race. A study evaluating this issue found that a wet suit did not adversely affect body temperature during the cycling and running stages, provided that the athlete maintained a good hydration state.[47] The importance of good hydration as it relates to triathlon performance is the theme of numerous studies, all of which state that hydration is one of two keys to a successful race (the other being maintenance of carbohydrate stores). Nevertheless, despite the importance of hydration, it appears that triathletes are rarely successful at maintaining good hydration during a competition, with a water-related weight loss that commonly exceeds 4 percent.[48] Triathletes may also be predisposed to hyponatremia (low blood-sodium level), which is a result of using replacement fluids (typically plain water) that contain no electrolytes.[49, 50] An assessment of athletes completing an Ironman triathlon found that athletes lose an average of 5.5 pounds (2.5 kilograms) in body weight, and athletes with hyponatremia had fluid overload despite modest fluid intakes.[51] These findings imply that even modest consumption of fluids that contain no sodium may increase the risk of hyponatremia. Both body water loss and hyponatremia are factors that influence performance, but these factors also place the athlete at health risk. Replacing sufficient fluids in the correct volume and of the right type is therefore critical for the athlete's safety and performance.[52]

Consumption of sufficient energy is needed. The energy requirement for carbohydrate in a triathlete exceeds the body's ability to store it. Therefore, triathletes should develop a strategy for adequate consumption of carbohydrate energy during a race (typically 1 to 1.5 grams of carbohydrate per kilogram of body weight per hour).[53] To do this, athletes should find sports beverages that contain carbohydrate in a form and concentration that are well tolerated. Some triathletes have found that carbohydrate gels, bananas, or crackers can be consumed during the cycle portion of the race (taken with a water chaser). If this is tolerated, it is an excellent way to boost the carbohydrate fuel level in the body before the beginning of the running portion of the race. Nutrition interventions capable of providing more fluids and carbohydrates to triathletes do work and lead to improvements in endurance performance.[54]

Triathletes run the risk of overtraining. Getting sufficient rest and tapering exercise before a race have been shown to be two of the best training strategies a triathlete can follow. By contrast, triathletes who increase the training frequency before an important race are not likely to do their best. Sufficient rest is just as important for a strong performance as sufficient training.

Planning a meal schedule for longer distances tends to take a back seat. The triathlon covers different distances, depending on whether it's a sprint, the Olympic distance, a long course, or the Ironman. The sprint can take as little as 45 minutes to complete, and the Ironman often takes longer than 10 hours. Regardless of the competition distance, triathletes train hard—and they find themselves juggling their training with work or school. Eating and drinking often take a back seat to all the other demands of life, yet they are critically important to the success an athlete can realize. The only solution is to sit down and develop a schedule that includes working, training, eating, resting, and drinking. All should be treated as having equal importance.

Many (if not most) triathletes have more than one workout each day, and some race weekly or every second week. This places a tremendous energy requirement on the athlete that is commonly not met. The more time an athlete takes to train, the less time there is to eat, so there is a natural conflict between the increased requirement for energy and the reduced time to supply what is needed. This problem makes a clear case for planning time for eating as much as planning time for training. If an athlete's training has a fixed schedule (it usually does) but the eating doesn't, the athlete will suffer.

Distance Swimming

Distance swimmers are unique people who must spend an enormous amount of time in the water to realize minuscule improvements in time. A key to performance appears to be the swimmer's capacity to go faster without increasing blood lactate levels or to go faster while utilizing a lower percentage of maximal aerobic capacity.[55] It appears that the endurance swimmer can work harder while maintaining a predominantly aerobic (oxidative) metabolic pathway. This translates into a terrific aerobic fitness, with the ability to maintain enough glycogen and oxygen in the system to ensure an efficient energy burn. Maintaining lower blood lactate concentrations may also be a function of maintaining a sufficient blood volume (lactate in a larger volume equals lower lactate concentration). Of course, this is largely dependent on adequate hydration and a good electrolyte status (sodium helps maintain blood volume).

Keeping this in mind, distance swimmers must consider the following nutritionally relevant factors for their sport.

Swimmers often have lower bone densities. Swimmers tend to have lower bone densities when compared with other athletes.[56] The reason is easy to understand: Swimming produces less impact stress than does running. However, it may also be related to spending many hours doing laps in an indoor pool while other athletes are running outside, where they can increase their exposure to sunlight and manufacture more vitamin D, a difference that may be enough to influence bone development. For long-distance swimmers lucky enough to live in areas warm enough for outdoor pools, this is not an issue. A study of female swimmers found inadequate calcium intakes, a

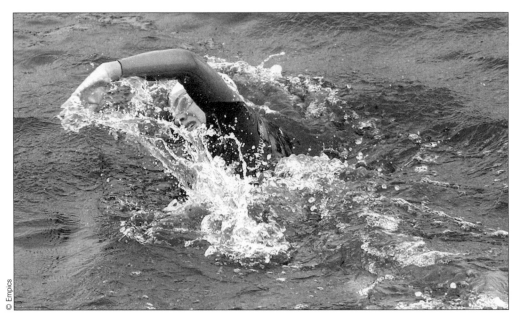

Long-distance swimmers who are lucky enough to train outdoors are less likely to suffer an insufficient intake of vitamin D.

factor that could clearly contribute to lower bone mineral density.[57] Clearly, having sufficient calcium (1,500 milligrams per day) is critical for maintaining strong bones, but swimmers should also make an effort to satisfy vitamin D needs, particularly if they have few opportunities for sunlight exposure.

Replacement of fluids needs to be more prevalent during all day events. The main focus for swimmers involved in a typical all-day meet is the replacement of adequate fluids to maintain blood volume and to provide a constant source of carbohydrate. It may not be the time in the water swimming that contributes to dehydration but the time out of the water (often in the sun) waiting for a turn to compete. Regardless of the source, a failure to drink sufficient fluids can lead to a serious performance detriment.

Consumption of carbohydrates during long competitions. Having a snacking plan is important to avoid hunger. Swimming competitions take many hours, making hunger an issue that must be addressed. It is a bad strategy to begin an endurance event in a hungry state. Athletes should sip on sports beverages and snack on crackers and other simple carbohydrate (mainly starchy) foods to get a constant trickle of carbohydrates into the system while they wait to compete.

Eating enough to support the activity. Swimming long distances uses a tremendous amount of energy, a deficit that must be matched with an appropriate energy delivery from food. Swimmers often complain that they can't keep their weights up during the long swim-competition season, and that means they're burning muscle to meet their needs.

Cycling

There are a number of cycling endurance events that take place over several days of competition. The Tour de France is notable for its extreme endurance demands on participating athletes, and each stage of the race places different physiological demands on the cyclists. They pedal approximately 4,000 kilometers over 3 weeks with only a single day of rest allowed! The energy expenditure ranges are the highest values ever reported for athletes over a period longer than 7 days.[58] The cyclists consume approximately 62 percent of their energy from carbohydrate, 15 percent from protein, and 23 percent from fat. More than 49 percent of total energy consumption takes place between meals. Some days have long hard hills, while other days have roads that are more level. Studies of Tour de France cyclists indicate that they consume approximately 30 percent of their total daily energy intake in the form of a liquid carbohydrate-enriched beverage.[59] So much time during the day is spent on the bike, there is perhaps no other way to adequately consume sufficient energy.

There may be a connection between cycling and asthma. In studies of athletes at the 1996 Olympic Games in Atlanta, U.S. athletes participating in cycling and mountain biking had the highest prevalence (45 percent) of asthma.[60] By contrast, 20 percent of the total U.S. team reported they had asthma. This suggests that asthma may be a contributing factor in determining the sport an athlete selects to participate in. For some athletes, it is possible that asthma might be triggered by an allergic response, and this could be an allergic response to food. Cyclists with asthma should

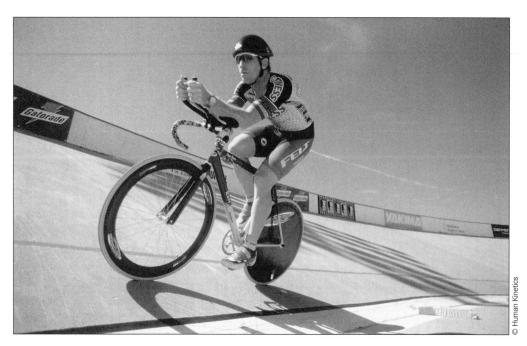

© Human Kinetics

Cyclists suffering from asthma must monitor their food intake carefully because certain foods may trigger an attack.

be extremely careful about avoiding foods or other substances that could trigger an asthmatic response.

Keeping this in mind, cyclists must consider the following nutritionally relevant factors for their sport.

Recovering from multiday events. The energy cost of multiday cycling events is enormous, and the meal planning of the athlete's team may make the difference between winning and losing. There is a clear requirement for carbohydrate, which conflicts with the huge requirement for energy because of carbohydrate's relatively low energy density. Although fats have a high energy density, they are not needed to the degree that carbohydrates are. Therefore, large amounts of carbohydrates should be consumed frequently, with the focus on starchy carbohydrates (e.g., pasta, bread, rice, potatoes).

Consumption of food and fluid during long rides. Cyclists have an advantage over other endurance athletes in that they can more easily carry fluids and foods on the bike frame or in jersey pockets. Since there is less bouncing while riding than while running, cyclists can consume solid foods without experiencing GI distress. Cyclists should take advantage of this on long rides by bringing along sports beverages to drink and some crackers, bananas, carbohydrate gel, or bread to eat. These high-carbohydrate foods should be well tolerated and can significantly boost the carbohydrate delivery to working muscles.

Training is very time and energy consuming. The longer athletes train, the more energy they need, but the less time available to them to consume it. Therefore, cyclists should consider the training period as a time to take in a proportion of their daily caloric requirements. To do this, cyclists should find foods that are well tolerated, such as bananas and crackers, and bring them along during the ride. Sports beverages are also an important source of energy, so these should be consumed instead of plain water as a rehydration beverage. A failure to eat during training will inevitably lead to inadequate energy consumption and a decrease in performance.

Endurance athletes spend many hours training and have enormous energy needs. However, these training times make it difficult to consume the needed foods. Athletes should plan multiple eating breaks throughout the day (consuming something high in carbohydrate every 3 hours) to ensure an adequate total energy consumption. Fluid intake is also critically important, and endurance athletes should develop the habit of drinking frequently (every 10 to 15 minutes) regardless of thirst. A large body of evidence suggests that lower levels of either carbohydrate or fluids inhibit endurance. Nevertheless, when high-carbohydrate diets impair an athlete's capacity to consume sufficient energy because of their relatively low energy density, consuming a higher fat intake to help the athlete meet energy needs should be considered.[61] Except to satisfy energy needs, however, fat is not the most desirable energy substrate for endurance athletes.

Carbohydrate after exercise stimulates muscle protein synthesis more favorably than an equivalent amount of fat, so athletes should be careful not to consume fats at the expense of carbohydrates.[62] Under certain circumstances (see chapter 4), caffeine ingestion coupled with adequate hydration and regular carbohydrate intake may aid endurance performance.[63] However, because some studies raise doubts as to caffeine's effectiveness,[64] athletes should determine for themselves whether a small amount of caffeine ingested in long-duration events is useful for enhancing performance.

Metabolic Needs for Both Power and Endurance

15

A number of team sports, including soccer, basketball, and volleyball, require a combination of power and endurance. The random intermittent fluctuations of exercise intensity in these sports result in a unique pattern of energy substrate utilization. Nutrition studies of athletes competing in these team sports indicate that a high carbohydrate intake (65 percent of total calories) results in improved performance. Nevertheless, surveys of soccer and basketball players have found that the typical intakes of these athletes provide a much lower carbohydrate level, suggesting there is great room for improvement. The periodic high bursts of activity in these sports also place a high reliance on PCr, signifying that protein intake (with adequate total calories) must also be consumed in amounts sufficient to synthesize the needed creatine, but surveys also indicate that many of these athletes don't consume sufficient calories, which could impede creatine synthesis. This chapter provides information on the nutrition requirements for team sport athletes, with techniques for optimizing glycogen storage and sustaining hydration state. In addition, strategies for achieving optimal nutriture during the precompetition, competition, and postcompetition periods are presented.

Nutrition Tactics for Sports Requiring Power and Endurance

This chapter provides nutrition information for sports where athletes have intermittent bouts of high-intensity activity followed by periods of lower-intensity activity. Team sports such as basketball, volleyball, rugby, team handball, and soccer all have combinations of high-intensity and lower-intensity activity interspersed throughout the competition. The mixed intensity of certain individual sports, such as figure skating and tennis, may also fall into this category. This differs from other sports, where the focus is either predominantly endurance or predominantly power or speed. There is nothing in artistic gymnastics training or competition that requires, for instance, a great deal of aerobic endurance; and marathon runners rarely require the explosive power exhibited by gymnasts. Team sport athletes must focus on speed, power, *and* endurance. Soccer players must run the field at a controlled pace until a sudden opening requires a quick burst of speed. Basketball players may jog back and forth in a steady aerobic pace, but each player must have the capacity for a powerful jump to grab a rebound or for a quick sprint to make a defensive play.

The intermittent high and low intensity of team sports creates a requirement for energy that is derived from a combination of aerobic and anaerobic means. Although the anaerobic metabolic processes are solely reliant on existing stores of ATP, phosphocreatine (PCr), and muscle glycogen, the aerobic processes derive energy from muscle glycogen, blood glucose, fat, and to a lesser extent, protein. As indicated in figure 15.1, there is a heavy reliance on muscle glycogen for the majority of muscle energy during team sport activity, with nearly an equal reliance on fat and blood glucose for most

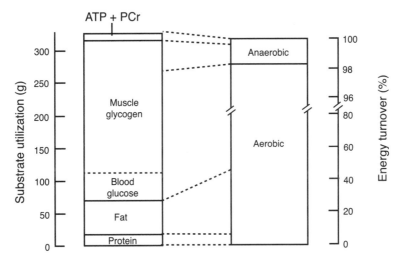

Figure 15.1   The relative anaerobic and aerobic substrate utilization in team sports, such as soccer.

Adapted from J. Bangsbo, 1994, "The physiology of soccer: With special reference to intense intermittent exercise," *Acta Physiologica Scandinavica* 151(Suppl 610): 1-156.

of the remaining source of energy. Fat is almost never in short supply. However, the amount of glucose energy in blood is small and requires constant vigilance by the athlete to ensure a continuing source of glucose during the competition.

The heavy reliance on muscle glycogen and blood glucose to fulfill the energy needs of working muscles demands a high level of consumed carbohydrates before exercise and carbohydrate-containing sports beverages during exercise. In a study of the performance outcomes of a moderate (39 percent of total calories) versus high (65 percent of total calories) carbohydrate intake, the higher-carbohydrate diet significantly improved intermittent exercise performance.[1]

Repeated sprint work is enhanced by consumption of a carbohydrate–electrolyte beverage.[2] Although it has been long established that consumption of a carbohydrate–electrolyte beverage enhances submaximal endurance performance, only recent studies have clearly shown the benefits of these beverages during high-intensity, short-duration efforts such as those found in football and basketball. Subjects performed seven additional 1-minute cycling sprints at 120 to 130 percent of peak $\dot{V}O_2$ when they consumed a 6 percent carbohydrate–electrolyte beverage, as compared with a water placebo. This finding suggests that a dramatic improvement in sprint capability during the last 5 to 10 minutes of a basketball game is possible if players methodically consume a sports beverage.

A similar study determined that sports drinks (i.e., carbohydrate–electrolyte beverages) can help maintain high-intensity efforts during high-intensity activities consisting of intermittent sprinting, running, and jogging.[3] Again, these findings have strong positive implications for sustaining high-intensity activity over the course of a typical basketball or soccer game.

The effects of consumption of the individual components of a sports beverage (electrolytes, water, or carbohydrate) and of the combination of all components have also been assessed. Compared with the electrolyte-only trial, performance during the water-only and carbohydrate-only trials was approximately 6 percent faster. However, the combination of carbohydrate and water caused a performance enhancement that was approximately 12 percent faster than the electrolyte trial and 5 to 6 percent faster than when water only or carbohydrate only were consumed.[4] These findings support the thesis that carbohydrate enhances water absorption and that the limited carbohydrate storage mandates consumption of carbohydrate during exercise. The high demands on circulating and stored carbohydrate during high-intensity work require a constant vigilance to ensure proper and speedy replacement. This study was based on earlier work that showed exercise performance improved significantly with carbohydrate feedings.[5] It has also been found that the optimal level of carbohydrate concentration during exercise is 6 to 7 percent. This concentration is best for fluid absorption and also helps to efficiently deliver carbohydrate. An 8 percent carbohydrate solution causes a slower fluid absorption.[6]

A basketball player leaping for the ball and a soccer player sprinting toward the ball and jumping high to kick it are activities comparable to certain forms of strength training. A study of resistance-trained athletes found that athletes tended to perform more repetitions of the same weight when carbohydrate was consumed versus a water placebo. Blood glucose and lactate concentrations were higher with the carbohydrate trial, suggesting that more carbohydrate was available and used to sustain the high-intensity exercise.[7] A study of head-to-head comparisons of Gatorade, Powerade, and All Sport found that Gatorade stimulates fluid absorption faster than either Powerade or All Sport.[8] This difference can be attributed to both the type of carbohydrate and the concentration of carbohydrate in the beverages. Gatorade has a carbohydrate concentration level that is consistent with the positive findings in virtually all the studies (6 percent) and contains an equal mixture of sucrose and glucose. Powerade and All Sport have higher carbohydrate concentrations, mainly from fructose. Fructose has been shown to cause gastrointestinal (GI) distress; it is also less efficient in sustaining blood glucose because it requires a secondary conversion in the liver after absorption.

Athletes who perform repeated or sustained high-power efforts experience a reduction in performance when they are dehydrated.[9] A 6 percent carbohydrate solution aids in fluid delivery, a fact that should be considered when team sport athletes select a rehydration beverage. The fluid-consumption guidelines established by the American College of Sports Medicine are summarized in table 15.1.[10]

Several general nutrition guidelines—covering what to do before, during, and after exercise and competition—are important for virtually all athletes involved in sports that have intermittent periods of maximal intensity. See table 15.2 for these guidelines.

The two keys to these guidelines are fluids and carbohydrates in the context of a generally varied diet. Athletes should explore workable strategies to consume both fluids and carbohydrates at every opportunity. Recent findings tend to contradict the traditional and commonly followed belief that carbohydrate-containing beverages are useful only for endurance (aerobic) activities lasting longer than 60 minutes. The best predictors of athletic performance are maintenance of blood volume and maintenance of glycogen and glucose. What follows are some strategies that might be useful for achieving both enhanced hydration and improved maintenance of system carbohydrate in different sports.

Table 15.1   **ACSM Fluid-Consumption Guidelines**

Timing	Amount	Adaptation
2 hr before exercise	Drink 500 ml (.5 L or approximately 17 oz).	None
During exercise	Drink 600 to 1,200 ml (.6 to 1.2 L or approximately 20 to 40 oz) per hour.	Drink 150 to 300 ml (about 5 to 10 oz) every 15 to 20 min.
After exercise	Based on pre- and postexercise body weight changes, drink enough fluid to restore body weight (16 oz fluid = 1 lb of body weight).	Drink 150% of the amount needed to restore body weight. This amount compensates for urine losses, which may induce hypohydration when only 100% of the weight-replacement fluid is consumed.

Table 15.2 General Guidelines for Athletes Involved in Sports That Include Intermittent Periods of High-Intensity Work

General nutrition	Maintain a diet high in complex carbohydrates, moderate in protein, and relatively low in fat. Strive for a varied consumption of foods to ensure exposure to all the nutrients that the body's cells need. Varying your intake also helps ensure that you don't overexpose your cells to substances in foods that may be, with frequent exposure, harmful to general health.
Preexercise or precompetition meal	Consume starchy, easy-to-digest, high-carbohydrate foods. Consume plenty of fluids with meals and during the period between the meal and the exercise session or competition. When possible, consume a high-carbohydrate meal about 3 hr before exercise.
During-exercise nourishment	Consume a sports drink that is approximately a 6 to 7 percent carbohydrate solution. The drink should also contain a small amount of salt to encourage drinking during the competition. Drink 20 to 40 oz (600 to 1,200 ml) of fluid per hour, depending on the environmental temperature and humidity and your predisposition to sweating. In some sports, there are no natural breaks in the action, which makes it difficult to consume fluids at this rate. In such cases, athletes and coaches should develop a clear strategy for fluid consumption that can take place during time-outs in the game. A good strategy will ensure that adequate personnel are available to provide fluids quickly and efficiently to every player whenever a break in the action occurs.
Postexercise or postcompetition replenishment	Drink a sports drink to ensure quick rehydration and replenishment of depleted glycogen stores. Consume approximately 24 oz per pound of body weight (1.5 L per kilogram of body weight) lost during the activity. Muscle glycogen stores are efficiently replaced if the athlete consumes carbohydrate immediately after the activity. For the 2 hr immediately after activity, consume high–glycemic index foods (i.e., foods high in natural sugars or foods that are quickly and easily digested into sugars). The goal is to consume at least 50 g (200 calories) of carbohydrate every hour until the next meal. In general, strive to consume approximately 4 g of carbohydrate per pound of body weight during the 24 hr after exercise or competition.

Adapted, by permission, from C. Williams and C.W. Nicholas, 1998, "Nutrition needs for team sport," *GSSI Sports Science Exchange* 11(3): 70.

A Sampling of Sports Relying on a Combination of Anaerobic and Aerobic Metabolism

Certain sports require a combination of aerobic and anaerobic metabolic processes. At times, these athletes work at maximal intensity (anaerobic), while at other times they work at submaximal intensity (aerobic). Imagine a soccer striker who is jogging to cover her area of the field, working to get an open position. At the moment the ball is passed to her, she sprints to the ball with maximal effort. This combination of anaerobic and aerobic effort has special nutrition considerations that are presented as examples in the following sports.

Basketball

Basketball combines many of the best aspects of team cooperation and individual effort, with two guards, two forwards, and one center, all of whom play both defense and offense during the 32 (high school) or 48 (professional) minutes of the game. Basketball is played around the world by both men's and women's teams and has been a highly visible part of the Olympic Games since the 1936 Olympics in Berlin. Among the most impressive winning streaks in basketball was the 10 national championships (7 won consecutively) by the John Wooden–coached UCLA men's teams. In a conversation many years later, one of John Wooden's players shared that Wooden was brilliant at making sure his team was the best conditioned on the floor, and part of that conditioning regimen was making certain the players worked harder during practice than would be needed during any game against any opponent. But he also made certain all the players ate and rested well enough to be ready to give a 100 percent effort.

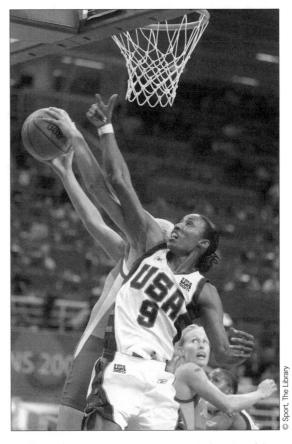

Studies of intermittent high-intensity sports imply that there are clear ergogenic benefits for basketball players who consume the right foods and fluids before, during, and after the game. A study surveying the nutrition knowledge of college basketball coaches and coaches in other sports found that only 33 percent of the coaches were confident that they responded correctly to questions related to nutrition.[11] In addition, this survey found that coaches believed college athletes had problems with the consumption of junk food, had generally poor eating habits, and generally

Basketball is a high-intensity sport often involving six days of practice and one full-speed game per week. This schedule creates a need for basketball players to continually fill their glycogen stores.

consumed unbalanced diets. This poor-quality diet affects vitamin and mineral intake. There is a high prevalence of iron depletion, anemia, and iron-deficiency anemia among both male and female basketball players.[12] Poor iron status will clearly have a negative impact on aerobic work capacity and, therefore, basketball performance. A survey of male and female basketball players revealed that the diet of the female players was lacking in a number of nutrients, and there was an excessive reliance on nutrient supplements.[13] Neither of these findings give confidence that basketball players are taking appropriate steps to compete at their conditioned capacity.

Intense physical activity is associated with the increase of free radicals, such as peroxide, which are created from the oxidation of intercellular lipids. Studies continue to evaluate whether the consumption of antioxidant supplements, including alpha-tocopherol (vitamin E), beta-carotene (pro-vitamin A), and ascorbic acid (vitamin C) might be useful in reducing the typical lipid peroxide production seen in basketball players during the season.[14, 15] Although there appears to be some benefit, taking high doses of antioxidant supplements also raises some concerns. Of very real concern is the potential for supplement contamination that may place athletes at risk of unknowingly consuming banned substances.[16] The best alternative for reducing the production of free radicals is likely the regular consumption of fresh fruits and vegetables, which have high concentrations of both carbohydrates and antioxidants.

Keeping this in mind, basketball players must consider the following nutritionally relevant factors for their sport.

Basketball games have a halftime that can be used to replenish fluids and carbohydrates. Basketball players have the advantage of a 10- to 20-minute halftime break. This is an excellent opportunity for players to sip on a sports beverage to replace lost fluids and carbohydrates. Some players may also find they do well by eating some plain crackers and drinking water. However, players should be cautioned against consuming candy bars and other foods that, although they contain some carbohydrate sugar, are high in fat. Players really need carbohydrate and water, and consuming anything else detracts from their ability to take in what they need most (see table 15.3).

Time spent on the bench should be used to maintain hydration state. Natural breaks in the game from official time-outs or substitutions should be taken advantage of by sipping on sports beverages, whether the players think they need it or not. Sipping on a carbohydrate-containing beverage should become part of the game plan, just as important as making the right team defensive or offensive plays.

Frequent practices and games can wear a player out. Basketball players typically practice 6 days each week and often have two practices in a single day. Add to that a match schedule that has them playing at least one game during the week, and it's easy to see why a typical basketball season can wear a player out. In general, players should eat enough carbohydrate to ensure an adequate total energy intake and to support optimal glycogen storage. Optimizing glycogen storage is critical for basketball performance, and meeting total energy needs helps maintain muscle mass. A common complaint of coaches is that they find it difficult to keep the weight of many players as high as they would like to, and this is a sure sign that the players are not eating enough to support the intense activity of practices and games. Teams that can make it through the season with muscle mass maintained are stronger and have better endurance than those who don't.

Table 15.3 Meeting Fluid and Carbohydrate Needs of Basketball Players

High-intensity training	For basketball players who train hard daily and need to maximize daily muscle glycogen recovery	7-10 g/kg body weight daily or 3.2-4.5 g/lb body weight daily (~500-700 g/day for a 155-lb player)	At least 10-12 cups/day (~2.5-3 L) plus fluids before, during, and after exercise
Moderate-intensity training	For basketball players who train less than 1 hr daily at a moderate intensity	5-7 g/kg body weight daily or 2.3-3.2 g/lb body weight daily	10-12 cups/day (~2.5-3 L) plus fluids before, during, and after exercise
Before exercise	To enhance fuel availability and prehydrate for a practice or game	1 g/kg body weight 1 hr before or 2 g/kg body weight 2 hr before or 3 g/kg body weight 3 hr before or 4 /kg body weight 4 hr before	16 oz or 2 cups (~.5 L) (noncaffeinated, nonalcoholic) 2 hr before exercise
During exercise	To provide an additional source of carbohydrate fuel during moderate- and high-intensity basketball practices and games	30-60 g/hr	At least 5-10 oz (150-300 ml) every 15 min to replace sweat losses
Recovery	To speed early recovery and rehydration after hard training or a game, especially during the season when there are back-to-back games and daily practices	1-1.5 g/kg body weight of high-glycemic carbohydrate beverages and foods immediately after exercise and every 2 hr after; total carbohydrate intake over the next 24 hr at 7-9 g/kg or approximately 500-600 g in 24 hr	~20 oz (~3 cups) per lb of body weight lost during exercise

Reprinted, with permission, from J. Burns, J.M. Davis, D.H. Craig and Y. Satterwhite, 1999, "Conditioning and nutrition tips for basketball," *GSSI Roundtable*, #38, 10(4).

Playing as well in the second half as in the first half wins games. Teams that can manage to sustain strength and endurance during the second half of the game tend to do better on the scoreboard than teams that don't. To do this, players should establish a pattern of frequent sipping on carbohydrate-containing beverages, whether they think they need to or not. Studies show that this frequent sipping pattern helps players keep their strength and endurance longer than if they drink water alone or fail to drink at all.

Figure Skating

Figure skating took its name from the "figures" that competitors were required to complete. These figures were, literally, outlined on the ice as two- or three-lobed figure eights that "figure" skaters had to skate over and match as closely as possible to receive a top score. In 1991, however, figures were removed from international competitive skating and eventually phased out of competition entirely, but the name "figure skating" has remained. Figure skaters aim to produce performances that are smooth, graceful, artistic, and seemingly effortless. The short, curved blades and toe picks used by figure skaters permit these athletes to create intricate spins and perform explosive jumps. Figure skaters have three separate events, and training is specialized for each of these: individual figure skating, pairs skating, and ice dancing. Singles skating is a single-gender competition (i.e., males compete against males, and females compete against females), and pairs skating and ice dancing are mixed-gender events.

In individual figure skating, there is an expectation of grace and effortlessness in the performance, but there is also a competitive premium placed on achieving difficult spins and jumps that favor stronger and smaller athletes. Since the density of air and the resistance of ice do not change for each athlete, large athletes have a greater ice resistance and are confronted with greater relative air resistance than are smaller competitors. Therefore, larger skaters require significantly greater strength to do the same skills as smaller skaters. The top flight of figure skaters appears to get smaller with each successive international competition.

In pairs skating, the male partner is usually considerably larger and stronger than the female.

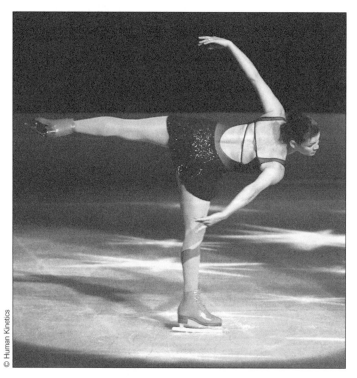

© Human Kinetics

Figure skaters need to consume sufficient energy before a competition in order to provide their muscles with the power needed for difficult techniques on the ice.

For anyone who has seen a pairs competition, the reason is obvious: The male must lift and throw his female partner frequently during the competition, and this is easier if he's lifting someone smaller. Finding the right physical match is difficult, and poorly matched pairs skaters have difficulty performing at the top level even if they are superb individual skaters.

In ice dancing, there is a much smaller premium on a large male and smaller female because there are no throws or overhead lifts in the competition. Given the intricacy of foot movement and grace found in ice dancing, the sport is well named. The constant movement coupled with a lower power requirement makes this the most aerobic of the three skating disciplines.

Studies have found that figure skaters possess an average aerobic capacity but have the ability to produce high power peaks.[17] That is, when they need to, they can call on their muscles to instantly produce a tremendous amount of power. Studies also indicate that young female skaters consume diets that are relatively high in fat and protein and relatively low in carbohydrate, calcium, and iron.[18] Dietary supplement intake in figure skaters is high, with 65 percent of the male skaters and 76 percent of the female skaters reporting regular supplement intake (mainly of multivitamin and multimineral supplements).[19] The three top reported reasons for taking the supplements were to prevent illness, provide more energy, and make up for an inadequate diet.

Although there has been a long-standing concern that competitive figure skaters do not consume sufficient energy, a recent study suggests that this concern may be unfounded for most skaters.[20] However, there remains a proportion of skaters who may be at risk for certain disordered eating patterns, and when this occurs, nutrient intake is likely to be low. The distribution of calories throughout the day in figure skaters does appear to be problematic, an issue that skaters should correct to optimize physical performance and mental concentration.[21]

As with any elite sport, injuries occur. The rate of injuries among pairs skaters is particularly alarming. In one study, female senior pairs skaters reported an average of 1.4 serious injuries over a 9-month period, while other skaters had injury rates averaging .5 serious injuries over this same time period.[22] Most of these injuries are lower-extremity injuries that might be related to boot design, but other researchers suggest that injuries might be related to poor conditioning.[23]

Keeping this in mind, figure skaters players must consider the following nutritionally relevant factors for their sport.

Many skaters are extremely concerned about their weight because appearance on the ice is important in this sport. Optimal weight is best achieved through the consumption of a low-fat, moderate-protein, high-complex-carbohydrate diet plus a good exercise and conditioning program. Although dieting is counterproductive, evidence suggests this is the weight-management strategy of choice among skaters. The consumption of adequate energy from carbohydrate is important for both performance and achievement of a desirable body composition. Inadequate energy intake may predispose the skater to nutrient deficiencies; low energy expenditure; and high body fat levels that can increase the risk of injury, create ill health, and reduce athletic performance.

The jumps in figure skating place a great deal of reliance on phosphocreatine and muscle glycogen. Adequate energy intake from carbohydrate, interspersed with a regular intake of meats (to provide creatine or sufficient protein to make creatine), is important for skaters. For vegetarian skaters, ensuring an adequate total protein and total energy consumption is critical for maintaining muscle mass and synthesizing creatine. The quick burst of muscular activity associated with the jumps required in competitive figure skating is not possible without sufficient storage of phosphocreatine and muscle glycogen. For ice dancing competitions, the fuel requirement involves more muscle glycogen than phosphocreatine, so these athletes are likely to do better with slightly less protein (or meat) but still require an adequate total energy intake to perform well.

Practices are considerably longer than performances. Although skating performances last only several minutes, practices may last for an hour or longer, they may occur more than once each day, and they may be very early in the morning or very late at night (ice time is hard to find). Practice schedules mandate that skaters must alter eating patterns to satisfy their practice needs. For very early morning practices, skaters should eat and drink something (even a slice of toast and a small glass of juice is better than nothing) before taking to the ice to be certain that muscles are well fueled. For late-night practices, a small dinner 2 hours before practice followed by another small dinner immediately after practice will help ensure that muscles are well fueled. Skating while "on empty" will not help the muscles become more conditioned and may actually be counterproductive in inducing a training benefit. There are clear benefits to ensuring a normal hydration state. A study of elite figure skaters found that plasma electrolyte concentrations were suggestive of a poor hydration state.[24]

Soccer

The popularity of soccer worldwide is enormous, and its popularity in the United States is on the rise. Soccer is a wonderful sport from a fitness standpoint because the average distance covered by a typical player during a match is approximately 6 miles (10 kilometers).[25] In addition, soccer players appear to have significantly greater bone mineral densities—likely from all the running stresses placed on the bones—than do age- and weight-matched controls.[26, 27] Although much of the activity is aerobic, a large proportion is anaerobic as players sprint for the ball. There is less activity in the second half of a typical soccer game compared with the first, likely the result of unsustained muscle glycogen stores. It was suggested long ago that the ingestion of carbohydrates immediately before, during, and after a game may play an important role in reducing player fatigue during a game.[28] Following this strategy would sustain available glucose and glycogen to working muscles.

In studies of professional soccer players' nutrient consumption, their energy and nutrient intake was similar to that of the general population, despite having a far higher energy and nutrient requirement.[29, 30] Although the recommended training diet for soccer players should include 55 to 65 percent carbohydrate, 12 to 15 percent protein, and less than 30 percent fat,[31] the athletes in this and other surveys consumed foods that were considerably lower in carbohydrate and higher in fat.[32] A survey of NCAA Division I female soccer players found that their carbohydrate consumption did not meet the minimum recommendations to promote glycogen repletion (7 to 10 grams per kilogram), but protein and fat intakes were above the recommended level.[33] It is generally believed that playing soccer places a high demand on glycogen stores, so glycogen depletion could cause premature fatigue and reduced performance during a match.[34]

The ergogenic benefit of carbohydrate for sports such as soccer was confirmed in a study assessing the combined and separate benefits of carbohydrate and chromium ingestion during intermittent high-intensity exercise to fatigue. Data from this study confirmed the benefit of carbohydrate but did not support the benefit of chromium.[35] Of course, adequate energy intake, estimated to be approximately 4,000 calories for males and 3,200 calories for females, is also important. Without sufficient energy intake, glycogen will become depleted regardless of the makeup of the diet. In addition, inadequate caloric intake makes optimal synthesis of phosphocreatine (needed for sudden, quick-burst activity) difficult. This point is emphasized in a study that demonstrated a performance benefit of creatine supplementation in young soccer players, a finding that would be unlikely with adequate energy consumption.[36]

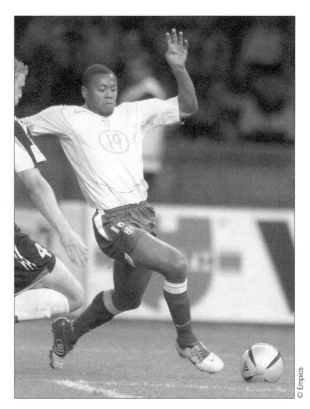

Professional soccer players need to consume approximately 4,000 calories per day during the competitive season to compensate for the massive amount of energy burned during play.

Keeping this in mind, figure skaters must consider the following nutritionally relevant factors for their sport.

Play in soccer is expected to be continuous, making it difficult for players to consume fluids. Since soccer players may not have an opportunity to regularly consume fluids during a game, pregame hydration status is particularly important. Whenever possible (between periods and during official breaks), players should consume a sports beverage to rehydrate and to replace carbohydrates. A study of soccer players found a wide variability in voluntary fluid intake patterns, with the conclusion that most players fail to adequately hydrate.[37]

Surveys suggest the consumption of carbohydrates is less than optimal for soccer players, yet carbohydrate consumption is critical for the achievement of optimal soccer performance. According to the surveys, soccer players typically consume diets that match those of the general public, with a carbohydrate intake of around 50 percent of total calories. Players should make a conscious effort to improve carbohydrate intake.

Pregame glycogen storage is critical. Soccer players spend a great deal of time running up and down the field, placing a tremendous drain on muscle glycogen. Players who begin the game with more stored glycogen will experience an endurance advantage. To achieve a higher glycogen storage, players should consistently consume plenty of carbohydrates and fluids and also focus mainly on carbohydrates during the pregame meal (see table 15.4).

Table 15.4   Fuel and Fluids for Soccer

Time	Recommendation
During routine training	• Consume 8-10 g of carbohydrate per kg body weight per day, or roughly 60-70% of total calories. • Drink sufficient fluids to sustain weight. Dark urine is a sign of dehydration.
Pregame	• Eat a high-carbohydrate meal of familiar, easy-to-digest foods 3-4 hr before match play. • Avoid high-fat (especially fried) foods. • Avoid high-fiber foods because they cause GI distress and gas. • Avoid solid foods just before the game because they are digested too slowly. • Nervous players should consider sipping on liquid meals.
During the game	• Consume a carbohydrate–electrolyte sports beverage at every opportunity. • At halftime drink enough sports beverage to maintain pregame weight.
Postgame	• Consume some sugar immediately after the game to help replace glycogen. • Consume 24 oz (720 ml) of fluid (preferably sports beverage) for every pound of weight lost over a 2- to 3-hr period after the game. • In 24 hr consume enough fluid and food to return weight to pregame level.

Adapted, by permission, from J. Lea, D. Richardson, H. O'Malley, Y. Satterwhite and M. Macedonio, 2000, "Maximizing performance and minimizing injuries in soccer," *GSSI Roundtable*, #39, 11(1).

Tennis

It is generally agreed that tennis has both aerobic and anaerobic components, but the majority of the energy supply appears to come from anaerobic systems.[38, 39] This heavy reliance on the anaerobic metabolic system is likely why carbohydrate supplementation improves the stroke quality during the final stages of a tennis match.[40] Since long-lasting, high-intensity exercise is highly dependent on carbohydrate as a fuel, it makes perfect sense that tennis players should ensure that carbohydrate is available to the muscles as a fuel.

Although carbohydrate consumption may be of concern, it appears that collegiate tennis players (Division I) have been well coached to consume sufficient fluids in hot environments. In a study evaluating fluid and electrolyte balance during multiday match play in a hot environment, the athletes successfully maintained overall balance, resulting in no occurrence of heat illness.[41]

It also appears, from data on young tennis players, that the adequacy of energy intake is better than that seen in other sports (gymnastics and swimming). It is well established that menstrual onset is, to a great degree, dependent on adequate energy intake. In general, females experience the first menses at age 13. Females who have energy deficits may have up to a 2-year delay in the age of menarche. Tennis players, however, appear to have only a slight delay (13.2 years) in the age of menarche, suggesting that energy consumption is good.[42] Typically, there is less concern in tennis about "making weight." The focus is on conditioning, regardless of where the weight ends up, and there is evidence that college women tennis players are no more at risk of eating disorders than any other young woman.[43]

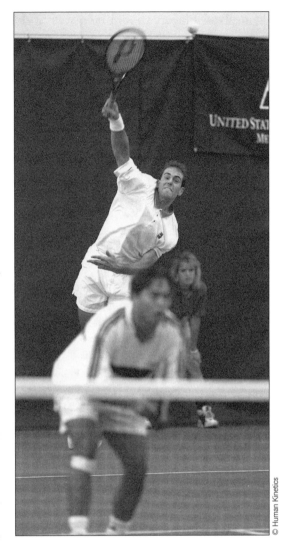

© Human Kinetics

Many tennis tournaments are played outside on courts that trap heat, a situation which unfortunately creates favorable conditions for heat-related illness. Hydration during breaks in the match is key for players to avoid this potential risk.

Keeping this in mind, tennis players must consider the following nutritionally relevant factors for their sport.

Tennis is commonly played outside on courts where the reflective temperature off the court is higher than the environmental temperature. The heat at courtside can quickly cause heat illness if tennis players fail to take steps to adequately hydrate themselves. Players should be aware of the signs of heat disorders (thirst, fatigue, vision problems, inability to speak normally) and take quick action if they, a partner, or an opponent appears to have any heat-related symptoms (see table 15.5).

Tennis has natural breaks after each odd game, when the opponents change sides. These natural breaks in a tennis match are, perhaps, why tennis players are in relatively good hydration state during and after a match. However, because carbohydrate supplementation has been found to improve end-of-game strokes, players should make certain that the beverage consumed contains carbohydrate. These sports beverages, if sipped during a match, will help ensure that high-intensity activity can be maintained for a longer period of time.

Table 15.5 Heat Disorder Symptoms

Heat cramps	Muscle spasms that occur involuntarily during or after exercise, typically in the muscles that did most of the work during the exercise.
Heat exhaustion	Weak and rapid heart rate with low blood pressure, headache, dizziness, and severe weakness. Body temperature is not elevated to dangerous levels, but sweat rate may be reduced, increasing the risk of high body temperature. Blood volume is typically low. At this stage, the athlete should stop exercising, go to a shady area or cool building, and consume fluids to rehydrate.
Heatstroke	A failure of the body's ability to maintain temperature. Characterized by a failure to sweat. Circulatory system collapse may lead to death. Immediate steps should be taken to cool the body by applying ice, placing the person in cold water, or applying alcohol rubs. This is an emergency condition, so medical assistance should be called immediately.

Sports that require a combination of power and endurance have only recently received the same level of scientific attention that endurance sports have enjoyed for many years. Studies on these sports indicate that carbohydrate consumption is useful for enhancing performance even if the activity lasts less than 1 hour. This is an important finding because the traditional thought has been that water is an appropriate hydration beverage for activities lasting less than 1 hour, whereas carbohydrate-containing sports beverages are important to consume for activities lasting longer than 1 hour. We now know that even for these shorter activities, carbohydrate consumption is performance enhancing. Since many of these sports (basketball, soccer, tennis) place an enormous caloric drain on the system, athletes should develop eating strategies (i.e., eating enough) that encourage maintenance of muscle mass during long and arduous seasons.

Part V

Nutritional Plans
for Specific Sports

16 | Sports Requiring Power and Speed

Power athletes are naturally focused on maximizing the strength-to-weight ratio so as to generate the greatest power at the lowest weight. To do this requires an eating strategy that will enable a maintenance or increase of the muscle mass, coupled with the lowest possible body fat percentage. Ideally, power athletes should sustain a protein intake of between 1.2 to 2.0 grams per kilogram of body weight, with the lower value for athletes seeking to sustain muscle mass and the higher value for athletes seeking to increase muscle mass. It is important to consider these two facts: (1) Most athletes (vegetarians are an exception) consume ample quantities of protein from food alone, often at levels well above 2.0 grams/kg of weight; and (2) a higher level of protein consumption by itself will not contribute to a larger muscle mass unless the higher protein intake is coupled with a higher total caloric intake. In essence, athletes should consume enough calories to sustain the current weight and muscle mass, plus enough additional calories to support a larger weight and muscle mass. This typically amounts to an additional 300 to 500 calories per day, coupled with enough of the right kind of resistance activity to stimulate the need for a larger mass.

A number of sports require the achievement of a specific competition weight (e.g., boxing, wrestling, horseracing), while other sports mandate the production of a high level of power at the lowest possible weight for both appearance and performance factors (e.g., gymnastics and diving). There is good evidence that both groups may follow eating strategies that either restrict calories or induce dehydration to achieve the desired weight. Neither of these strategies is appropriate or healthful. Importantly, restrained eating is likely to cause a significant catabolism of the lean body mass, which negatively influences the strength-to-weight ratio, and dehydration causes negative performance outcomes. Because restrained eating and induced dehydration are counterproductive to the athletes' ultimate goals, may be dangerous, and may lead to more serious eating disorders, they are inappropriate strategies for power athletes to follow. Instead, athletes should consider eating strategies that optimize performance and hydration state. To do so requires a meal pattern that includes 6 or more eating opportunities. This is a distinct separation from the usual three-meals-per-day eating pattern and, because of this, may be difficult to accomplish (people tend to eat in the way that most around them eat). Nevertheless, the rewards of having smaller and more frequent meals are real. Athletes who practice eating smaller and more frequent meals and drink frequently are likely to feel better and do better, a fact that is likely to encourage them to continue eating in this way.

About the Eating Plans in This Chapter

This chapter includes three eating plans for intakes of 2,500, 3,500, and 4,000 calories. To help athletes understand how to best integrate the eating plan into their exercise schedule, the plans include differently timed practice sessions. You will note that the right-hand column of each eating plan includes a "food exchange" list, which can be found in the appendix. The food exchange will allow you to make food substitutions with foods that have similar (but not identical) caloric and nutrient contents. For instance, if a roast beef sandwich is listed for lunch and you don't like roast beef, you can look at the food exchange list to find a near equivalent substitute for a food you do like. The goal here is to provide a *guide* for eating that gives the athlete a starting point for developing the best possible eating strategy for them. It is important to note that the caloric level of these diets is *not* likely to be perfect for anyone. Weight stability and a healthy body fat level are the best guides that an appropriate level of calories are being consumed at the right times. Athletes should find a caloric intake level that works for them as individuals. It is also important to note that fluid intakes are likely to be much higher than the fluids listed here. Athletes should consume ample quantities of water with meals and may also need to consume more sports beverages during bouts of physical activity. Athletes should drink enough to sustain optimal body water, an indication of which is nearly clear urine.

2,500 Calorie Intake

Meal/event	Foods	Amount	Calories	Food exchange
Early-morning snack	Bagel, whole wheat	1/2	145	2 starch
	Jam	2 tsp	37	1 fruit
	Grapefruit	1/2	60	1/2 fruit
			Meal calories: 242	
AM workout	Sports drink (6%)	16 oz	120	2 fruit
			Meal calories: 120	
Breakfast	Corn flakes	3/4 cup	98	1 starch
	All-bran cereal	1/4 cup	39	1/2 starch
	Blueberries	1/2 cup	41	1/2 fruit
	Flaxseed, ground	1 tbsp	36	1 fat
	Milk (1%)	8 oz	110	1 dairy
			Meal calories: 324	
Midmorning snack	Almonds	6	42	1 fat
	Raisins	4 tbsp	108	2 fruit
	Apple, fresh, med.	1	72	1 fruit
			Meal calories: 222	
Lunch	*Burrito*			
	Lean ground beef, 5% fat	2 oz	109	2 lean protein
	Refried beans, fat-free	1/4 cup	55	1/2 starch
	Cheddar cheese, shredded	2 tbsp	50	1/2 high-fat protein
	Salsa	1/4 cup	20	1 vegetable
	Tortilla, flour (7-8 in.)	1	159	2 starch
	Shredded carrot salad with	1 cup	50	2 vegetable
	lemon juice	2 tbsp	8	–
	Pear, fresh	1	96	1 fruit
			Meal calories: 547	
Afternoon snack	Yogurt, fruit, nonfat	1/2 cup	115	1 dairy
	Vanilla wafers	5	88	1 starch
			Meal calories: 203	
Late afternoon workout	Sports drink (6%)	16 oz	120	2 fruit
			Meal calories: 120	
Dinner	Chicken breast, broiled (no skin)	1 (3 oz)	142	3 lean meat
	Baked potato	1 large	188	2 starch
	Sour cream	2 tbsp	60	2 fat
	Green beans, steamed	1 cup	44	1 cup
	Cabbage slaw with	1 cup	21	1 vegetable
	Canola oil	1 tsp	41	1 fat
	Vinegar and salt	To taste	0	–
			Meal calories: 496	
Evening snack	Cottage cheese (4% fat)	1/2 cup	120	2 lean protein
	Peach slices in juice	1 cup	96	2 fruit
			Meal calories: 216	
Meal totals	Total calories: 2,490	FE (mg): 25	Vit C (mg): 198	Vit A (IU): 18,963
	Carb (g): 647 (67%)	ZN (mg): 12	Vit B$_1$ (mg): 1.35	Vit D (IU): 125
	Prot (g):145 (17%)	CA (mg): 1,156	Vit B$_2$ (mg): 1.79	Vit E (mg): 6.9
	Fat (g): 99 (16%)	NA (mg): 3,402	Niacin (mg): 41.0	Vit K (mcg): 136
	Dietary fiber (g): 53.3	MG (mg): 412	Vit B$_6$ (mg): 3.18	
		K (mg): 4,663	Vit B$_{12}$ (mcg): 6.0	
			Folate (mcg): 595	

This 2,500-calorie meal plan is for an athlete who has an early-morning workout and a late-afternoon workout, much like an elite gymnast. [The meal plan represents the approximate energy requirement for a very active female, age 17, who weighs 100 lb and is 5 ft tall.]

3,500 Calorie Intake

Meal/event	Foods	Amount	Calories	Food exchange
Breakfast	Whole wheat cereal	1.5 cups	175	2 starch
	Milk (1%)	1.5 cups	165	1.5 dairy
	Strawberries	1 cup	49	10 fruit
	Roll (whole wheat)	1 roll (small)	75	1 starch
	Orange juice	1.5 cups	165	3 fruit
	Margarine	1 tsp	35	1 fat
	Jam	1 tsp	19	1/2 fruit
			Meal calories: 683	
Midmorning snack	Bagel, plain	1/2 bagel (medium)	160	2 starch
	Cream cheese	1 tbsp	50	1 fat
	Apple juice	8 oz	110	2 fruit
			Meal calories: 420	
Lunch	*Roast beef sandwich*			
	Roast beef sliced (lean)	4 slices (2 oz total)	100	2 medium-fat protein
	Whole wheat bread	2 slices	138	2 starch
	Mayonnaise	1.5 tsp	52	1.5 fat
	Lettuce	1 leaf	0	Free exchange
	Potato salad	1 cup	325	3 starch; 3 fat
	Cranberry juice	1 cup	144	2.5 fruit
	Peach	1 medium (fresh)	40	1 fruit
			Meal calories: 799	
Afternoon snack	Saltine crackers	10 squares	130	1.5 starch
	Apple	1 medium	72	1 fruit
	Sports drink (6% carb)	16 oz	120	2 fruit
			Meal calories: 322	
Late afternoon workout	Sports drink (6% carb)	16 oz	120	2 fruit
			Meal calories: 120	
Dinner	Chicken chow mein	2 cups	365	3 starch; 3 lean protein; 1 fat
	Rice, white	2 cups	411	4 starch
	Orange	1 fresh	62	1 fruit
	Tea	1 cup	0	Free exchange
	Sugar (for tea)	1 tsp	23	1/3 fruit
			Meal calories: 861	
Evening snack	Milk (1%)	1 cup	110	1 dairy
	Graham crackers, chocolate coated	5 squares	339	1 starch
			Meal calories: 449	
Meal totals	Total calories: 3,654	FE (mg): 23	Vit C (mg): 446	Vit A (IU): 3,072
	Carb (g): 604 (67.2%)	ZN (mg): 6.2	Vit B_1 (mg): 1.99	Vit D (IU): 270
	Prot (g):107 (11.9%)	CA (mg): 1,278	Vit B_2 (mg): 1.1	Vit E (mg): 2.38
	Fat (g): 83 (20.9%)	NA (mg): 7,066	Niacin (mg): 15.59	Vit K (mcg): 12.98
	Dietary fiber (g): 53	MG (mg): 324	Vit B_6 (mg): 1.48	
		K (mg): 2,902	Vit B_{12} (mcg): 0.41	
			Folate (mcg): 552	

This 3,500-calorie meal plan is for an athlete who has a single late-afternoon workout, much like a football player.

[The meal plan represents the approximate energy requirement for a very active male, age 25, who weighs 170 lb and is 5 ft, 11 in. tall.]

4,000 Calorie Intake

Meal/event	Foods	Amount	Calories	Food exchange
Early-morning snack	Toast (whole wheat)	1 slice	70	1 starch
	Grape Juice	9 oz	170	1.5 fruit
			Meal calories: 240	
AM workout	Sport drink (6% carb)	18 oz	135	3 fruit
			Meal calories: 135	
Breakfast	Orange juice	4 oz	60	1 fruit
	Honeydew melon (fresh)	1/4 melon, cubed	115	2 fruit
	Unsweetened cereal	2 cups	320	2.75 starch
	Milk (1%)	1.5 cups	165	1.5 dairy
	Toast (whole wheat)	2 slice	140	2 starch
	Margarine	2 tsp	70	2 fat
	Jam	1 tsp	17	1/4 fruit
			Meal calories: 887	
Midmorning snack	Bagel (whole wheat)	1 medium	320	4 starch
	Margarine	1 tsp	35	1 fat
	Jam	2 tsp	35	1/2 fruit
	Coffee or tea	1 cup	0	Free exchange
	Sport drink (6% carb)	18 oz	135	3 fruit
			Meal calories: 525	
Lunch	*Hamburger*			
	Hamburger	3 oz	215	3 very lean protein
	Hamburger roll	1 roll	230	2 starch
	Ketchup	2 tsp	10	2 fat
	Lettuce	1 leaf	0	—
	Tomato	2 slices	12	1/2 vegetable
	French fries	1/2 cup	290	2 starch; 2 fat
	Banana	1 medium	100	1 fruit
	V-8 juice cocktail	8 oz	50	2.5 fruit
			Meal calories: 907	
Afternoon snack	Cheddar cheese	1 oz	115	1 medium-fat protein
	Saltine crackers	6 small	80	1 starch
	Grapes	1 cup	60	1 fruit
			Meal calories: 255	
Late-afternoon workout	Sport drink (6% carb)	18 oz	135	3 fruit
			Meal calories: 135	
Dinner	Broiled salmon filet	4 oz	185	4 very lean protein
	Broccoli	2 cup	90	4 vegetable
	Margarine	2 tsp	70	2 fat
	Baked potato	1 medium	190	1 starch
	Sour cream	1 tbsp	30	1 fat
	Fruit cocktail	1 cup fresh	120	1 fruit
			Meal calories: 685	
Evening snack	Milk (1%)	1 cup	110	1 dairy
	Popcorn	3 cups microwaved	92	1 starch
			Meal calories: 202	
Meal totals	Total calories: 3,971	FE (mg): 23	Vit C (mg): 345	Vit A (IU): 11,749
	Carb (g): 647 (63.8%)	ZN (mg): 15	Vit B_1 (mg): 1.53	Vit D (IU): 635
	Prot (g):145 (14.3%)	CA (mg): 1,399	Vit B_2 (mg): 2.04	Vit E (mg): 11
	Fat (g): 99 (21.9%)	NA (mg): 4,829	Niacin (mg): 31.17	Vit K (mcg): 461
	Dietary fiber (g): 52.8	MG (mg): 491	Vit B_6 (mg): 6.21	
		K (mg): 4,689	Vit B_{12} (mcg): 5.58	
			Folate (mcg): 595	

This 4,000-calorie meal plan is for an athlete who has an early-morning workout and a late-afternoon workout, much like a swimmer.

[The meal plan represents the approximate energy requirement for a very active male, age 25, who weighs 190 lb and is 6 ft tall.]

17 | Sports Requiring Endurance

Endurance athletes spend long hours in training and competition, a fact that underlines the importance they place on consumption of adequate calories to fuel the activity and sufficient fluids to sustain body temperature. While endurance-trained athletes have a wonderful capacity to burn fat as a source of energy and use fat as the *primary* source of energy during endurance events, it is their ability to stay well hydrated and store carbohydrate, as glycogen, that are the critical factors in endurance. While athletes have a phenomenally high capacity to store fat (and have all the necessary aerobic enzymes to metabolize it), there is an inherent limit to how much glycogen (stored carbohydrate) a human can store. Since this stored carbohydrate enables a more complete oxidation of fat for energy and is the primary fuel for higher intensity work (as with the high speed "kick" successful endurance runners have at the end of a race), endurance athletes can't afford to let it run out. This is precisely the reason so many endurance athletes consume large volumes of pasta and other carbohydrates before a race. However, *how* the carbohydrate is provided can influence how well the glycogen is stored. While endurance athletes can effectively process carbohydrates into stored glycogen, this process takes time and water.

Water is necessary because for every gram of stored glycogen 3 grams of water are needed. Because there is a limit to how quickly a cell can convert excess glucose to stored glycogen, endurance athletes should focus on consuming carbohydrates frequently over the course of several days rather than relying on a belly-busting high-carbohydrate meal on the day before an event.

About the Eating Plans in This Chapter

This chapter includes three eating plans for intakes of 2,500 (vegetarian), 3,000, and 4,000 calories. To help athletes understand how to best integrate the eating plan into their exercise schedule, the plans include differently timed practice sessions. You will note that the right-hand column of each eating plan includes a "food exchange" list, which can be found in the appendix. The food exchange will allow you to make food substitutions with foods that have similar (but not identical) caloric and nutrient contents. For instance, if a roast beef sandwich is listed for lunch and you don't like roast beef, you can look at the food exchange list to find a near equivalent substitute for a food you do like. The goal here is to provide a *guide* for eating that gives the athlete a starting point for developing the best possible eating strategy for them. It is important to note that the caloric level of these diets is *not* likely to be perfect for anyone. Weight stability and a healthy body fat level are the best guides that an appropriate level of calories are being consumed at the right times. Athletes should find a caloric intake level that works for them as individuals. It is also important to note that fluid intakes are likely to be much higher than the fluids listed here. Athletes should consume ample quantities of water with meals and may also need to consume more sports beverages during bouts of physical activity. Athletes should drink enough to sustain optimal body water, an indication of which is nearly clear urine.

2,500 Calorie Vegetarian (Lacto-Ovo) Intake

Meal/event	Foods	Amount	Calories	Food exchange
Early-morning snack	Bagel, whole wheat Jam Grapefruit	1/2 2 tsp 1/2	145 37 60 *Meal calories: 242*	2 starch 1 fruit 1/2 fruit
AM workout	Sports drink (6%)	16 oz	120 *Meal calories: 120*	2 fruit
Breakfast	Corn flakes All-bran cereal Blueberries Milk (1%)	3/4 cup 1/4 cup 1/2 cup 8 oz	98 39 41 110 *Meal calories: 288*	1 starch 1/2 starch 1/2 fruit 1 dairy
Midmorning snack	Almonds Raisins Apple, fresh, med.	6 4 tbsp 1	42 108 72 *Meal calories: 222*	1 fat 2 fruit 1 fruit
Lunch	*Burrito* Refried beans, fat-free Rice, cooked Cheddar cheese, shredded Salsa Tortilla, flour (7-8 in.) Shredded carrot salad 　with lemon juice Grapes, fresh	 1/2 cup 1/3 cup 4 tbsp 1/4 cup 1 1 cup 2 tbsp 10	 110 68 100 20 159 50 8 55 *Meal calories: 570*	 1 very lean protein = 1 starch 1 starch 1 high-fat protein 1 vegetable 2 starch 2 vegetable – 1 fruit
Afternoon snack	Yogurt, fruit, nonfat Vanilla wafers	1/2 cup 5	115 88 *Meal calories: 203*	1 dairy 1 starch
Late-afternoon workout	Sports drink (6%)	16 oz	120 *Meal calories: 120*	2 fruit
Dinner	Eggs, poached Tomatoes, canned, diced Olive oil Baked potato Sour cream Spinach, cooked Lemon juice	2 1 cup 2 tsp 1 med 1 tbsp 1 cup To taste	147 50 80 188 30 41 6 *Meal calories: 542*	2 medium-high-fat protein 2 vegetable 2 fat 2 starch 1 fat 2 vegetable –
Evening snack	Cottage cheese (1% fat) Peach slices in juice	3/4 cup 1/2 cup	120 60 *Meal calories: 180*	3 lean protein 1 fruit
Meal totals	Total calories: 2,487 Carb (g): 444 (69%) Prot (g): 93 (14%) Fat (g): 47 (17%) Dietary fiber (g): 50	Iron (mg): 30 Zinc (mg): 9 Calcium (mg): 1,672 Sodium (mg): 4,806 Magnesium (mg): 461 Potassium (mg): 4,413	Vit C (mg): 203 Vit B_1 (mg): 1.47 Vit B_2 (mg): 2.53 Niacin (mg):14 Vit B_6 (mg): 2.8 Vit B_{12} (mcg): 5.8 Folate (mcg): 734	Vit A (IU): 38,399 Vit D (IU): 160 Vit E (mg): 10.8 Vit K (mcg): 947

This 2,500-calorie vegetarian meal plan is for an athlete who has an early-morning workout and a late-afternoon workout, much like a marathon runner. [The meal plan represents the approximate energy requirement for a very active female, age 30, who weighs 105 lb and is 5 ft, 3 in. tall.]

3,000 Calorie Intake

Meal/event	Foods	Amount	Calories	Food exchange
Early-morning snack	Toast (whole wheat)	1 slice	69	1 starch
	Jam	1 tsp	17	1/4 fruit
	Apple juice	4 oz	55	1 fruit
			Meal calories: 141	
AM workout	Sport drink (6% carb)	12 oz	90	1.5 fruit
			Meal calories: 90	
Breakfast	Orange juice	4 oz	55	1 fruit
	Strawberries (fresh)	1 cup	53	1 fruit
	Egg, hard-cooked	1	78	1 medium-fat protein
	All-bran cereal	1.5 cups	184	2 starch
	Milk (1%)	8 oz	110	1 dairy
	Toast (whole wheat)	1 slice	69	1 starch
	Margarine, soft	1 tsp	34	1 fat
	Jam	1 tsp	17	1/4 fruit
			Meal calories: 600	
Midmorning snack	Bagel (whole wheat)	1 medium	320	4 starch
	Margarine	1 tsp	34	1 fat
	Jam	2 tsp	33	1/2 fruit
	Coffee or tea	1 cup	0	Free exchange
			Meal calories: 387	
Lunch	*Turkey sandwich*			
	Turkey, deli sliced	4 oz	126	4 very lean protein
	Bread (whole wheat)	2 slices	138	2 starch
	Mayonnaise	2 tsp	70	2 fat
	Lettuce	1 leaf	0	–
	Tomato	2 thick slices	8	1/3 vegetable
	Potato salad (deli type)	1/3 cup	107	1 starch; 1 fat
	Apple	1 medium	80	1 fruit
	Cranberry juice cocktail	8 oz	144	2.5 fruit
			Meal calories: 673	
Afternoon workout	Sport drink (6% carb)	12 oz	90	1.5 fruit
			Meal calories: 90	
Afternoon snack	String cheese	1 oz	80	1 medium-fat protein
	Pretzels	1 oz	108	1.3 starch
	Grapes	1 cup	60	1 fruit
			Meal calories: 248	
Dinner	*Chicken vegetable stir-fry*			
	Chicken breast, cooked	4 oz	170	4 lean protein
	Broccoli	1 cup	44	2 vegetable
	Red pepper, carrots, celery, bean sprouts	1/4 cup each	59	2 vegetable
	Vegetable oil	2 tsp	80	2 fat
	Soy sauce	To taste	137	Free exchange
	Rice	2/3 cup cooked	62	2 starch
	Orange	1 medium fresh	0	1 fruit
	Tea	1 cup	0	Free exchange
			Meal calories: 552	

Meal/event	Foods	Amount	Calories	Food exchange
Evening snack	Milk (1%) Graham crackers	8 oz 5 squares	110 75 *Meal calories: 185*	1 dairy 1 starch
Meal totals	Total calories: 2,966 Carb (g): 483 (63%) Protein (g):139 (18%) Fat (g): 64 (19%) Dietary fiber (g): 44	FE (mg): 56 ZN (mg): 37 CA (mg): 1,211 NA (mg): 4,934 MG(mg): 393 K (mg): 3,105	Vit C (mg) : 666 Vit B_1 (mg) : 4.6 Vit B_2 (mg): 4.8 Niacin (mg): 61 Vit B_6 (mg): 5.7 Vit B_{12} (mcg): 12.9 Folate (mcg): 1,287	Vit A (IU): 15,581 Vit D (IU): 320 Vit E (mg): 61 Vit K (mcg): 32

This 3,000-calorie meal plan is for an athlete who has an early-morning workout and an afternoon workout, much like a high school runner at summer camp.

[The meal plan represents the approximate energy requirement for a very active female, age 16, who weighs 125 lb and is 5 ft, 8 in. tall.]

4,000 Calorie Intake

Meal/event	Foods	Amount	Calories	Food exchange
Breakfast	Orange juice	12 oz	180	3 fruit
	Honeydew melon (fresh)	1/4 melon, cubed	115	2 fruit
	Unsweetened cereal	2 cups	320	2.75 starch
	Milk (1%)	1.5 cups	165	1.5 dairy
	Toast (whole wheat)	3 slice	210	3 starch
	Margarine	2 tsp	70	2 fat
	Jam	1 tsp	17	1/4 fruit
			Meal calories: 1,077	
Midmorning snack	Bagel (whole wheat)	1 medium	320	4 starch
	Margarine	1 tsp	35	1 fat
	Jam	2 tsp	35	1/2 fruit
	Coffee or tea	1 cup	0	Free exchange
	Sport drink (6% carb)	18 oz	135	3 fruit
			Meal calories: 525	
Lunch	*Hamburger*			
	Hamburger	3 oz	215	3 very lean protein
	Hamburger roll	1 roll	230	2 starch
	Ketchup	2 tsp	10	2 fat
	Lettuce	1 leaf	0	—
	Tomato	2 slices	12	1/2 vegetable
	French fries	1/2 cup	290	2 starch; 2 fat
	Banana	1 medium	100	1 fruit
	V-8 juice cocktail	8 oz	50	2.5 fruit
			Meal calories: 907	
Afternoon snack	Cheddar cheese	1 oz	115	1 medium-fat
	Saltine crackers	6 small	80	protein
	Grapes	1 cup	60	1 starch
	Sport drink (6% carb)	18 oz	135	1 fruit
			Meal calories: 390	3 fruit
Late-afternoon workout	Sport drink (6% carb)	18 oz	135	3 fruit
			Meal calories: 135	
Dinner	Broiled salmon filet	4 oz	185	4 very lean protein
	Broccoli	2 cups	90	4 vegetable
	Margarine	2 tsp	70	2 fat
	Baked potato	1 medium	190	1 starch
	Sour cream	1 tbsp	30	1 fat
	Fruit cocktail	1 cup fresh	120	1 fruit
			Meal calories: 685	
Evening snack	Milk (1%)	1 cup	110	1 dairy
	Popcorn	3 cups microwaved	92	1 starch
			Meal calories: 202	
Meal totals	Total calories: 3,921	FE (mg): 23	Vit C (mg): 345	Vit A (IU): 11,749
	Carb (g): 647 (63.8%)	ZN (mg): 15	Vit B_1 (mg): 1.53	Vit D (IU): 635
	Prot (g):145 (14.3%)	CA (mg): 1,399	Vit B_2 (mg): 2.04	Vit E (mg): 11
	Fat (g): 99 (21.9%)	NA (mg): 4,829	Niacin (mg): 31.17	Vit K (mcg): 461
	Dietary fiber (g): 52.8	MG (mg): 491	Vit B_6 (mg): 6.21	
		K (mg): 4,689	Vit B_{12} (mcg): 5.58	
			Folate (mcg): 595	

This 4,000-calorie meal plan is for an athlete who has a single late-afternoon workout, much like a triathlete.

[The meal plan represents the approximate energy requirement for a very active male, age 35, who weighs 190 lb and is 6 ft, 2 in. tall.]

18

Sports Requiring Combined Power and Endurance

Team sports such as soccer and basketball, and individual sports such as tennis, have a combined requirement for power *and* endurance. These sports require the ultimate balance in conditioning and often have an additional requirement for a high level of skill that is sports specific. The nutritional demands on athletes involved in team sports are high, with a need for sufficient calories to endure long and frequent practices, and a high need for fluids to sustain hydration state. Unlike many other sports, team sports often have natural "breaks" during practices and competitions that should be considered by the participating athlete as a golden opportunity to replenish carbohydrate stores and fluids. The ideal training regimen would be one that gives athletes constant practice in understanding how much fluid they can tolerate during these breaks, so that drinking during competitions will be performance enhancing rather than performance detracting. Athletes should understand, however, that humans are highly adaptable to food and nutrient intake, so practicing fluid consumption should lead to an enhanced capacity to consume more fluids over time without any GI distress. Given what we now know to be true from well-designed research studies, athletes who drink plain water during the natural breaks in practice and competition are missing a valuable opportunity to sustain blood volume, sustain sweat rates, and sustain carbohydrate delivery to working muscles. Only carbohydrate-electrolyte containing beverages have the potential of fulfilling these during-exercise needs, while plain water may actually have the opposite effect. Combined power and endurance sports often have periods or halftime breaks interspersed during the competition. These should also be considered valuable opportunities for consuming fluids and carbohydrates. Consumption of anything else, such as protein bars, simply detracts from what working muscles really need: carbohydrate and fluid. There is a place for meal-replacement bars that contain vitamins, minerals, and protein, but halftime during a basketball game is not one of those times. In some cases, athletes have adapted to eating a banana, crackers, or bread during halftime, but these should be well practiced *before* a competition to be certain they are well tolerated and leave the stomach before the game restarts.

About the Eating Plans in This Chapter

This chapter includes three eating plans for intakes of 2,000 (vegetarian), 3,000, and 3,500 calories. To help athletes understand how to best integrate the eating plan into their exercise schedule, the plans include differently timed practice sessions. You will note that the right-hand column of each eating plan includes a "food exchange" list, which can be found in the appendix. The food exchange will allow you to make food substitutions with foods that have similar (but not identical) caloric and nutrient contents. For instance, if a roast beef sandwich is listed for lunch and you don't like roast beef, you can look at the food exchange list to find a near equivalent substitute for a food you do like. The goal here is to provide a *guide* for eating that gives the athlete a starting point for developing the best possible eating strategy for them. It is important to note that the caloric level of these diets is *not* likely to be perfect for anyone. Weight stability and a healthy body fat level are the best guides that an appropriate level of calories are being consumed at the right times. Athletes should find a caloric intake level that works for them as individuals. It is also important to note that fluid intakes are likely to be much higher than the fluids listed here. Athletes should consume ample quantities of water with meals and may also need to consume more sports beverages during bouts of physical activity. Athletes should drink enough to sustain optimal body water, an indication of which is nearly clear urine.

2,000 Calorie Vegetarian (Lacto-Ovo) Intake

Meal/event	Foods	Amount	Calories	Food exchange
Early-morning snack	English muffin, whole wheat	1/2	67	1 starch
	Orange juice	4 oz	55	1 fruit
			Meal calories: 122	
AM workout	Sports drink (6%)	16 oz	120	2 fruit
			Meal calories: 120	
Breakfast	All-bran cereal	3/4 cup	119	1 starch
	Milk (1%)	6 oz	82	3/4 dairy
	Blueberries	1/2 cup	41	1 fruit
			Meal calories: 242	
Midmorning snack	Banana, small	1	90	1.5 fruit
	Soy nuts, unsalted	1 oz	120	2 very lean protein + 1/2 starch
			Meal calories: 210	
Lunch	*Salad*			
	Chick peas	1/2 cup	110	1 very lean protein + 1 starch
	Cheddar cheese, diced	1 oz	114	1 high-fat protein
	Tomatoes, chopped	1/2 cup	19	1/2 vegetable
	Corn, yellow	1/4 cup	33	1/2 starch
	Carrots, raw, grated	1/2 cup	23	1/2 vegetable
	Romaine lettuce, chopped	2 cups	19	1 vegetable
	Salsa	1/2 cup	40	2 vegetable
	Pita, toasted, whole wheat	1/2	60	1 starch
	Melon cubes	1/2 cup	54	1 fruit
			Meal calories: 472	
Afternoon snack	Milk (1%)	8 oz	110	1 dairy
	Graham crackers, 2.5 in. square	3	89	1 starch
			Meal calories: 199	
Late-afternoon workout	Sports drink	16 oz	120	2 fruit
			Meal calories: 120	
Dinner	*Stir-fry*			
	Tofu, extra firm, cubed	1/2 cup	80	1 medium-fat protein
	Broccoli	1 cup	44	2 vegetable
	Mushrooms, sliced	1/2 cup	8	1 vegetable
	Red bell peppers	1/2 cup	12	1 vegetable
	Scallions, chopped	2 tbsp	4	—
	Peanut oil	2 tsp	80	2 fat
	Soy sauce	To taste	137	Free exchange
	Brown rice, cooked	3/4 cup	163	2 starch
			Meal calories: 528	
Evening snack	Applesauce, unsweetened	1/2 cup	52	1 fruit
	Cottage cheese (1% fat)	1/2 cup	82	3 very lean protein
			Meal calories: 134	
Meal totals	Total calories: 2,027	FE (mg): 19	Vit C (mg): 431	Vit A (IU): 26,123
	Carb (g): 324 (64%)	ZN (mg): 7	Vit B$_1$ (mg): 1.5	Vit D (IU): 205
	Prot (g): 335 (18%)	CA (mg): 1,315	Vit B$_2$ (mg): 1.7	Vit E (mg): 5.8
	Fat (g): 43 (18%)	NA (mg): 3,119	Niacin (mg): 19	Vit K (mcg): 149
	Dietary fiber (g): 31	MG (mg): 383	Vit B$_6$ (mg): 2.4	
		K (mg): 4,087	Vit B$_{12}$ (mcg): 2.9	
			Folate (mcg): 562	

This 2,000-calorie vegetarian meal plan is for an athlete who has an early-morning workout and a late-afternoon workout, much like a young tennis player at summer camp.

[The meal plan represents the approximate energy requirement for a moderately active female, age 11, who weighs 70 lb and is 4 ft, 6 in. tall.]

3,000 Calorie Intake

Meal/event	Foods	Amount	Calories	Food exchange
Early-morning snack	Toast (whole wheat)	1 slice	69	1 starch
	Jam	1 tsp	17	1/4 fruit
	Apple juice	4 oz	55	1 fruit
			Meal calories: 141	
Breakfast	Orange juice	4 oz	55	1 fruit
	Strawberries (fresh)	1 cup	53	1 fruit
	Egg, hard-cooked	1	78	1 medium-fat protein
	All-bran cereal	1.5 cups	184	2 starch
	Milk (1%)	8 oz	110	1 dairy
	Toast (whole wheat)	1 slice	69	1 starch
	Margarine, soft	1 tsp	34	1 fat
	Jam	1 tsp	17	1/4 fruit
			Meal calories: 600	
Midmorning snack	Bagel (whole wheat)	1 medium	320	4 starch
	Margarine	1 tsp	34	1 fat
	Jam	2 tsp	33	1/2 fruit
	Coffee or tea	1 cup	0	Free exchange
			Meal calories: 387	
Lunch	*Turkey sandwich*			
	Turkey, deli sliced	4 oz	126	4 very lean protein
	Bread (whole wheat)	2 slices	138	2 starch
	Mayonnaise	2 tsp	70	2 fat
	Lettuce	1 leaf	0	1/3 vegetable
	Tomato	2 thick slices	8	1 starch; 1 fat
	Potato salad (deli type)	1/3 cup	107	1 fruit
	Apple	1 medium	80	2.5 fruit
	Cranberry juice cocktail	8 oz	144	
			Meal calories: 673	
Afternoon workout	Sport drink (6% carb)	24 oz	180	3 fruit
			Meal calories: 180	
Afternoon snack	String cheese	1 oz	80	1 medium-fat protein
	Pretzels	1 oz	108	1.3 starch
	Grapes	1 cup	60	1 fruit
			Meal calories: 248	
Dinner	*Chicken vegetable stir-fry*			
	Chicken breast, cooked	4 oz	170	4 lean protein
	Broccoli	1 cup	44	2 vegetable
	Red pepper, carrots, celery, bean sprouts	1/4 cup each	59	2 vegetable
	Vegetable oil	2 tsp	80	2 fat
	Soy sauce	To taste	137	Free exchange
	Rice	2/3 cup cooked	62	2 starch
	Orange	1 medium fresh	0	1 fruit
	Tea	1 cup	0	Free exchange
			Meal calories: 552	
Evening snack	Milk (1%)	8 oz	110	1 dairy
	Graham crackers	5 squares	75	1 starch
			Meal calories: 185	
Meal totals	Total calories: 2,966	FE (mg): 56	Vit C (mg): 666	Vit A (IU): 15,581
	Carb (g): 483 (63%)	ZN (mg): 37	Vit B$_1$ (mg): 4.6	Vit D (IU): 320
	Protein (g):139 (18%)	CA (mg): 1,211	Vit B$_2$ (mg): 4.8	Vit E (mg): 61
	Fat (g): 64 (19%)	NA (mg): 4,934	Niacin (mg): 61	Vit K (mcg): 32
	Dietary fiber (g): 44	MG (mg): 393	Vit B$_6$ (mg): 5.7	
		K (mg): 3,105	Vit B$_{12}$ (mcg): 12.9	
			Folate (mcg): 1,287	

This 3,000-calorie meal plan is for an athlete who has a single afternoon workout, much like a high school soccer player.

[The meal plan represents the approximate energy requirement for a very active female, age 16, who weighs 125 lb and is 5 ft, 8 in. tall.]

3,500 Calorie Intake

Meal/event	Foods	Amount	Calories	Food exchange
Pre-exercise snack	Toast	1 slice	70	1 starch
	Apple juice	1/2 cup	55	1 fruit
			Meal calories: 125	
AM workout	Sports drink (6% carb)	16 oz	120	2 fruit
			Meal calories: 120	
Breakfast	Whole wheat cereal	1.5 cups	175	2 starch
	Milk (1%)	1.5 cups	165	1.5 dairy
	Strawberries	1 cup	49	10 fruit
	Roll (whole wheat)	1 roll (small)	75	1 starch
	Orange juice	1.5 cups	165	3 fruit
	Margarine	1 tsp	35	1 fat
	Jam	1 tsp	19	1/2 fruit
			Meal calories: 683	
Midmorning snack	Bagel, plain	1/2 bagel (medium)	160	2 starch
	Cream cheese	1 tbsp	50	1 fat
	Apple juice	8 oz	110	2 fruit
			Meal calories: 320	
Lunch	*Roast beef sandwich*			
	Roast beef sliced (lean)	4 slices (2 oz total)	100	2 medium-fat protein
	Whole wheat bread	2 slices	138	2 starch
	Mayonnaise	1.5 tsp	52	1.5 fat
	Lettuce	1 leaf	0	Free exchange
	Potato salad	1 cup	325	3 starch; 3 fat
	Cranberry juice	1 cup	144	2.5 fruit
	Peach	1 medium (fresh)	40	1 fruit
			Meal calories: 799	
Afternoon snack	Saltine crackers	10 squares	130	1.5 starch
	Apple	1 medium	72	1 fruit
			Meal calories: 202	
Late-afternoon workout	Sports drink (6% carb)	16 oz	120	2 fruit
			Meal calories: 120	
Dinner	Chicken chow mein	2 cups	365	3 starch; 3 lean protein; 1 fat
	Rice, white	2 cups	411	4 starch
	Orange	1 fresh	62	1 fruit
	Tea	1 cup	0	Free exchange
	Sugar (for tea)	1 tsp	23	1/3 fruit
			Meal calories: 861	
Evening snack	Milk (1%)	1 cup	110	1 dairy
	Graham crackers, chocolate coated	5 squares	339	1 starch
			Meal calories: 449	
Meal totals	Total calories: 3,679	Iron (mg): 23	Vit C (mg): 446	Vit A (IU): 3,072
	Carb (g): 604 (67.2%)	Zinc (mg): 6.2	Vit B$_1$ (mg): 1.99	Vit D (IU): 270
	Prot (g):107 (11.9%)	Calcium (mg): 1,278	Vit B$_2$ (mg): 1.1	Vit E (mg): 2.38
	Fat (g): 83 (20.9%)	Sodium (mg): 7,066	Niacin (mg): 15.59	Vit K (mcg): 12.98
	Dietary fiber (g): 53	Magnesium (mg): 324	Vit B$_6$ (mg): 1.48	
		Potassium (mg): 2,902	Vit B$_{12}$ (mcg): 0.41	
			Folate (mcg): 552	

This 3,500-calorie meal plan is for an athlete who has an early-morning and a late-afternoon workout, much like a lacrosse player.

[The meal plan represents the approximate energy requirement for a very active male, age 25, who weighs 170 lb and is 5 ft, 11 in. tall.]

Food Exchange Lists

Dairy (approximately 110 calories per serving of fat-free or very low-fat dairy products)	
Serving size	**Food**
1 cup (8 oz)	Milk (fat free or 1% fat)
1/2 cup	Yogurt (sweetened plain, nonfat or lowfat)
1 cup	Yogurt (artificially sweetened, nonfat or lowfat)

Very lean protein (approximately 35 calories and 1 gram of fat per serving)	
Serving size	**Food**
1/2 cup	Beans, cooked (black, kidney, chick peas, lentils); also contain carbohydrate equivalent to 1 starch: Example: 1/2 cup lentils = 1 very lean protein + 1 starch
1 oz	Canned tuna (packed in water)
1 oz	Cheese (nonfat)
¼ cup	Cottage cheese (nonfat or 1% fat)
2	Egg whites
1 oz	Fish fillet (flounder, sole, scrod, cod, etc.—either baked, broiled, or boiled)
1 oz	Shellfish (clams, lobster, scallop, shrimp either steamed, boiled, or baked)
1 oz	Turkey breast or chicken breast, deli-sliced

Lean protein (approximately 55 calories and up to 3 grams of fat per serving)	
Serving size	**Food**
1 oz	Cheese (low fat—3 grams or less of fat per ounce)
1 oz	Chicken or turkey, white meat (no skin)
1/4 cup	Cottage cheese (4% fat)
1 oz	Fish (salmon, swordfish, or herring)
1 oz	Lamb (roasted or lean chop)
1 oz	Lean beef (flank, ground beef [5%], London broil, tenderloin, roast beef)
1 oz	Luncheon meat (low fat)
2 tbsp	Parmesan cheese, grated
1 oz	Pork (tenderloin or fresh ham)
2 medium	Sardines
1 oz	Veal (roasted or lean chop)

Medium-fat protein (approximately 75 calories and 5 grams of fat per serving)	
Serving size	**Food**
1 oz	Beef (any prime cut, corned beef, ground beef [10%])
1 oz	Cheese (mozzarella or other cheese with ≤ 5 g fat per oz)
1 oz	Chicken or turkey, dark meat (no skin)
1 egg	Egg (boiled, poached, or scrambled without fat)
1 oz	Pork chop
1/4 cup (2 oz)	Ricotta cheese
4 oz	Tofu

High-fat protein (approximately 100 calories and 8 grams of fat per serving)	
Serving size	Food
3 slices	Bacon (20 slices per lb)
1 oz	Cheese (regular cheeses: American, cheddar, Monterey Jack, or Swiss)
1 oz	Pork (spare ribs, ground pork, pork sausage)
1 oz	Processed sandwich meats (bologna, salami, or other with ≤ 8 g fat per oz)
1 oz	Sausage or hot dogs
Count as one high-fat protein plus one fat exchange	
2 tbsp	Peanut butter

Fruit (approximately 60 calories and 15 grams of carbohydrate per serving)	
Serving size	Food
3-4	Apricots or prunes, dried
1/2	Banana
1 cup	Berries
1/2 cup	Canned fruit (unsweetened)
1.5	Figs, dried
1 medium	Fresh fruit (your choice)
4 oz	Fruit juice (unsweetened)
1/2	Grapefruit
1/8	Honeydew melon
4 tsp	Jelly or jam
1 cup	Melon
2 tbsp	Raisins or dried cranberries
8 oz	Sports drink (6% carbohydrate solution)

Vegetables (approximately 25 calories and 5 grams of carbohydrate per serving)

Serving size	Food
1/2 cup	Cooked vegetables (prepared without fat: boiled or steamed)
1 cup	Raw vegetables or salad greens
1/4 cup	Salsa
1/2 cup	Vegetable juice

Starches (80 calories and 15 grams of carbohydrate per serving)	
Serving size	**Food**
1/4	Bagel
1/2 cup	Barley or couscous (cooked)
1/2 cup	Bran cereals
1 slice	Bread
1/2 cup	Bulgar
3/4 cup	Cereal (flakes)
1/2 cup	Cereal, hot (oatmeal, grits, etc.)
1.5 cup	Cereal, puffed
1/2 cup	Corn, sweet potato, or green peas
1/2	English muffin
3	Graham crackers (2.5 in. squares)
1/4 cup	Grape nuts, low-fat granola
1/2	Hamburger bun
1/3 cup	Legumes (dried beans, peas, or lentils prepared)
1/4 cup	Muesli
1/2 cup	Pasta, cooked
3 cups	Popcorn (microwaved [80% lite] or air-popped)
1 small	Potato (baked)
3/4 ounce	Pretzels
1/3 cup	Rice, cooked
2	Rice cakes (4 in.)
6	Saltine-type crackers
1 cup	Squash, winter (acorn, butternut)
1/2	Tortilla, corn (6 in.) or flour (7-8 in.)
5	Vanilla wafers

Fats (45 calories and 5 grams of fat per serving)	
Serving size	**Food**
6	Almonds, cashews
1/8	Avocado
1 slice	Bacon
8 large	Black olives
1 tsp	Butter or margarine
1 tbsp	Cream cheese
1 tbsp	Flax seed, ground
2 tbsp	Lite cream cheese
1 tsp	Mayonnaise
1 tsp	Oil, vegetable
6 large	Olives, black
6 nuts	Peanuts
1 tbsp	Reduced-fat margarine or mayonnaise
1 tbsp	Salad dressing
10 large	Stuffed green olives
4 halves	Walnuts, pecans

Endnotes

Chapter 1

1 Hultman E and Nilsson LH. Liver glycogen in man: Effects of different diets and muscular exercise. *Muscle metabolism during intense exercise* (Ed. Pernow B and Saltin B). London: Plenum Press. 1971: pp. 143-151.

2 Hultman E and Greenhaff PL. Carbohydrate metabolism in exercise. *Nutrition in sport* (Ed. Maughan RJ). London: Blackwell Science. 2000: pp. 90-91.

3 Pate TD and Brunn JC. Fundamentals of carbohydrate metabolism. *Nutrition in exercise and sport* (Ed. Hickson JF and Wolinsky I). Boca Raton, FL: CRC Press. 1989: pp. 37-49.

4 Karlsson J and Saltin B. Diet, muscle glycogen, and endurance. *Journal of Applied Physiology* 1971; 31(2): 203-206.

5 Sahlin K, Katz A, and Broberg S. Tricarboxylic cycle intermediates in human muscle during submaximal exercise. *American Journal of Physiology* 1990; 259: C834-C841.

6 Fitts RH. Cellular mechanisms of muscle fatigue. *Physiological Reviews* 1994; 74: 49-94.

7 The branched-chain amino acids are leucine, isoleucine, and valine.

8 Newsholme EA and Castell LM. Amino acids, fatigue and immunodepression in exercise. In: *Nutrition in sport* (Ed. Maughan RJ). London: Blackwell Science. 2000: pp. 156-158.

9 Davis JM, Alderson NL, and Welsh RS. Serotonin and central nervous system fatigue: nutritional considerations. *American Journal of Clinical Nutrition* 2000; 72(2) Suppl: 573S-8S.

10 Davis JM, Zhao Z, Stock HS, Mehl KA, Buggy J & Hand GA. Central nervous system effects of caffeine and adenosine on fatigue. *American Journal of Physiology: Regulatory, Integrative and Comparative Physiology* 2003; 284(2): R399-404.

11 Institute of Medicine. Dietary Reference Intakes for energy, carbohydrate, fiber, fat, fatty acids, cholesterol, protein and amino acids. Food and Nutrition Board. Washington, DC: National Academies Press. 2002.

12 Position of the American Dietetic Association, Dietitians of Canada, and the American College of Sports Medicine. Nutrition and athletic performance. *Journal of the American Dietetic Association* 2000; 100: 1543-1556.

13 USDA/HHS. Nutrition and your health: Dietary guidelines for Americans. Home and Garden Bulletin no. 232. Washington DC: Government Printing Office. 2000.

14 Costill DL, Sherman WM, Fink WJ, Maresh C, Witten M, and Miller JM. The role of dietary carbohydrate in muscle glycogen synthesis after strenuous running. *American Journal of Clinical Nutrition* 1981; 34: 1831-1836.

15 Sherman WM. Metabolism of sugars and physical performance. *American Journal of Clinical Nutrition* 1995; 62(suppl.): S228-S241.

16 Burke LM, Kiens B, and Ivy JL. Carbohydrate and fat for training and recovery. *Journal of Sports Sciences* 2004; 22: 15-30.

17 Coutts A, Reaburn P, Mummery K, & Holmes M. The effect of glycerol hyperhydration on Olympic distance triathlon performance in high ambient temperatures. *International Journal of Sport Nutrition and Exercise Metabolism* 2002; 12(1): 105-19.

18 Magal, M, Webster MJ, Sistrunk LE, Whitehead MT, Evans RK, & Boyd JC. Comparison of glycerol and water hydration regimens on tennis-related performance. *Medicine & Science in Sports & Exercise* 2003; 35(1): 150-6.

19 The typical energy cost of walking or running 1 mile (1.6 km) is approximately 100 calories.

20 Coyle EF. Fat metabolism during exercise. *Sports Science Exchange* (59) 1995; 8(6).

21 Kiens B and Helge JW. Adaptations to a high fat diet. In: *Nutrition in sport* (Ed. Maughan RJ). London: Blackwell Science. 2000: pp. 192-202.

22 Bach AS & Babayan VK. Medium-chain triglycerides: An update. *American Journal of Clinical Nutrition* 1982; 36(5): 950-62.

23 Seaton TB, Welle SL, Warenko MK, & Campbell RG. Thermic effect of medium-chain and long-chain triglycerides in man. *American Journal of Clinical Nutrition* 1986; 44(5): 630-4.

24 Geliebter A, Torbay N, Bracco EF, Hashim SA, & Van Itallie TB. Overfeeding with medium-chain triglyceride diet results in diminished deposition of fat. *American Journal of Clinical Nutrition* 1983; 37(1): 1-4.

25 Scalfi L, Coltorti A, & Contaldo F. Postprandial thermogenesis in lean and obese subjects after meals supplemented with medium-chain and long-chain triglycerides. *American Journal of Clinical Nutrition* 1991; 53(5): 1130-3.

26 Angus DJ, Hargreaves M, Dancey J, and Febbraio MA. Effect of carbohydrate or carbohydrate plus medium-chain triglyceride ingestion on cycling time trial performance. *Journal of Applied Physiology* 2000; 88(1): 113-119.

27 Lambert EV, Goedecke JH, Zyle C, Murphy K, Hawley JA, Dennis SC, and Noakes TD. High-fat diet versus habitual diet prior to carbohydrate loading: Effects of exercise metabolism and cycling performance. *International Journal of Sport Nutrition and Exercise Metabolism* 2001; 11(2): 209-225.

28 Misell LM, Lagomarcino ND, Schuster V, and Kern M. Chronic medium-chain triacylglycerol consumption and endurance performance in trained runners. *Journal of Sports Medicine and Physical Fitness* 2001; 41(2): 210-215.

29 Kern M, Lagomarcino ND, Misell LM, and Schuster V. The effect of medium-chain triacylglycerols on the blood lipid profile of male endurance runners. *Journal of Nutritional Biochemistry* 2000; 11(5): 288-292.

30 Kasai M, Nosaka N, Maki H, Suzuki Y, Takeuchi H, Aoyama T, Ohra A, Harada Y, Okazaki M, and Kondo K. *Journal of Nutritional Science and Vitaminology* 2002; 48(6): 536-240.

31 St-Onge MP, Ross R, Parsons WD, and Jones PJ. Medium-chain triglycerides increase energy expenditure and decrease adiposity in overweight men. *Obesity Research* 2003; 11(3): 395-402.

32 Jukendrup AE, Saris WHM, Schrauwen P, Brouns F, and Wagermakers AJM. Metabolic availability of medium-chain triglycerides coingested with carbohydrate during prolonged exercise. *Journal of Applied Physiology* 1995; 79: 756-762.

33 Bucci L. "Nutrients as Ergogenic Aids for Sports and Exercise." Boca Raton, FL: CRC Press, © 1993, pg 20.

34 Brilla LF & Landerholm TE. Effect of fish oil supplementation and exercise on serum lipids and aerobic fitness. *Journal of Sports Medicine* 1990; 30(2): 173.

35 Huffman DM, Altena TS, Mawhinney TP, & Thomas TR. Effect on n-3 fatty acids on free tryptophan and exercise fatigue. *European Journal of Applied Physiology* 2004; 92(4-5): 584-91.

36 Lenn J, Uhl T, Mattacola C, Boissonneault G, Yates J, Ibrahim W, & Bruckner G. The effects of fish oil and isoflavones on

delayed onset muscle soreness. *Medicine & Science in Sports & Exercise* 2002; 34(10): 1605-13.

37 Meredith CN, Zackin MJ, Frontera WR, & Evans WJ. Dietary protein requirements and body protein metabolism in endurance-trained men. *Journal of Applied Physiology* 1989; 66(6): 2850-2856.

38 Butterfield GE & Calloway DH. Physical activity improves protein utilization in young men. *British Journal of Nutrition* 1984; 51: 171-184.

39 Butterfield G, Cady C & Moynihan S. Effect of increasing protein intake on nitrogen balance in recreational weight lifters. *Medicine & Science in Sports & Exercise* 1992; 24: S71.

40 Amphoteric substances can behave as either an acid or a base, with the capacity to donate or take up hydrogen atoms to control wide shifts in pH.

41 USDA/HHS. Dietary guidelines for Americans, 2005. Washington, DC: Government Printing Office. 2005.

42 Tarnopolsky MA, MacDougall JD, and Atkinson SA. Influence of protein intake and training status on nitrogen balance and lean body mass. *Journal of Applied Physiology* 1988; 64(1): 187-193.

43 Steen SN. Precontest strategies of a male bodybuilder. *International Journal of Sport Nutrition* 1991; 1: 69-78.

44 Kleiner SM, Bazzarre TL, and Ainsworth BE. Nutritional status of nationally ranked elite body-builders. *International Journal of Sport Nutrition* 1994; 4: 43-69.

45 Gibala M. Regulation of skeletal muscle amino acid metabolism during exercise. *International Journal of Sport Nutrition and Exercise Metabolism* 2001; 11: 87-108.

46 Gibala MJ. Dietary protein, amino acid supplements, and recovery from exercise. *GSSI Sports Science Exchange* 2002; 15(4): 1-4.

47 Gibala MJ. Dietary protein, amino acid supplements, and recovery from exercise. *GSSI Sports Science Exchange* 2002; 15(4).

48 Gibala MJ. Dietary protein, amino acid supplements, and recovery from exercise. *GSSI Sports Science Exchange* 2002; 15(4).

49 Zawadzki KM, Yaspelkis BB, and Ivy JL. Carbohydrate-protein complex increases the rate of muscle glycogen storage after exercise. *Journal of Applied Physiology* 1992; 72(5): 1854-1859.

Chapter 2

1 Institute of Medicine. "Dietary Reference Intakes for Thiamin, Riboflavin, Niacin, Vitamin B_6, Folate, Vitamin B_{12}, Pantothenic Acid, Protein, and Choline." Food and Nutrition Board. Washington DC: National Academies Press. 1999. pp 150-195.

2 Belko, A.Z., Obarzanek, E., Kalkwarf, J.H., Rotter, M.A., Bogusz, S., Miller, D., Haas, J.D., and Roe, D.A. 1983. Effects of exercise on riboflavin requirements of young women. *Am. J. Clin. Nutr.* 37: 509-517.

3 Belko, A.Z., Obarzanek, M.P., Rotter, B.S., Urgan, G., Weinberg, S., and Roe, D.A. 1984. Effects of aerobic exercise and weight loss on riboflavin requirements of moderately obese, marginally deficient young women. *Am. J. Clin. Nutr.* 40: 553.

4 Belko, A.Z., Meredith, M.P., Kalkwarf, H.J., Obarzanek, E., Weinberg, S., Roach, R., McKeon, G., and Roe, D.A. 1985. Effects of exercise on riboflavin requirements: Biological validation in weight-reducing young women. *Am. J. Clin. Nutr.* 41: 270.

5 Tremblay, A., Boiland, F., Breton, M., Bessette, H., and Roberge, A.G. 1984. The effects of a riboflavin supplementation on the nutritional status and performance of elite swimmers. *Nutr. Res.* 4: 201.

6 Manore M and Thompson J. "Sports Nutrition for Health and Performance." Champaign IL: Human Kinetics, © 2000, pg 252.

7 Carlson, L.A., Havel, R.J., Ekelund, L.G., and Holmgren, A. 1963. Effect of nicotinic acid on the turnover rate and oxidation

of the free fatty acids of plasma in man during exercise. *Metab. Clin. Exp.* 12: 837.

8 Bergstrom, J., Hultman, E., Jorfeldt, L., Pernow, B., and Wahnen, J. 1969. Effect of nicotinic acid on physical working capacity and on metabolism of muscle. *J. Appl. Physiol.* 26: 170.

9 Hilsendager, D., and Karpovich, P.V. 1964. Ergogenic effect of glycine and niacin separately and in combination. *Res. Q.* 35: 389.

10 Dalton, K., and Dalton, M.J.T. 1987. Characteristics of pyridoxine overdose neuropathy syndrome. *Acta. Neurol. Scand.* 76: 8-11.

11 Schaumberg, H., Kaplan, J., Windebank, A., Vick, N., Ragmus, S., Pleasure, D., and Brown, M.J. 1983. Sensory neuropathy from pyridoxine abuse. *New Engl. J. Med.* 309: 445-448.

12 Manore, M.M. 1994. Vitamin B-6 and exercise. *Int. J. Sport Nutr.* 4: 89-103.

13 Fogelholm, M., Ruokonen I., Laakso, J.T., Vuorimaa, T., and Himberg, J.J. 1993. Lack of association between indices of vitamin B-1, B-2, and B-6 status and exercise-induced blood lactate in young adults. *Int. J. Sport Nutr.* 3: 165-176.

14 Guilland, J.C., Penarand, T., Gallet, C., Boggio, V., Fuchs, F., and Klepping, J. 1989. Vitamin status of young athletes including the effects of supplementation. *Med. Sci. Sports Exerc.* 21: 441-449.

15 Telford, R.D., Catchpole, E.A., Deakin, V., McLeay, A.C., and Plank, A.W. 1992. The effect of 7 to 8 months of vitamin/mineral supplementation on the vitamin and mineral status of athletes. *Int. J. Sport Nutr.* 2: 123-134.

16 Suboticanec, K., Stavljenic, A., Schalch, W., and Buzina, R. 1990. Effects of pyridoxine and riboflavin supplementation of physical fitness in young adolescents. *Int. J. Vit. Nutr. Res.* 60: 81-88.

17 Delitala, G., Masala, A., Alagna, S., and Devilla, L. 1976. Effect of pyridoxine on human hypophyseal trophic hormone release: A possible stimulation of hypothalamic dopaminergic pathway. *J. Clin. Endocr. Metab.* 42: 603-606.

18 Dunton, N., Virk, R., Young, J., Leklem, J. 1992. Effect of vitamin B-6 supplementation and exhaustive exercise on vitamin B-6 metabolism and growth hormone. [Abstract]. *FASEB Journal* 6: A1374.

19 Moretti, C., Fabbri, A., Gnessi, L., Bonifacio, V., Fraioli, F., and Isidori, A. 1982. Pyridoxine (B_6) suppresses the rise in prolactin and increases the rise in growth hormone induced by exercise. *New Engl. J. Med.* 307 (7): 444-445.

20 Manore, M.M. 1994. Vitamin B-6 and exercise. *Int. J. Sport Nutr.* 4: 89-103.

21 Dreon, D.M., and Butterfield, G.E. 1986. Vitamin B-6 utilization in active and inactive young men. *Am. J. Clin. Nutr.* 43: 816-824.

22 Rokitzki, L., Sagredos, A.N., F., BŸchner, M., and Keul, J. 1994. Acute changes in vitamin B-6 status in endurance athletes before and after a marathon. *Int. J. Sport Nutr.* 4: 154-165.

23 Albert, M.J., Mathan, V.I., and Baker, S.J. 1980. Vitamin B-12 synthesis by human small intestinal bacteria. *Nature* 283: 781-782.

24 Ryan, A. 1977. Nutritional practices in athletics abroad. *Physician Sports Med.* 5: 33.

25 U.S. Senate. 1973. Proper and improper use of drugs by athletes. June 18 and July 12-13. Hearing Washington, DC: U.S. Government Printing Office.

26 Montoye, H.J., Spata, P.J., Pincney, V., and Barron, L. 1955. Effects of vitamin B-12 supplementation on physical fitness and growth of young boys. *J. Appl. Physiol.* 7: 589.

27 Tin-May Than Ma-Win-May, Khin-Sann-Aung, and Mya-Tu, M. 1978. The effect of vitamin B-12 on physical performance capacity. *Br. J. Nutr.* 40: 269.

28 Read, M., and McGuffin, S. 1983. The effect of B-complex supplementation on endurance performance. *J. Sports Med. Phys. Fitness* 23: 178.

29 McNulty, H. 1995. Folate requirements for health in different population groups. *Br. J. Biomed. Sci.* 52: 110-112.

30 Baily, L.B. 1995. Folate requirements and dietary recommendations. *Folate in health and disease,* ed. Baily, L.B. New York: Marcel Dekker, 123.

31 Matter, M., Stittfall, T., Graves, J., Myburgh, K., Adams, B., Jacobs, P., and Noakes, T.D. 1987. The effect of iron and folate therapy on maximal exercise performance in female marathon runners with iron and folate deficiency. *Clin. Sci.* 72Z: 415-420.

32 Weight, L.M., Noakes, T.D., Labadarios, D., Graves, J., Jacobs, P., and Berman, P.A. 1988. Vitamin and mineral status of trained athletes including the effects of supplementation. *Am. J. Clin. Nutr.* 47: 186-192.

33 Institute of Medicine. "Dietary Reference Intakes for Vitamin C, Vitamin E, Selenium, and Carotenoids." Food and Nutrition Board. Washington DC: National Academies Press. 2000.

34 Hickson, J.F., and Wolinsky, I., eds. 1989. *Nutrition in exercise and sport.* Boca Raton, FL: CRC Press, 121.

35 Bramich, K., and McNaughton, L. 1987. The effects of two levels of ascorbic acid on muscular endurance, muscular strength, and on $\dot{V}O_2$max. *Int. Clin. Nutr. Rev.* 7: 5.

36 Schwartz, P.L. 1970. Ascorbic acid in wound healing: A review. *J. Am. Diet. Assoc.* 56: 497.

37 Kanter, M.M. 1994. Free radicals, exercise, and antioxidant supplementation. *Int. J. Sport Nutr.* 4: 205-220.

38 Herbert, V. 1993. Does mega-C do more good than harm, or more harm than good? *Nutr. Today* Jan/Feb: 28-32.

39 Peake JM. Vitamin C: Effects of exercise and requirements with training. *International Journal of Sport Nutrition and Exercise Metabolism* 2003; 13: 125-151.

40 Institute of Medicine. "Dietary Reference Intakes for Vitamin A, Vitamin K, Arsenic, Boron, Chromium, Copper, Iodine, Iron, Manganese, Molybdenum, Nickel, Silicon, Vanadium, and Zinc." Food and Nutrition Board. Washington DC: National Academies Press. 2002.

41 Institute of Medicine. "Dietary Reference Intakes for Calcium, Phosphorus, Magnesium, Vitamin D, and Fluoride." Food and Nutrition Board. Washington DC: National Academies Press. 2000.

42 Murray, R., and Horsun II, C.A. 1998. Nutrient requirements for competitive sports. In *Nutrition in Exercise and Sport*, 3rd ed., ed. Ira Wolinsky. Boca Raton, FL: CRC Press, 550.

43 Barr, S.I., Prior, J.C., and Vigna, Y.M. 1994. Restrained eating and ovulatory disturbances: Possible implications for bone health. *Am. J. Clin. Nutr.* 59: 92-97.

44 Chesnut, C.H. 1991. Theoretical overview: Bone development, peak bone mass, bone loss, and fracture risk. *Am. J. Medicine* 91(Suppl 5B): 2-4.

45 Heaney, R.P. 1991. Effect of calcium on skeletal development, bone loss, and risk of fractures. *Am. J. Medicine* 91(Suppl 5B): 23-28.

46 Benardot, D. 1997. Unpublished data from USOC research project on national team gymnasts. Laboratory for Elite Athlete Performance.

47 The symbol for beta-tocopherol that you will often see on labels is β, as in β-tocopherol.

48 The symbol for alpha-tocopherol that you will often see on labels is α, as in α-tocopherol.

49 Talbot, D., and Jamieson, J. 1977. An examination of the effect of vitamin E on the performance of highly trained swimmers. *Can. J. Appl. Sport Sci.* 2: 67.

50 Bunnell, R.H., DeRitter, E., and Rubin, S.H. 1975. Effect of feeding polyunsaturated fatty acids with a low vitamin E diet on blood levels of tocopherol in men performing hard physical labor. *Am. J. Clin. Nutr.* 28: 706.

51 Sharman, I.M., Down, M.G., and Sen, R.N. 1971. The effect of vitamin E and training on physiological function and athletic performance in adolescent swimmers. *Br. J. Nutr.* 26: 265.

52 Sharman, I.M., Down, M.B., and Norgan, N.G. 1976. The effects of vitamin E on physiological function and athletic performance of trained swimmers. *J. Sports Med.* 16: 215.

53 Brady, P.S., Brady, L.J., and Ullrey, D.E. 1979. Selenium, vitamin E, and the response to swimming stress in the rat. *J. Nutr.* 109: 1103.

54 Dillard, C.J., Liton, R.E., Savin, W.M., Dumelin, E.E., and Tappel, A.L. 1978. Effects of exercise, vitamin E, and ozone on pulmonary function and lipid peroxidation. *J. Appl. Physiol.* 45: 927.

55 Shephard, R.J., Campbell, R., Pimm, P., Stuart, D., and Wright, G.R. 1974. Vitamin E, exercise, and the recovery from physical activity. *J. Appl. Physiol.* 33: 119-126.

56 Weber P. Vitamin K and bone health. *Nutrition* 2001; 17: 880-887

57 Feskanich D, Weber P, Willett WC, Rockett H, Booth SL, and Colditz GA. Vitamin K intake and hip fractures in women: A prospective study. *American Journal of Clinical Nutrition* 1999; 69: 74-79

58 Booth SL, Tucker KL, Chen H, et al. Dietary vitamin K intakes are associated with hip fracture but not with bone mineral density in elderly men and women. *American Journal of Clinical Nutrition* 2000; 71: 1201-1208

59 Booth SL, Pennington JA, and Sadowski JA. Food sources and dietary intakes of vitamin K-1 (phylloquinone) in the American diet: Data from the FDA Total Diet Study. *Journal of the American Dietetic Association* 1996; 96: 149-154

60 Lukaski, H.C. 1995. Micronutrients (magnesium, zinc, and copper): Are mineral supplements needed for athletes? *Int. J. Sport Nutr.* 5: S74-S83.

61 Benardot, D. 1999. Nutrition for gymnasts. *The Athlete Wellness Book,* ed. Marshall, N.T. Indianapolis, IN: USA Gymnastics, 12-13.

62 Lotz, M., Zisman, E., and Bartter, F.C. 1968. Evidence for a phosphorus-depletion syndrome in man. *New Engl. J. Med.* 278: 409-415.

63 National Research Council. 1989. *Recommended Dietary Allowances,* 10th ed. Washington, DC: National Academy of Sciences.

64 Bucci, L. 1993. *Nutrients as ergogenic aids for sports and exercise.* Boca Raton, FL: CRC Press.

65 Keller, W.D., and Kraut, H.A. 1959. Work and nutrition. *World Rev. Nutr. Diet* 3: 65.

66 Cade, R., Conte, M., Zauner, C., Mars, D., Peterson, J., Lunne, D., Hommen, N., and Packer, D. 1984. Effects of phosphate loading on 2,3-diphosphoglycerate and maximal oxygen uptake. *Med. Sci. Sports Exerc.* 12: 263.

67 Duffy, D.J., and Conlee, R.K. 1986. Effects of phosphate loading on leg power and high intensity treadmill exercise. *Med. Sci. Sports Exerc.* 18: 674.

68 Shils, M.E. Magnesium. 1993. *Modern nutrition in health and disease,* 8th ed., ed. Shils, M.E., Olson, J.A., and Shike, M., Philadelphia: Lea & Febiger, 164-184.

69 Steinacker, J.M., Grunert-Fuchs, M., Steininger, K., and Wodick, R.E. 1987. Effects of long-time administration of magnesium on physical capacity. *Int. J. Sports Med.* 8: 151.

70 Golf, S.W., Bohmer, D., and Nowacki, P.E. 1993. Is magnesium a limiting factor in competitive exercise? A summary of relevant scientific data. In *Magnesium,* ed. Golf, S., Dralle, D., and Vecchiet, L., 209-220. London: John Libbey.

71 Brilla, L.R., and Haley, T.F. 1992. Effect of magnesium supplementation on strength training in humans. *J. Am. Coll. Nutr.* 11: 326-329.

72 Terblanche S, Noakes TD, Dennis SC, Marais D, and Eckert M. Failure of magnesium supplementation to influence marathon running performance or recovery. *International Journal of Sport Nutrition* 1992; 2(2): 154-164.

73 Hickson, J.F., Schrader, J., and Trischler, L.C. 1986. Dietary intake of female basketall and gymnastics athletes. *J. Am. Diet. Assoc.* 86: 251-254.

74 Lukaski, H.C. 1995. Prevention and treatment of magnesium deficiency in athletes. In *Magnesium and physical activity,* ed. Vecchiet, L., 211-226. Carnforth, UK: Parthenon.

75 Table salt is 40 percent sodium and 60 percent chloride. To obtain 1.5 grams of sodium, an individual would require an intake of approximately 3.8 grams of table salt.

76 Institute of Medicine. *Dietary Reference Intakes for water, potassium, sodium, chloride, and sulfate.* Washington, DC: National Academies Press. 2004: p. 6.

77 Pivarnik, J.M. Water and electrolytes during exercise 1989. In *Nutrition in exercise and sport*, ed. Hickson, J.F., and Wolinsky, I. Boca Raton, FL: CRC Press, 185-200.

78 Craig, S. "Hyponatremia." eMedicine, January 20, 2005. http://www.emedicine.com/EMERG/topic275.htm/.

79 Pivarnik, J.M. 1989. Water and electrolytes during exercise. In *Nutrition in exercise and sport*, ed. Hickson J.F., and Wolinsky, I. Boca Raton: CRC Press. 185-200.87 Clarkson, P. 1991. Vitamins, iron, and trace minerals. In *Ergogenics: Enhancement of performance in exercise and sport*, ed. Lamb, D., and Williams, M. Indianapolis: Benchmark Press.

80 Clarkson, P. 1991. Vitamins, iron, and trace minerals. In *Ergogenics Enhancement of performance in exercise and sport*, ed. Lamb, D., and Williams, M. Indianapolis: Benchmark Press.

81 Shaskey DJ and Green GA. Sports haematology. *Sports Medicine* 2000; 29(1): 27-38.

82 Selby GB and Eichner ER. Endurance swimming, intravascular hemolysis, anemia, and iron depletion. *American Journal of Medicine* 1986; 81: 791-794.

83 Waller M and Haymes E. The effects of heat and exercise on sweat iron loss. *Medicine and Science in Sports and Exercise* 1996; 28: 197-203.

84 Brune M, Magnusson B, Persson H, and Hallberg L. Iron losses in sweat. *American Journal of Clinical Nutrition* 1986; 43: 438-443.

85 Baska RS, Moses FM, Graeber G, and Kearney G. Gastrointestinal bleeding during an ultramarathon. *Digestive Diseases and Sciences* 1990; 35: 276-279.

86 Balaban EP. Sports anemia. *Clinical Sports Medicine* 1992; 11(2): 313-325.

87 Gleeson M, Nieman DC, and Pedersen BK. Exercise, nutrition and immune function. *Journal of Sports Sciences* 2004; 22(1): 115-125.

88 Cook JD, Finch CA, and Smith NJ. Evaluation of the iron status of a population. *Blood* 1976; 48: 449-455.

89 Wolinsky, I., and Driskell, J.A. 1997. *Sports nutrition: Vitamins and trace elements.* Boca Raton, FL: CRC Press, 148.

90 Lampe JW, Slavin JL, and Apple FS. Iron status of active women and the effect of running a marathon on bowel function and gastrointestinal blood loss. *International Journal of Sports Medicine* 1991; 12: 173-179.

91 Haymes EM and Spillman DM. Iron status of women distance runners, sprinters, and control women. *International Journal of Sports Medicine* 1989; 10: 430-433.

92 Bucci, L. 1993. *Nutrients as ergogenic aids for sports and exercise.* Boca Raton, FL: CRC Press.

93 Stephenson, L.S. 1995. Possible new developments in community control of iron-deficiency anemia. *Nutrition Reviews* 53(2): 23-30.

94 Zoller H and Vogel W. Iron supplementation in athletes: First do no harm. *Nutrition* 2004; 20(7/8): 615-619.

95 Zotter H, Robinson N, Zorzoli M, Schattenberg L, Saugy M, and Mangin P. Abnormally high serum ferritin levels among professional road cyclists. *British Journal of Sports Medicine* 2004; 38(6): 704-708.

96 Gleeson M, Lancaster GI, and Bishop NC. Nutritional strategies to minimize exercise-induced immunosuppression in athletes. *Canadian Journal of Applied Physiology* 2001; 26(suppl.): S23-S35.

97 Dressendorfer, R.H., and Sockolov, R. 1980. Hypozincemia in runners. *Physician Sports Med.* 8: 97-100.

98 Haralambie, G. 1981. Serum zinc in athletes during training. *Int. J. Sports Med.* 2: 135-138.

99 Singh, A., Deuster, P.A., and Moser, P.B. 1990. Zinc and copper status of women by physical activity and menstrual status. *J. Sports Med. Phys. Fitness* 30: 29-35.

100 Krotkiewski, M., Gudmundsson, M., Backstrom, P., and Mandroukas, K. 1982. Zinc and muscle strength and endurance. *Acta Physiol. Scand.* 116: 309-311.

101 Koury JC, de Olilveria AV Jr., Portella ES, de Olilveria CF, Lopes GC, and Donangelo CM. Zinc and copper biochemical indices of antioxidant status in elite athletes of different modalities. *International Journal of Sport Nutrition and Exercise Metabolism* 2004; 14(3): 358-372.

102 Brun JF, Dieu-Cambrezy C, Charpiat A, Fons C, Fedou C, Micallef JP, Fussellier M, Bardet L, and Orsetti A. Serum zinc in highly trained adolescent gymnasts. *Biological Trace Element Research* 1995; 47(1-3): 273-278.

103 Fischer, P.W.F., Giroux, A. and L'Abbe, M.R. 1984. Effect of zinc supplementation on copper status in adult man. *Am. J. Clin. Nutr.* 40: 743-746.

104 Hooper, P.L., Visconti, L., Garry, P.J., and Johnson, G.E. 1980. Zinc lowers high-density lipoprotein cholesterol levels. *JAMA* 244: 1960-1961.

105 Spencer, H. 1986. Minerals and mineral interactions in human beings. *J. Am. Diet. Assoc.* 86: 864-867.

106 Zamora, A.J., Tessier, F., Marconnet, P., Margaritis, I., and Marini, J.F. Mitochondria changes in human muscle after prolonged exercise, endurance training, and selenium supplementation. *Eur. J. Appl. Physiol.* 71(6): 505-511.

107 Bucci, L. 1993. *Nutrients as ergogenic aids for sports and exercise.* Boca Raton, FL: CRC Press.

108 Tessier, F., Margaritis, I., Richard, M.-J., Moynot, C., and Marconnet, P. 1995. Selenium and training effects on the glutathione system and aerobic performance. *Med. Sci. Sports Exerc.* 27 (3): 390-396.

109 Lukaski, H.C. 1995. Micronutrients (magnesium, zinc, and copper): Are mineral supplements needed for athletes? *Int. J. Sports Med.* 5: S74-S83.

110 Lukaski, H.C., Hoverson, B.S., Gallagher, S.K., and Bolonchuk, W.W. 1990. Physical training and copper, iron, and zinc status of swimmers. *Am. J. Clin. Nutr.* 53: 1093-1099.

111 Wolinsky, I., and Driskell, J.A. 1997. *Sports nutrition: Vitamins and trace elements.* Boca Raton, FL: CRC Press.

112 Wolinsky, I., and Driskell, J.A. 1997. *Sports nutrition: Vitamins and trace elements.* Boca Raton, FL: CRC Press.

113 Evans, G.W. 1989. The effect of chromium picolinate on insulin controlled parameters in humans. *Int. J. Biosocial Res.* 11: 163.

114 Clancy, S.P., Clarkson, P.M., DeCheke, M.E., Nosaka, K., Freedson, P.S., Cunningham, J.J., and Valentine, J.J. 1994. Effects of chromium picolinate supplementation on body composition, strength, and urinary chromium loss in football players. *Int. J. Sport Nutr.* 4: 142.

115 Hasten, D.L., Rome, E.P., Franks, B.D., and Hegsted, M. 1992. Effects of chromium picolinate on beginning weight training students. *Int. J. Sport Nutr.* 2: 343.

116 Stearns, D., Wise, J., Paterno, S., and Wetterhahn. 1995. Chromium (III) picolinate produces chromosome damage in Chinese hamster ovary cells. *FASEB J* 9: 1643-8.

Chapter 3

1 Poortmans J. Exercise and renal function. *Sports Medicine* 1984; 1: 125-153.

2 Zambraski EJ. Renal regulation of fluid homeostasis during exercise. In: *Perspectives in exercise science and sports medicine, volume 3: Fluid homeostasis during exercise* (Ed. Gisolfe CV and Lamb CV). Carmel, IN: Benchmark Press. 1990: pp. 247-280.

3 It is necessary to excrete metabolic by-products. This excretion can take place via the production of dilute or concentrated urine, depending on hydration state.

4 Sawka MN, Latzka WA, and Montain SJ. Effects of dehydration and rehydration on performance. In: *Nutrition in sport* (Ed. Maughan RJ). London: Blackwell Science. 2000: pp. 216-217.

5 Maughan RJ. Water and electrolyte loss and replacement in exercise. In: *Nutrition in sport* (Ed. Maughan RJ). London: Blackwell Science. 2000: p. 226.

6 This assumes a mechanical efficiency conversion rate of 25%.

7 There is a loss of approximately 620 calories of heat energy for each liter of water evaporated from the skin's surface.

8 Leithead CS and Lind AR. *Heat stress and heat disorders*. London: Casell. 1964.

9 Maughan RJ. Thermoregulation and fluid balance in marathon competition at low ambient temperature. *International Journal of Sports Medicine* 1985; 6: 15-19.

10 Costill DL. *Sweating: Its composition and effects on body fluids*. Annals of the New York Academy of Sciences 1977; 301: 160-174.

11 Kenney WL. Body fluid and temperature regulation as a function of age: In: *Perspectives in exercise science and sports medicine, volume 8: Exercise in older adults* (Ed. Lamb DR, Gisolfi CV, and Nadel ER). Indianapolis: Benchmark Press. 1995: pp. 305-352.

12 Hubbard RW, Szlyk PC, and Armstrong LE. Influence of thirst and fluid palatability on fluid ingestion during exercise. In: *Perspectives in exercise science and sports medicine, volume 3: Fluid homeostasis during exercise* (Ed. Gisolfi CV and Lamb DR). Indianapolis: Benchmark Press. 1990: pp. 39-95.

13 Fitzsimons JT. Evolution of physiological and behavioural mechanism in vertebrate body and homeostasis. In: *Thirst: Physiological and psychological aspects* (Ed. Ramsay DJ and Booth DA). ILSI Human Nutrition Reviews. London: Springer-Verlag. 1990: pp. 3-22.

14 Rehrer NJ. Factors influencing fluid bioavailability. *Australian Journal of Nutrition and Dietetics* 1996; 53 (suppl. 4): S8-S12.

15 Hubbard RW, Szlyk PC, and Armstrong LE. Influence of thirst and fluid palatability on fluid ingestion during exercise. In: *Perspectives in exercise science and sports medicine, volume 3: Fluid homeostasis during exercise* (Ed. Gisolfi CV and Lamb DR). Carmel, IN: Benchmark Press, 1990: pp. 39-95.

16 Davis JM, Burgess WA, Slentz CA, Bartoli WP, and Pate RR. Effects of ingesting 6% and 12% glucose-electrolyte beverages during prolonged intermittent cycling in the heat. *European Journal of Applied Physiology* 1988; 57: 563-569.

17 Rehrer JN, Beckers EJ, Brouns F, ten Hoor F, and Saris WHM. Exercise and training effects on gastric emptying of carbohydrate beverages. *Medicine and Science in Sports and Exercise* 1989; 21: 540-549.

18 American College of Sports Medicine. Position paper: Nutrition and athletic performance. *Medicine and Science in Sports and Exercise* 2000; 32(12): 2130-2145.

19 Glucose is also referred to as dextrose on package labels.

20 Rehrer JN, Brouns F, Beckers EJ, and Saris WHM. The influence of beverage composition and gastrointestinal function on fluid and nutrient availability during exercise. *Scandinavian Journal of Medicine and Science in Sports* 1994; 4: 159-172.

21 Noakes TD, Rehrer NJ, and Maughan RJ. The importance of volume in regulating gastric emptying. *Medicine and Science in Sports and Exercise* 1991; 23: 307-313.

22 American College of Sports Medicine. Position paper: Nutrition and athletic performance. *Medicine and Science in Sports and Exercise* 2000; 32(12): 2130-2145.

23 Sun WM, Houghton LA, Read NW, Grundy DG, and Johnson AG. Effect of meal temperature on gastric emptying of liquids in man. *Gut* 1988; 29: 302-305.

24 Costill DL and Saltin B. Factors limiting gastric emptying. *Journal of Applied Physiology* 1974; 37: 679-683.

25 Ryan AJ, Navarne AE, and Gisolfi CV. Consumption of carbonated and noncarbonated sports drinks during prolonged treadmill exercise in the heat. *International Journal of Sport Nutrition* 1991; 1: 225-139.

26 Lambert GP, Bleiler TL, Chang R, Johnson AK, and Gisolfi CV. Effects of carbonated and noncarbonated beverages at specific intervals during treadmill running in the heat. *International Journal of Sport Nutrition* 1993; 3: 177-193.

27 Rehrer JN, Brouns F, Beckers EJ, and Saris WHM. The influence of beverage composition and gastrointestinal function on fluid and nutrient availability during exercise. *Scandinavian Journal of Medicine and Science in Sports* 1994; 4: 159-172.

28 Wolf S. The psyche and the stomach. *Gastroenterology* 1981; 80: 605-614.

29 Rehrer NJ. Factors influencing fluid bioavailability. *Australian Journal of Nutrition and Dietetics* 1996; 53(suppl. 4): S8-S12.

30 Rehrer NJ. Factors influencing fluid bioavailability. *Australian Journal of Nutrition and Dietetics* 1996; 53(suppl. 4): S8-S12.

31 Bar-Or O. Children's responses to exercise in hot climates: Implications for performance and health. *GSSI Sports Science Exchange* 1994; 7(2): 1-4.

32 Gisolfi CV, Summers R, and Schedl H. Intestinal absorption of fluids during rest and exercise. In: *Perspectives in exercise science and sports medicine, volume 3: Fluid homeostasis during exercise* (Ed. Gisolfi CV and Lamb DR). Carmel, IN: Benchmark Press, 1990: pp. 39-95.

33 Maughan RJ and Noakes TD. Fluid replacement and exercise stress: A brief review of studies on fluid replacement and some guidelines for the athlete. *Sports Medicine* 1991; 12: 16-31.

34 Kenney WL. Heat flux and storage in hot environments. *International Journal of Sports Medicine* 1998; 19: S92-S95.

35 Kenefick R et al. Hypohydration adversely affects lactate threshold in endurance athletes. *Journal of Strength and Conditioning Research* 2002; 16: 38-43.

36 Naghii M. The significance of water in sport and weight control. *Nutrition and Health* 2000; 14: 127-132.

37 Bergeron M. Averting muscle cramps. *Physician and Sportsmedicine* 2002; 30(11): 14.

38 Bergeron M. Sodium: The forgotten nutrient. *GSSI Sports Science Exchange* 2000; 13(3): 1-4.

39 Eichner E. Heat stroke in sports: Causes, prevention, and treatment. *GSSI Sports Science Exchange* 2002; 15(3): 1-4.

40 Hyponatremia is descriptive of low blood sodium.

41 USA Track & Field is the national governing body (NGB) for the following events: track and field, long-distance running, and race walking.

42 Noakes T. The hyponatremia of exercise. *International Journal of Sport Nutrition* 1992; 2: 205-228.

43 Gisolfi C. Fluid balance for optimal performance. *Nutrition Revue* 1996; 54: S159-S168.

44 Rehrer N. Fluid and electrolyte balance in ultra-endurance sport. *Sports Medicine* 2001; 31: 701-715.

45 Speedy D, Noakes TD, and Schneider C. Exercise-associated hyponatremia: A review. *Emergency Medicine* 2001; 13: 17-27.

46 May Clinic staff. "Low blood sodium in endurance athletes." MayoClinic.com, July 28, 2003. http://www.mayoclinic.com/.

47 Hargreaves M. Physiological benefits of fluid and energy replacement during exercise. *Australian Journal of Nutrition and Dietetics* 1996; 53(suppl. 4): S3-S7.

48 Burke LM. Rehydration strategies before and after exercise. *Australian Journal of Nutrition and Dietetics* 1996; 53(suppl. 4): S22-S26).

49 Nadel ER, Mack GW, and Nose H. Influence of fluid replacement beverages on body fluid homeostasis during exercise and recovery. In: *Perspectives in exercise science and sports medicine, volume 3: Fluid homeostasis during exercise* (Ed. Gisolfi CV and Lamb DR). Carmel, IN: Benchmark Press, 1990: pp. 181-205.

50 Kristal-Boneh E, Glusman JG, Shitrit R, Chaemovitz C, and Cassuto Y. Physical performance and heat tolerance after chronic water loading and heat acclimation. *Aviation, Space and Environmental Medicine* 1995; 66: 733-738.

51 Burke LM. Rehydration strategies before and after exercise. *Australian Journal of Nutrition and Dietetics* 1996; 53(suppl. 4): S22-S26.

52 Sawka MN, Montain SJ, and Lazka WA. Body fluid balance during exercise: Heat exposure. In *Body fluid balance: Exercise and sport* (Ed. Buskirk ER and Puhl SM). Boca Raton, FL: CRC Press. 1996: pp. 143-161.

53 Lyons TP, Riedesel ML, Meuli LE, and Chick TW. Effects of glycerol-induced hyperhydration prior to exercise in the heat on sweating and core temperatures. *Medicine and Science in Sports and Exercise* 1990; 22: 477-483.

54 Burke LM. Rehydration strategies before and after exercise. *Australian Journal of Nutrition and Dietetics* 1996; 53(suppl. 4): S22-S26.

55 Montner P, Stark DM, Riedesel ML, Murata G, Robergs R, Timms M, et al. Pre-exercise glycerol hydration improves cycling endurance time. *International Journal of Sports Medicine* 1996; 17: 27-33.

56 Rehrer NJ. Fluid and electrolyte balance in ultra-endurance sport. *Sports Medicine* 2001; 31(10): 701-715.

57 Shirreffs SM, Armstrong LE, and Cheuvront SN. Fluid and electrolyte needs for preparation and recovery from training and competition. *Journal of Sports Sciences* 2004; 22(1): 57-63.

58 Lyle DM, Lewis PR, Richards DAB, Richards R, Bauman AE, Sutton JR, et al. Heat exhaustion in the Sun-Herald city to surf fun run. *Medical Journal of Australia* 1994; 161: 361-365.

59 McConnell G, Burge CM, Skinner SL, and Hargreaves M. Ingested fluid volume and physiological responses during prolonged exercise in a mild environment. *Medicine and Science in Sports and Exercise* 1995; 27: S19 (abstract).

60 Walsh RM, Noakes TD, Hawley JA, and Dennis SC. Impaired high-intensity cycling performance time at low levels of dehydration. *International Journal of Sports Medicine* 1994; 15: 392-398.

61 Maughan RJ, Fenn CE, and Leiper JB. Effects of fluid, electrolyte and substrate ingestion on endurance capacity. *European Journal of Applied Physiology* 1989; 58: 481-486.

62 Mitchell JB, Costill DL, Houmard JA, Fink WJ, Pascoe DD, and Pearson DR. Influence of carbohydrate dosage on exercise performance and glycogen metabolism. *Journal of Applied Physiology* 1989; 67: 1843-1849.

63 Tsintzas OK, Liu R, Williams C, Campbell I, and Gaitanos G. The effect of carbohydrate ingestion on performance during a 30-km race. *International Journal of Sport Nutrition* 1993; 3: 127-139.

64 Coggan AR and Coyle EF. Reversal of fatigue during prolonged exercise by carbohydrate infusion or ingestion. *Journal of Applied Physiology* 1987; 63: 2388-2395.

65 Coyle EF, Hagberg JM, Hurley BF, Martin WH, Ehami AA, and Holloszy JO. Carbohydrate feeding during prolonged strenuous exercise can delay fatigue. *Journal of Applied Physiology* 1983; 55: 230-235.

66 Coyle EF, Coggan AR, Hemmert MK, and Ivy JL. Muscle glycogen utilization during prolonged, strenuous exercise when fed carbohydrate. *Journal of Applied Physiology* 1986; 61: 165-172.

67 Tsintzas OK, Williams C, Boobis L, and Greenhaff P. Carbohydrate ingestion and glycogen utilization in different muscle fibre types in man. *Journal of Physiology* 1995; 489: 243-250.

68 Hargreaves M, Costill DL, Coggan AR, Fink WJ, and Nishibata I. Effect of carbohydrate feedings on muscle glycogen utilization and exercise performance. *Medicine and Science in Sports and Exercise* 1984; 16: 219-222.

69 Yaspelkis BB, Patterson JG, Anderla PA, Ding Z, and Ivy JL. Carbohydrate supplementation spares muscle glycogen during variable-intensity exercise. *Journal of Applied Physiology* 1993; 75: 1477-1485.

70 Below PR, Mora-Rodriquez R, Gonzalez-Alonso J, and Coyle EF. Fluid and carbohydrate ingestion independently improve performance during 1 h of intense exercise. *Medicine and Science in Sports and Exercise* 1995; 27: 200-210.

71 Nicholas CW, Williams C, Lakomy HKA, Phillips G, and Nowitz A. Influence of ingesting a carbohydrate-electrolyte solution on endurance capacity during intermittent, high intensity shuttle running. *Journal of Sports Sciences* 1995; 13: 283-290.

72 Simard C, Tremblay A, and Jobin M. Effects of carbohydrate intake before and during an ice hockey match on blood and muscle energy substrates. *Research Quarterly for Exercise and Sport* 1988; 59: 144-147.

73 Coyle EF, Coggan AR, Hemmert MK, and Ivy JL. Muscle glycogen utilization during prolonged, strenuous exercise

when fed carbohydrate. *Journal of Applied Physiology* 1986; 61: 165-172.

74 Murray R, Paul GL, Seifert JG, Eddy DE, and Halaby GA. The effects of glucose, fructose, and sucrose ingestion during exercise. *Medicine and Science in Sports and Exercise* 1989; 21: 275-282.

75 Owen MD, Kregel KC, Wall PT, and Gisolfi CV. Effects of ingesting carbohydrate beverages during exercise in the heat. *Medicine and Science in Sports and Exercise* 1986; 18: 568-575.

76 Murray R, Paul GL, Seifert JG, Eddy DE, Halaby GA. The effects of glucose, fructose, and sucrose ingestion during exercise. *Medicine and Science in Sports and Exercise* 1989; 21: 275-282.

77 Bjorkman O, Sahlin K, Hagenfeldt L, and Wahren J. Influence of glucose and fructose ingestion on the capacity for long-term exercise in well-trained men. *Clinical Physiology* 1984; 4: 483-494.

78 Hargreaves M. Physiological benefits of fluid and energy replacement during exercise. *Australian Journal of Nutrition and Dietetics* 1996; 53(suppl. 4): S3-S7.

79 Mason WL, McConell GK, and Hargreaves M. Carbohydrate ingestion during exercise: Liquid vs. solid feedings. *Medicine and Science in Sports and Exercise* 1993; 25: 966-969.

80 A 1 percent carbohydrate solution is 1 gram of carbohydrate per 100 milliliters of water. One liter of water is 1,000 milliliters, so consumption of 1 liter of a 6 percent carbohydrate solution will provide 240 calories from carbohydrate (6 × 4 kilocalories per gram × 10).

81 Coggan AR and Coyle EF. Reversal of fatigue during prolonged exercise by carbohydrate infusion or ingestion. *Journal of Applied Physiology* 1987; 63: 2388-2395.

82 Coyle EF and Montain SJ. Benefits of fluid replacement with carbohydrate during exercise. *Medicine and Science in Sports and Exercise* 1992; 24(suppl.): S324-S330.

83 Wagenmakers AJM, Brouns F, Saris WHM, and Halliday D. Oxidation rates of orally ingested carbohydrates during prolonged exercise in men. *Journal of Applied Physiology* 1993; 75: 2774-2780.

84 Broad EM, Burke LM, Gox GR, Heeley P, and Riley M. Body weight changes and voluntary fluid intakes during training and competition sessions in team sports. *International Journal of Sport Nutrition* 1996; 6: 307-320.

85 Noakes TD, Adams BA, Myburgh KH, Greff C, Lotz T, and Nathan M. The danger of inadequate water intake during prolonged exercise. *European Journal of Applied Physiology* 1988; 57: 210-219.

86 Rothstein A, Adolph EF, and Wills JH. Voluntary dehydration. In: *Physiology of man in the desert* (Ed. Adolph EF). New York: Interscience. 1947: pp. 254-270.

87 Carter JE and Gisolfi CV. Fluid replacement during and after exercise in the heat. *Medicine and Science in Sports and Exercise* 1989; 21: 532-539.

88 Gonzalez-Alonso J, Heaps CL, and Coyle EF. Rehydration after exercise with common beverages and water. *International Journal of Sports Medicine* 1992; 13: 399-406.

89 Maughan RJ and Leiper JB. Sodium intake and post-exercise rehydration in man. *European Journal of Applied Physiology* 1995; 71: 311-319.

90 Maughan RJ, Leiper JB, and Shirreffs SM. Restoration of fluid balance after exercise-induced dehydration: Effects of food and fluid intake. *European Journal of Applied Physiology* 1996; 73: 317-325.

91 Burke LM. Rehydration strategies before and after exercise. *Australian Journal of Nutrition and Dietetics* 1996; 53(suppl. 4): S22-S26.

Chapter 4

1 Greenhaff, P.L., Casey, A., Short, A.H., Harris, R., Soderlund, K., and Hultman, E. 1993. Influence of oral creatine supplementation of muscle torque during repeated bouts of maximal voluntary exercise in man. *Clin. Sci.* 84: 565-571.

2 Harris, R.C., Soderlund, K., and Hultman, E. 1992. Elevation of creatine in resting and exercised muscle of normal subjects by creatine supplementation. *Clin. Sci.* 83: 367-374.

3 Maughan, R.J. 1995. Creatine supplementation and exercise performance. *Intl. J. Sport Nutr.* 5: 94-101.

4 Walker, J.B. 1979. Creatine biosynthesis, regulation, and function. *Adv. Enzmmol.* 50: 117-142.

5 Butterfield, G., Cady, C., and Moynihan, S. 1992. Effect of increasing protein intake on nitrogen balance in recreational weight lifters. *Med. Sci. Sports Exerc.* 24: S71.

6 Ahrendt DM. Ergogenic aids: Counseling the athlete. *American Family Physician* 2001; 63(5): 913-922.

7 Gurley BJ, Gardner SF, White LM, and Wang PL. Ephedrine pharmacokinetics after the ingestion of nutritional supplements containing ephedra sinica (ma huang). *Therapeutic Drug Monitoring* 1998; 20: 439-45.

8 Maughan RJ. Dietary supplements: Contamination may cause failed drug tests. *GSSI Hot Topics* 2001 (May).

9 Nagle, F.J., and Bassett, D.R. 1989. Energy metabolism. In *Nutrition in exercise and sport*, ed. Hickson, J.F., and Wolinsky, I. Boca Raton, FL: CRC Press, 87-106.

10 Costill, D.L., and Hargreaves, M. 1992. Carbohydrate nutrition and fatigue. *Sports Med.* 13 (2): 86

11 Valeriani, A. 1991. The need for carbohydrate intake during endurance exercise. *Sports Med.* 12 (6): 349.

12 Tarnopolsky MA, Atkinson SA, Phillips SM, and MacDougall JD. Carbohydrate loading and metabolism during exercise in men and women. *Journal of Applied Physiology* 1995; 78: 1360-1368.

13 Nagle, F.J., and Bassett, D.R. 1989. Energy metabolism. In *Nutrition in exercise and sport*, ed. Hickson, J.F., and Wolinsky, I. Boca Raton, FL: CRC Press, 87-106.

14 Coyle, E.F. 1983. Effects of glucose polymer feedings on fatigability and the metabolic response to prolonged strenuous exercise. In *Ross symposium on nutrient utilization during exercise*, ed. Fox, E.L. Columbus, OH: Ross Laboratories, 4-11.

15 Berning JR, Leenders MM, Ratliff K, Clem KL, and Troup JP. The effects of a high carbohydrate pre-exercise meal on the consumption of confectioneries of different glycemic indices. *Medicine and Science in Sports and Exercise* 1993; 25(5): S125.

16 Anantaraman R, Carmines AA, Gaesser GA, and Weltman A. The effects of carbohydrate supplementation on maximal effort endurance performance. *Medicine and Science in Sports and Exercise* 1994; 26(5): S34.

17 Coyle EF. Timing and method of increased carbohydrate intake to cope with heavy training, competition and recovery. *Journal of Sports Sciences* 1991; 9: 18-37.

18 Roy BD, Tamopolsky MA, MacDougall JD, Fowles J, and Yarasheski KE. The effect of oral glucose supplements on muscle protein synthesis following resistance training. *Medicine and Science in Sports and Exercise* 1996; 28(5): S769.

19 Nagle, F.J., and Bassett, D.R. 1989. Energy metabolism. In *Nutrition in exercise and sport*, ed. Hickson, J.F., and Wolinsky, I. Boca Raton, FL: CRC Press, 87-106.

20 Greenhaff, P.L. 1995. Creatine and its application as an ergogenic aid. *Intl. J. Sport Nutr.* 5: S100-S110.

21 Greenhaff, P.L., Casey, A., Short, A.H., Harris, R., Soderlund, K., and Hultman, E. 1993. Influence of oral creatine supplementation on muscle torque during repeated bouts of maximal voluntary exercise in man. *Clin. Sci.* 84: 565-571.

22 Maughan, R.J. 1995. Creatine supplementation and exercise performance. *Intl. J. Sport Nutr.* 5: 94-101.

23 Volek JS and Rawson ES. Scientific basis and practical aspects of creatine supplementation for athletes. *Nutrition* 2004; 20: 609-614.

24 Kozak, C.J., Benardot, D., Cody, M., Doyle, J.A., and Thompson, W.R. 1996. The effect of creatine monohydrate supplementation on anaerobic power and anaerobic endurance in elite female gymnasts. Master's thesis, Georgia State University.

25 Koenig C, Benardot D, Cody M, and Thompson W. The influence of creatine monohydrate and carbohydrate supplements on repeated jump height. *Medicine and Science in Sports and Exercise* 2004; 36(5): S347.

26 Harris, R.C., Soderlund, K., and Hultman, E. 1992. Elevation of creatine in resting and exercised muscle of normal subjects by creatine supplementation. *Clin. Sci.* 83: 367-374.

27 Maughan, R.J. 1995. Creatine supplementation and exercise performance. *Intl. J. Sport Nutr.* 5: 94-101.

28 Walker, J.B. 1979. Creatine biosynthesis, regulation, and function. *Adv. Enzmmol.* 50: 117-142.

29 Maughan, R.J. 1995. Creatine supplementation and exercise performance. *Intl. J. Sport Nutr.* 5: 94-101.

30 Robergs RA. Glycerol hyperhydration to beat the heat? *Sportscience Training and Technology* 1988 (January).

31 Montner P, Stark DM, Riedesel ML, Murata G, Robergs RA, Timms M, and Chick TW. Pre-exercise glycerol hydration improves cycling endurance time. *International Journal of Sports Medicine* 1996; 17: 27-33.

32 Montgomery, D.L, and Beaudin, P.A. 1982. Blood lactate and heart rate response of young females during gymnastic routines. *J. Sports Med.* 22: 358-365.

33 Hyland PJ, MacConnie SE, and Meigs RA. The effect of sodium bicarbonate ingestion on work output during a 2,000 meter rowing ergometer time trial. *Medicine and Science in Sports and Exercise* 1993; 25(5): S1085.

34 Webster MJ, Webster MN, Crawford RE, and Gladden LB. Effect of sodium bicarbonate ingestion on exhaustive resistance exercise performance. *Medicine and Science in Sports and Exercise* 1993; 25(5): S1086.

35 Avedisian L, Guerra A, Wilcox A, and Fox S. The effect of selected buffering agents on performance in the competitive 1600 meter run. *Medicine and Science in Sports and Exercise* 1995; 27(5): S133.

36 Butterfield, G., Cady, C., and Moynihan, S. 1992. Effect of increasing protein intake on nitrogen balance in recreational weight lifters. *Med. Sci. Sports Exerc.* 24: S71.

37 Tarnopolsky, M.A., MacDougall, J.D., and Atkinson, S.A. 1988. Influence of protein intake and training status on nitrogen balance and lean body mass. *J. Appl. Physiol.* 64 (1): 187-193.

38 Spriet, L.L. 1995. Caffeine and performance. *Int. J. Sport Nutr.* 5: S84-S99.

39 Bucci, L. 1993. *Nutrients as ergogenic aids for sports and exercise.* Boca Raton, FL: CRC Press.

40 Graham TE and Spriet LL. Performance and metabolic responses to a high caffeine dose during prolonged exercise. *Journal of Applied Physiology* 1991; 71: 2292-2298.

41 Silver MD. Use of ergogenic aids by athletes. *Journal of the American Academy of Orthopaedic Surgeons* 2001; 9(1): 61-70.

42 Kalmar JM and Cafarelli E. Effects of caffeine on neuromuscular function. *Journal of Applied Physiology* 1999; 87: 801-808.

43 Paluska SA. Caffeine and exercise. *Current Sports Medicine Reports* 2003; 2(4): 213-219.

44 Kanter, M.M., and Williams, M.H. 1995. Antioxidants, carnitine, and choline as putative ergogenic aids. *Int. J. Sport Nutr.* 5: S120-S131.

45 Clarkson PM. Nutrition for improved sports performance: Current issues on ergogenic aids. *Sports Medicine* 1996; 21: 393-401.

46 Juhnson WA and Landry GL. Nutritional supplements: Fact vs. fiction. *Adolescent Medicine* 1998; 9: 501-513.

47 Bucci, L. 1993. *Nutrients as ergogenic aids for sports and exercise.* Boca Raton, FL: CRC Press, 6; 20.

48 Oostenbrug GS, Mensink RP, Hardeman MR, DeVries T, Brouns F, and Hornstra G. Exercise performance, red blood cell deformability, and lipid peroxidation: Effects of fish oil and vitamin E. *Journal of Applied Physiology* 1997; 83(3): 746-752.

49 Raastad T, Hostmark AT, and Stromme SB. Omega-3 fatty acid supplementation does not improve maximal aerobic power, anaerobic threshold and running performance in well-trained soccer players. *Scandinavian Journal of Medicine and Science in Sports* 1997; 7: 25-31

50 Babayan, V.K. 1967. Medium-chain triglycerides: Their composition, preparation, and application. *J. Am. Oil Chem. Soc.* 45: 23.

51 Bach, A.S., and Babayan, V.K. 1982. Medium-chain triglycerides: An update. *Am. J. Clin. Nutr.* 36: 950.

52 Misell LM, Lagomarcino ND, Schuster V, and Kern M. Chronic medium-chain triacylglycerol consumption and endurance performance in trained runners. *Journal of Sports Medicine and Physical Fitness* 2001; 41(2): 210-215.

53 Horowitz JF, Mora-Rodriguez R, Byerley LO, and Coyle EF. Preexercise medium-chain triglyceride ingestion does not alter muscle glycogen use during exercise. *Journal of Applied Physiology* 2000; 88(1): 219-225.

54 Goedecke JH, Elmer-English R, Dennis SC, Schloss I, Noakes TD, and Lambert EV. Effects of medium-chain triacylglycerol ingested with carbohydrate on metabolism and exercise performance. *International Journal of Sport Nutrition* 1999; 9(1): 35-47.

55 Avakian, E.V., and Sugimoto, B.R. 1980. Effect of Panax ginseng extract on blood energy substrates during exercise. *Fed. Proc.* 39: 287.

56 Morris AC, Jacobs I, Klugerman A, and McLellan, TM. No ergogenic effect of ginseng extract ingestion. *Medicine and Science in Sports and Exercise* 1994; 26(5): S35.

Chapter 5

1 This common bacterium is the cause of the majority of all stomach ulcers. Eighty percent of people in developing countries are infected, and in the United States about 20 percent of young adults and 50 percent of adults older than age 60 are infected. H. pylori appears to be transmitted from person to person by close contact. Most people become infected with H. pylori in childhood, and that infection remains throughout life unless eliminated through antibiotics.

2 Shi X, Bartoli W, Horn M, and Murray R. Gastric emptying of cold beverages in humans: Effect of transportable carbohydrates. *International Journal of Sport Nutrition and Exercise Metabolism* 2000; 10: 394-403.

3 Maughan RJ and Leiper JB. Limitations to fluid replacement during exercise. *Canadian Journal of Applied Physiology* 1999; 24(2): 173-187.

4 The pancreatic duct and bile duct meet to form a single duct, referred to as the common bile duct.

5 Emulsifying agents are unique chemicals, water soluble on one end and fat soluble on the other. The fat-soluble end attaches itself to fat droplets, and the water-soluble end surrounds the fat droplet. This allows the fat to mix (and stay mixed) in a water-based environment.

6 Bile has an interesting feature in that it is 50 percent cholesterol. Higher intakes of fat stimulate a higher production of bile, which is absorbed with the fats it has emulsified. This higher bile production–absorption cycle increases circulating cholesterol, even if the intake of dietary cholesterol is zero. Therefore, dietary fat intake is more of a culprit in high circulating cholesterol levels than dietary cholesterol intake.

7 Vitamin B$_{12}$ requires intrinsic factor, which is produced by the parietal cells of the stomach, for absorption. A failure to produce intrinsic factor will cause vitamin B$_{12}$ deficiency disease (pernicious anemia), regardless of the amount of B$_{12}$ consumed.

8 Yogurt is made from pasteurized milk using one of these bacterial strains.

Chapter 6

1 Ziegler PJ, Jonnalagadda SS, Nelson JA, Lawrence C, & Baciak B. Contribution of meals and snacks to nutrient intake of male and female elite figure skaters during peak competitive season. *Journal of the American College of Nutrition* 2002; 21(2): 115-119.

2 Burke LM. Energy needs of athletes. *Canadian Journal of Applied Physiology* 2001; 26(suppl.): S202-S219.

3 Hubbard RW, Szlyk PC, and Armstrong LE. Influence of thirst and fluid palatability on fluid ingestion during exercise. In: *Perspectives in exercise science and sports medicine, volume 3:*

Fluid homeostasis during exercise (Ed. Gisolfi CV and Lamb DR). Carmel, IN: Benchmark Press. 1990: pp. 39-95.

4 Hawley JA and Burke LM. Meal frequency and physical performance. *British Journal of Nutrition* 1997; 77: S91-S103.

5 Deutz B, Benardot D, Martin D, and Cody M. Relationship between energy deficits and body composition in elite female gymnasts and runners. *Medicine and Science in Sports and Exercise* 2000; 32(3): 659-668.

6 Iwao S, Mori K, and Sato Y. Effects of meal frequency on body composition during weight control in boxers. *Scandinavian Journal of Medicine and Science in Sports* 1996; 6(5): 265-272.

7 Dulloo AG and Girardier C. Adaptive changes in energy expenditure during refeeding following low-calorie intake: Evidence for a specific metabolic component favoring fat storage. *American Journal of Clinical Nutrition* 1990; 52: 415-420.

8 Saltzman E and Roberts SB. The role of energy expenditure in regulation: Findings from a decade of research. *Nutrition Reviews* 1995; 53(8): 209-220.

9 Benardot D and Thompson WR. Energy: The importance of getting enough and getting it on time. *ACSM's Health and Fitness Journal* 1999; 3(4): 14-18.

10 Heshka S, Yank M-U, Wang J, Burt P, and Pi-Sunyer FX. Weight loss and change in resting metabolic rate. *American Journal of Clinical Nutrition* 1990; 52: 981-986.

11 Deutz B, Benardot D, Martin D, and Cody M. Relationship between energy deficits and body composition in elite female gymnasts and runners. *Medicine and Science in Sports and Exercise* 2000; 32(3): 659-668.

12 Hawley JA and Burke LM. Meal frequency and physical performance. *British Journal of Nutrition* 1997; 77: S91-S103.

13 Jenkins DJA et al. Nibbling versus gorging: Metabolic advantages of increased meal frequency. *New England Journal of Medicine* 1989; 321(14): 929-934.

14 Metzner HL, Lamphiear DE, Wheeler NC, and Larkin FA. The relationship between frequency of eating and adiposity in adult men and women in the Tecumseh Community Health Study. *American Journal of Clinical Nutrition* 1977; 30: 712-715.

15 Steen SN, Oppliger RA, and Brownell KD. Metabolic effects of repeated weight loss and regain in adolescent wrestlers. *Journal of the American Medical Association* 1988; 260(1): 47-50.

16 Benardot D, Martin DE, Thompson WR, and Roman S. Between-meal energy intake effects on body composition, performance, and total caloric consumption in athletes. *Medicine and Science in Sports and Exercise* 2005; 37(5): S339.

17 deCastro JM. Genetic influences on daily intake and meal patterns of humans. *Physiology and Behavior* 1993; 53(4): 777-782.

18 LeBlanc J, Mercier I, and Nadeau A. Components of postprandial thermogenesis in relation to meal frequency in humans. *Canadian Journal of Physiology and Pharmacology* 1993; 71(12): 879-883.

19 Luke A and Schoeller DA. Basal metabolic rate, fat-free mass, and body cell mass during energy restriction. *Metabolism* 1992; 41(4): 450-456.

20 Tuschl RJ, Platte P, Laessle RG, Stichler W, and Pirke KM. Energy expenditure and everyday eating behavior in healthy young women. *American Journal of Clinical Nutrition* 1990; 52(1): 81-86.

21 Heshka S, Yang MU, Wang J, Burt P, and Pi-Sunyer FX. Weight loss and change in resting metabolic rate. *American Journal of Clinical Nutrition* 1990; 52(6): 981-986.

22 Farshchi HR, Taylor MA, and Macdonald IA. Decreased thermic effect of food after an irregular compared with a regular meal pattern in healthy lean women. *International Journal of Obesity and Related Metabolic Disorders* 2004; 28(5): 653-660.

23 Jenkins DJA, Wolever TM, Vuksan V, Brighenti F, Cunnane SC, Rao AV, Jenkins AL, Buckley G, Patten R, Singer W, et al. Nibbling versus gorging: Metabolic advantages of increased meal frequency. *New England Journal of Medicine* 1989; 321(14): 929-934.

24 Kassab SE, Abdul-Ghaffar T, Nagalla DS, Sachdeva U, and Nayar U. Serum leptin and insulin levels during chronic diurnal fasting. *Asia Pacific Journal of Clinical Nutrition* 2003; 12(4): 483-487.

25 Hubbard RW, Szlyk PC, and Armstrong LE. Influence of thirst and fluid palatability on fluid ingestion during exercise. In: *Perspectives in exercise science and sports medicine, volume 3: Fluid homeostasis during exercise* (Ed. Gisolfi CV and Lamb DR). Carmel, IN: Benchmark Press. 1990: pp. 39-95.

26 Sandor RP. Heat illness: On-site diagnosis and cooling. *Physician and Sportsmedicine* 1997; 25(6).

27 Benardot D. *Nutrition for serious athletes: An advanced guide to foods, fluids, and supplements for training and performance.* Champaign, IL: Human Kinetics. 2000: pp. 77-78.

28 Williams MH. *Nutrition for health, fitness and sport.* 5th ed. New York: WCB McGraw-Hill: pp. 276-277.

29 Maughan RJ and Noakes TD. Fluid replacement and exercise stress: A brief review of studies on fluid replacement and some guidelines for the athlete. *Sports Medicine* 12: 16-31.

30 Levey JM. Runner's diarrhea. *American Medical Association Quarterly* 2000; 14(1): 6-7.

31 Osmolality is determined by the number of particles in a solution, not the size of the particles. Therefore, you can deliver more carbohydrate with a lower osmolality when polymers (strands of attached glucose) are used instead of individual glucose molecules.

32 Blom PCS, Hostmark AT, Vaage O, Kardel KR, and Maehlum S. Effect of different post-exercise sugar diets on the rate of muscle glycogen synthesis. *Medicine and Science in Sports and Exercise* 1987; 19: 491-496.

33 Welsh RS, Davis JM, Burke JR, and Williams HG. Carbohydrates and physical/mental performance during intermittent exercise to fatigue. *Medicine and Science in Sports and Exercise* 2002; 34: 723-731.

34 Walberg-Rankin J, Ocel JV, and Craft LL. Effect of weight loss and refeeding diet composition on anaerobic performance in wrestlers. *Medicine and Science in Sports and Exercise* 1996; 28: 1292-1299.

35 Conley M and Stone M. Carbohydrate ingestion/ supplementation for resistance exercise and training. *Sports Medicine* 1996; 21: 7-17.

36 Jeukendrup A, Brouns F, Wagenmakers AJ, and Saris WH. Carbohydrate-electrolyte feedings improve 1 h time trial cycling performance. *International Journal of Sports Medicine* 1997; 18(2): 125-129.

37 Davis JM, Jackson DA, Broadwell MS, Queary JL, and Lambert CL. Carbohydrate drinks delay fatigue during intermittent, high-intensity cycling in active men and women. *International Journal of Sport Nutrition* 1997; 7: 261-273.

38 Kimber N, Ross JJ, Mason SL, and Speedy DB. Energy balance during an ironman triathlon in male and female triathletes. *International Journal of Sport Nutrition and Exercise Metabolism* 2002; 12: 47-62.

39 Glycogen storage requires extra fluid in a 3: 1 ratio (water: glycogen).

40 Sherman WM, Costill DL, Fink W, Hagerman F, Armstrong L, and Murray T. Effect of a 42.2-km footrace and subsequent rest or exercise on muscle glycogen and enzymes. *Journal of Applied Physiology* 1983; 55: 1219-1224.

41 Bergstrom J, Hermansen L, Hultman E, and Saltin B. Diet, muscle glycogen and physical performance. *Acta Physiologica Scandinavica* 1967; 71: 140-150.

Chapter 7

1 Maughan RJ. Role of micronutrients in sport and physical activity. *British Medical Bulletin* 1999; 55(3): 683-690.

2 Weiler JM, Metzger WJ, Donnelly AL, Crowley ET, and Sharath MD. Prevalence of bronchial hyperresponsiveness in highly trained athletes. *Chest* 1986; 90(1): 23-28.

3 Larsson K, Ohlsen P, Larsson L, Malmberg P, Rydstrom PO, and Ulriksen H. High prevalence of asthma in cross country skiers. *British Medical Journal* 1993; 307(6915): 1326-1329.

4 Columbini L. Exercise-induced asthma in children. *Canadian Journal of Continuing Medical Education* 1998; 10(8): 67-81.

5 Lacroix VJ. Exercise-induced asthma. *Physician and Sportsmedicine* 1999; 27(12).

6 Schumacher YO, Schmid A, Grathwohl D, Bultermann D, and Berg A. Hematological indices and iron status in athletes of various sports and performances. *Medicine and Science in Sports and Exercise* 2002; 34(5): 869-875.

7 Beard J and Tobin B. Iron status and exercise. *American Journal of Clinical Nutrition* 2000; 72(2): S594-S597.

8 Portal S, Epstein M, and Dubnov G. Iron deficiency and anemia in female athletes: Causes and risks. *Harefuah* 2003; 142(10): 698-703, 717.

9 Lukaski HC. Vitamin and mineral status: Effects on physical performance. *Nutrition* 2004; 20(7/8): 632-644.

10 Jones GR and Newhouse I. Sport-related hematuria: A review. *Clinical Journal of Sport Medicine* 1997; 7(2): 119-125.

11 Fallon KE and Bishop G. Changes in erythropoiesis assessed by reticulocyte parameters during ultralong distance running. *Clinical Journal of Sport Medicine* 2002; 12(3): 172-178.

12 Shaskey DJ and Green GA. Sports haematology. *Sports Medicine* 2000; 29(1): 27-38.

13 Opara EC. Oxidative stress, micronutrients, diabetes mellitus and its complications. *Journal of the Royal Society of Health* 2002; 122(1): 28-34.

14 Shephard RJ and Shek PN. Immunological hazards from nutritional imbalance in athletes. *Exercise Immunology Review* 1998; 4: 22-48.

Chapter 8

1 Zone JJ. Skin manifestations of celiac disease. *Gastroenterology* 2005; 128(4) (suppl. 1): S87-S91.

2 Dewar DH and Ciclitira PJ. Clinical features and diagnosis of celiac disease. *Gastroenterology* 2005; 128(4) (suppl. 1): S19-S24.

3 Kupper C. Dietary guidelines and implementation for celiac disease. *Gastroenterology* 2005; 128(4) (suppl. 1): S121-S127.

4 Dube C, Rostom A, Sy R, Cranney A, Saloojee N, Garritty C, Sampson M, Zhang L, Yazdi F, Mamaladze V, Pan I, Macneil J, Mack D, Patel D, and Moher D. The prevalence of celiac disease in average-risk and at-risk Western European populations: A systematic review. *Gastroenterology* 2005; 128(4) (suppl. 1): S57-S67.

5 Kupper C. Dietary guidelines and implementation for celiac disease. *Gastroenterology* 2005; 128(4) (suppl. 1): S121-S127.

6 Wells RW and Blennerhassett MG. The increasing prevalence of Crohn's disease in industrialized societies: The price of progress? *Canadian Journal of Gastroenterology* 2005; 19(2): 89-95.

7 Nayar M and Rhodes JM. Management of inflammatory bowel disease. *Postgraduate Medical Journal* 2004; 80(942): 206-213.

8 Ikeuchi H, Yamamura T, Nakano H, Kosaka T, Shimoyama T, and Fukuda Y. Efficacy of nutritional therapy for perforating and non-perforating Crohn's disease. *Hepatogastroenterology* 2004; 51(58): 1050-1052.

9 Faloon WW, Paes IC, Woolfolk D, Nankin H, Wallace K, and Haro EN. Effect of neomycin and kanamycin upon intestinal absorption. *Annals of the New York Academy of Sciences* 1966; 132(2): 879-887.

10 Mahan LK and Escott-Stump S (Eds.). *Krause's Food, Nutrition, & Diet Therapy.* Philadelphia: Saunders. 2000. p. 403.

11 Faucheron JL and Parc R. Non-steroidal anti-inflammatory drug induced colitis. *International Journal of Colorectal Disease* 1996; 11: 99.

12 Haber P. Magnesium update. *Acta Medica Austriaca* 2004; 31(2): 37-39.

13 El-Sayed MS, Ali N, and El-Sayed Ali Z. Interaction between alcohol and exercise: Physiological and haematological implications. *Sports Medicine* 2005; 35(3): 257-269.

14 Review article: Alcohol, vitamin A, and β-carotene: Adverse interactions, including hepatotoxicity and carcinogenicity. *American Journal of Clinical Nutrition* 1999; 69(6): 1071-1085.

15 Peretti-Watel P, Guagliardo V, Verger P, Pruvost J, Mignon P, and Obadia Y. Sporting activity and drug use: Alcohol, cigarette and cannabis use among elite student athletes. *Addiction* 2003; 98(9): 1249-1256.

16 Miller KE, Hoffman JH, Barnes GM, Farrell MP, Sabo D, and Melnick MJ. Jocks, gender, race, and adolescent problem drinking. *Journal of Drug Education* 2003; 33(4): 445-462.

17 Lorente FO, Souville M, Griffet J, and Grelot L. Participation in sports and alcohol consumption among French adolescents. *Addictive Behaviors* 2004; 29(5): 941-946.

Chapter 9

1 Gayton WF, Broida J, and Elgee L. An investigation of coaches perceptions of the causes of home advantage. *Perceptual Motor Skills* 2001; 92(3): 933-936.

2 Nevill AM and Holder RL. Home advantage in sport: An overview of studies on the advantage of playing at home. *Sports Medicine* 1999; 28(4): 221-236.

3 Loat E and Rhodes EC. Jet-lag and human performance. Sports Medicine 1989; 8(4): 226-238.

4 Pace A and Carron AV. Travel and the home advantage. Canadian Journal of Sport Sciences 1992; 17(1): 60-64.

5 Bishop D. The effects of travel on team performance in the Australian national netball competition. *Journal of Science and Medicine in Sport* 2004; 7(1): 118-122.

6 Reilly T, Atkinson G, and Waterhouse J. Travel fatigue and jet-lag. *Journal of Sports Sciences* 1997; 15(3): 365-369.

7 Atkinson G and Reilly T. Circadian variation in sports performance. *Sports Medicine* 1996; 21(4): 292-312.

8 Hill DW, Hill CM, Fields KL, and Smith JC. Effects of jet lag on factors related to sport performance. *Canadian Journal of Applied Physiology* 1993; 18(1): 91-103.

9 Straub WF, Spino MP, Alattar MM, Pfleger B, Downes JW, Belizaire MA, Heinonen OJ, and Vasankari T. The effect of chiropractic care on jet lag of Finnish junior elite athletes. *Journal of Manipulative and Physiological Therapeutics* 2001; 24(3): 191-198.

10 Nieman DC. Current perspective on exercise immunology. *Current Sports Medicine Reports* 2003; 5: 239-242.

11 So SC, Ko J, Yuan YW, Lam JJ, and Louie L. Severe acute respiratory syndrome and sport: Facts and fallacies. *Sports Medicine* 2004; 34(15): 1023-1033.

12 Gatorade Sports Nutrition Advisory Board. "Eating on the Road." Chicago, IL: Gatorade Sports Science Institute. 1996.

13 Mielcarek J & Kleiner S. "Time Zone Changes." *Sports Nutrition: A Guide for Professionals Working with Active People.* Ed: Benardot D. Chicago: American Dietetic Association. 1993.

Chapter 10

1 National Academy of Sciences. *Nutritional needs in cold and high-altitude environments: Applications for military personnel in field operations.* Washington DC: National Academy Press. 1996: p. 1.

2 Horvath SM. Exercise in a cold environment. *Exercise Sport Science Review* 1981; 9: 221-263.

3 Webb P. Temperature of skin, subcutaneous tissue, muscle and core in resting men in cold, comfortable and hot conditions. *European Journal of Applied Physiology* 1992; 64: 471-476.

4 Vallerand AL and Jacobs I. Rates of energy substrates utilization during human cold exposure. *European Journal of Applied Physiology* 1989; 58: 873-878.

5 Young AJ, Muza SR, Sawka MN, Gonzalez RR, and Pandolf KB. Human thermoregulatory responses to cold air are altered by repeated cold water immersion. *Journal of Applied Physiology* 1986; 60: 1542-1548.

6 Febbraio MA. Exercise in climatic extremes. In: *Nutrition in sport* (Ed. Maughan RJ). London: Blackwell Science. 2000. p. 498.

7 Young AJ. Effects of aging on human cold tolerance. *Experimental Aging Research* 1991; 17(3): 205-213.

8 Freund BJ and Sawka MN. Influence of cold stress on human fluid balance. In: *Nutritional needs in cold and high altitude environments.* Washington DC: National Academy Press. 1996: p. 161.

9 Jefferson JA, Simoni J, Escudero E, Hurtado ME, Swenson ER, Wesson DE, Schreiner GF, Schoene RB, Johnson RJ, and Hurtado A. Increased oxidative stress following acute and chronic high altitude exposure. *High Altitude Medicine and Biology* 2004; 5(1): 61-69.

10 Altitude illness. NOLS Wilderness First Aid. Available: www.elbrus.org/eng1/high_altitude1.htm [March 21, 2005].

11 Askew EW. Nutrition at high altitude. Wilderness Medical Society. Available: www.wms.org/pubs/altitude.html [March 21, 2005].

12 Rodway GW, Hoffman LA, and Sanders MH. High-altitude-related disorders, part I: Pathophysiology, differential diagnosis, and treatment. *Heart Lung* 2003; 32(6): 353-359.

13 Leppk JA, Icenogle MV, Maes D, Riboni K, Hinghofer-Szalkay H, and Roach C. Early fluid retention and severe acute mountain sickness. *Journal of Applied Physiology* 2005; 98(2): 591-597.

14 Talbot TS, Townes DA, and Wedmore IS. To air is human: Altitude illness during an expedition length adventure race. *Wilderness and Environmental Medicine* 2004; 15(2): 90-94.

15 Gallagher SA and Hackett PH. High-altitude illness. *Emergency Medicine Clinics of North America* 2004; 22(2): 329-355.

16 Hackett PH and Roach RC. High altitude cerebral edema. *High Altitude Medicine and Biology* 2004; 5(2): 136-146.

17 High altitude medicine guide. Available: www.high-altitude-medicine.com/AMS.html [March 25, 2005].

18 Ri-Li G, Chase PJ, Witkowski S, Wyrick BL, Stone JA, Levine BD, and Babb TG. Obesity: Associations with acute mountain sickness. *Annals of Internal Medicine* 2003; 139(4): 253-257.

19 Beidleman BA, Muza SR, Fulco CS, Cymerman A, Ditzler D, Stulz D, Staab JE, Skrinar GS, Lewis SF, and Sawka MN. Intermittent altitude exposures reduce acute mountain sickness at 4300 m. *Clinical Science* 2004; 106(3): 321-328.

20 Dumont L, Lysakowski C, Tramer MR, Junod JD, Mardirosoff C, Tassonyi E, and Kayser B. Magnesium for the prevention and treatment of acute mountain sickness. *Clinical Science* 2004; 106(3): 269-277.

21 Bartsch P, Bailey DM, Berger MM, Knauth M, and Baumgartner RW. Acute mountain sickness: Controversies and advances. *High Altitude Medicine and Biology* 2004; 5(2): 110-124.

22 Major C and Doucet E. Energy intake during a typical Himalayan trek. *High Altitude Medicine and Biology* 2004; 5(3): 355-363.

23 Rose MS, Houston CS, Fulco CS, Coates G, Sutton JR, and Cymerman A. Operation Everest II: Nutrition and body composition. *Journal of Applied Physiology* 1988; 65: 2545.

24 Butterfield GE. Maintenance of body weight at altitude: In search of 500 kcal/day. In: *Nutritional needs in cold and high altitude environments* (Ed. Marriott BM and Carlson SJ). Washington DC: National Academy Press. 1996: p. 357.

25 Freund BJ and Sawka MN. Influence of cold stress on human fluid balance. In: *Nutritional needs in cold and high altitude environments* (Ed. Marriott BM and Carlson SJ). Washington DC: National Academy Press. 1996: p. 167.

26 Freund BJ and Sawka MN. Influence of cold stress on human fluid balance. In: *Nutritional needs in cold and high altitude environments* (Ed. Marriott BM and Carlson SJ). Washington DC: National Academy Press. 1996: p. 170.

27 Reynolds RD, Lickteig JA, Deuster PA, Howard MP, Conway JM, Pietersma A, deStoppelaar J, and Deurenberg P. Energy metabolism increases and regional body fat decreases while regional muscle mass is spared in humans climbing Mt. Everest. *Journal of Nutrition* 1999; 129(7): 1307-1314.

28 Westerterp-Plantenga MS. Effects of extreme environments on food intake in human subjects. *Proceedings of the Nutrition Society* 1999; 58(4): 791-798.

29 Nutritional advice for military operations in a high-altitude environment. Available: http://www.usariem.army.mil/nutri/nuadalti.htm [March 21, 2005].

30 Reynolds RD, Lickteig JA, Howard MP, and Deuster PA. Intakes of high fat and high carbohydrate foods by humans increased with exposure to increasing altitude during an expedition to Mt. Everest. *Journal of Nutrition* 1998; 128(1): 50-55.

31 Askew EW. Environmental and physical stress and nutrient requirements. *American Journal of Clinical Nutrition* 1995; 61(3): S632-S637.

32 Chao WH, Askew EW, Roberts DE, Wood SM, and Perkins JB. Oxidative stress in humans during work at moderate altitude. *Journal of Nutrition* 1999; 129(11): 2009-2012.

33 Freund BJ and Sawka MN. Influence of cold stress on human fluid balance. In: *Nutritional needs in cold and high altitude environments* (Ed. Marriott BM and Carlson SJ). Washington DC: National Academy Press. 1996: p. 175.

34 Freund BJ and Sawka MN. Influence of cold stress on human fluid balance. In: *Nutritional needs in cold and high altitude environments* (Ed. Marriott BM and Carlson SJ). Washington DC: National Academy Press. 1996: pp. 170-171.

35 Murray R. Fluid needs in hot and cold environments. *International Journal of Sport Nutrition* 1995; 5: S62-S73.

Chapter 11

1 Unnithan VB and Goulopoulou S. Nutrition for the pediatric athlete. *Current Sports Medicine Reports* 2004; 3(4): 206-211.

2 Petrie HJ, Stover EA, and Horswill CA. Nutritional concerns for the child and adolescent competitor. *Nutrition* 2004; 20(7/8): 620-631.

3 Bass M, Turner L, and Hunt S. Counseling female athletes: Application of the stages of change model to avoid disordered eating, amenorrhea, and osteoporosis. *Psychol Rep* 2001; 88(3), pt. 2: 1153-1160.

4 Warren MP and Perlroth NE. The effects of intense exercise on the female reproductive system. *Journal of Endocrinology* 2001; 170(1): 3-11.

5 Korpelainen R, Orava S, Karpakka J, Siira P, and Hulkko A. Risk factors for recurrent stress fractures in athletes. *American Journal of Sports Medicine* 2001; 29(3): 304-310.

6 Nattiv A. Stress fractures and bone health in track and field athletes. *Journal of Science and Medicine in Sport* 2000; 3(3): 268-279.

7 Tarnopolsky LJ, MacDougall JD, Atkinson SA, Tarnopolsky MA, and Sutton JR. Gender differences in substrate for endurance exercise. *Journal of Applied Physiology* 1990; 68: 302-308.

8 Gabel KA. The female athlete. In: *Nutrition in sport* (Ed. Maughan RJ). London: Blackwell Science. 2000: pp. 417-428.

9 Burke LM, Cox GR, Culmmings NK, and Desbrow B. Guidelines for daily carbohydrate intake: Do athletes achieve them? *Sports Medicine* 2001; 31(4): 267-299.

10 Lemon PWR. Do athletes need more dietary protein and amino acids? *International Journal of Sport Nutrition* 1995; 5: S39-S61.

11 Perry AC, Crane LS, Applegate B, Marquez-Sterling S, Signorile JF, and Miller PC. Nutrient intake and psychological and physiological assessment in eumenorrheic and amenorrheic female athletes: A preliminary study. *International Journal of Sport Nutrition* 1996; 6: 3-13.

12 Manore MM. Vitamin B_6 and exercise. *International Journal of Sport Nutrition* 1994; 4: 89-103.

13 Huang YC, Chen W, Evans MA, Mitchell ME, and Shultz TD. Vitamin B-6 requirement and status assessment of young women fed a high-protein diet with various levels of vitamin B-6. *American Journal of Clinical Nutrition* 1998; 67: 208-220.

14 Pate RR, Miller BJ, Davis JM, Slentz CA, and Kling-Shirn LA. Iron status of female runners. *International Journal of Sport Nutrition* 1993; 6: 3-13.

15 Fogelholm M. Indicators of vitamin and mineral status in athletes blood: A review. *International Journal of Sport Nutrition* 1995; 5: 267-284.

16 Dueck CA, Manore MM, and Matt KS. Role of energy balance in athletic menstrual dysfunction. *International Journal of Sport Nutrition* 1996; 6(2): 165-190.

17 Van de Loo DA and Johnson MD. The young female athlete. *Clinical Sports Medicine* 1995; 14(3): 687-707.

18 Nelson Steen S. Nutrition for the school-aged child athlete. In: *The child and adolescent athlete* (Ed. Bar-Or O). Oxford: Blackwell Science. 1996: pp. 260-273.

19 Unnithan VB and Baxter-Jones ADG. The young athlete. In: *Nutrition in sport* (Ed. Maughan RJ). London: Blackwell Science. 2000: p. 430.

20 Chumlea WC, Schubert CM, Roche AF, Kulin HE, Lee PA, Himes JH, and Sun SS. Age at menarche and racial comparisons in US girls. *Pediatrics* 2003; 111(1): 110-113.

21 American Academy of Pediatrics, Committee on Sports Medicine and Fitness. Intensive training and sports specialization in young athletes. *Pediatrics* 2000; 106(1): 154-157.

22 Kurz KM. Adolescent nutritional status in developing countries. *Proceedings of the Nutrition Society* 1996; 55: 321-331.

23 Beard J and Tobin B. Iron status and exercise. *American Journal of Clinical Nutrition* 2000; 72(2): S594-S597.

24 Hebestreit H, Meyer F, Htay-Htay, Heigenhauser GJF, and Bar-Or O. Plasma metabolites, volume and electrolytes following 30-s high-intensity exercise in boys and men. *European Journal of Applied Physiology* 1996; 72: 563-569.

25 Martinez LR and Haymes EM. Substrate utilization during treadmill running in prepubertal girls and women. *Medicine and Science in Sports and Exercise* 1992; 24: 975-983.

26 Petrie HJ, Stover EA, and Horswill CA. Nutritional concerns for the child and adolescent competitor. *Nutrition* 2004; 20(7/8): 620-631.

27 American Academy of Pediatrics, Committee on Sports Medicine and Fitness. Intensive training and sports specialization in young athletes. *Pediatrics* 2000; 106(1): 154-157.

28 Bompa T. *From childhood to champion athlete*. Toronto: Veritas. 1995.

29 Bar-Or O, Dotan R, Inbar O, Rothstein A, and Zonder H. Voluntary hypohydration in 10- to 12-year-old boys. *Journal of Applied Physiology* 1980; 48: 104-108.

30 Bar-Or O. Nutrition for child and adolescent athletes. *Sports Science Exchange* 2000; 12(2): #77.

31 Bar-Or O. Nutrition for child and adolescent athletes. *Sports Science Exchange* 2000; 13(2): #77.

32 Campbell WW and Geik RA. Nutritional considerations for the older athlete. *Nutrition* 2004; 20(7/8): 603-608.

33 Miller KK. Mechanisms by which nutritional disorders cause reduced bone mass in adults. *Journal of Womens Health* 2003; 12(2): 145-150.

34 Kenney WL. The older athlete: Exercise in hot environments. *Sports Science Exchange* 1993; 6(3): #44.

35 Kenney WL and Hodgson JL. Heat tolerance, thermoregulation and aging. *Sports Medicine* 1987; 4: 446-456.

36 Kenney WL, Tankersley CG, Newswanger DL, Hyde DE, and Turner NL. Age and hypohydration independently influence the peripheral vascular response to heat stress. *Journal of Applied Physiology* 1990; 68: 1902-1908.

37 Kenney WL and Fowler SR. Methylcholine-activated eccrine sweat gland density and output as a function of age. *Journal of Applied Physiology* 1988; 65: 1082-1086.

38 Thompson J and Manore M. *Nutrition: An applied approach*. New York: Pearson-Benjamin Cummings. 2005: p. 600.

39 Nieman DC. Exercise immunology: Future directions for research related to athletes, nutrition, and the elderly. *International Journal of Sports Medicine* 2000; 21(suppl. 1): S61-S68.

Chapter 12

1 Okely AD, Booth ML, and Chey T. Relationships between body composition and fundamental movement skills among children and adolescents. *Research Quarterly for Exercise and Sport* 2004; 75(3): 238-247.

2 Augestad LB, Saether B, and Gotestam KG. The relationship between eating disorders and personality in physically active women. *Scandinavian Journal of Medicine and Science in Sports* 1999; 9: 304-312.

3 Williams, M.H. 1999. *Nutrition for health, fitness, and sport.* (New York: WCB McGraw-Hill). 317-318.

4 Saltzman, E., and Roberts, S.B. 1995. The role of energy expenditure in energy regulation: findings of a decade of research. *Nutr. Rev.* 53(8): 209-220.

5 Forbes, G.F., Brown, M.R., Welle, S.L., and Lipinski, B.A. 1986. Deliberate overfeeding in women and men: energy cost and composition of the weight gain. *Brit. J. of Nutr.* 56: 1-9.

6 Roberts, S.B., Young, V.R., Fuss, P., et al. 1990. Energy expenditure and subsequent nutrient intakes in overfed young men. *Am. J. Clin. Nutr.* 259: R461-9.

7 Diaz, E.O., Prentice, A.M., Goldberg, G.R., Murgatroyd, P.R., and Coward, W.A. 1992. Metabolic response to experimental overfeeding in lean and overweight healthy volunteers. *Am. J. Clin. Nutr.* 56: 641-55.

8 Leibel, R.L., Rosenbaum, M., and Hirsch, J. 1995. Changes in energy expenditure resulting from altered body weight. *New Eng. J. Med.* 332: 621-8.

9 Archimedes was a Greek mathematician, engineer, and physicist. He discovered formulas for determining the area and volume of different shapes the principal of buoyancy.

10 Rhea DJ. Eating disorder behaviors of ethnically diverse urban female adolescent athletes and non-athletes. *Journal of Adolescence* 1999; 22(3): 379-388.

11 Sundgot-Borgen J and Torstveit MK. Prevalence of eating disorders in elite athletes is higher than in the general population. *Clinical Journal of Sport Medicine* 2004; 14(1): 25-32.

12 Weimann E. Gender-related differences in elite gymnasts: The female athlete triad. *Journal of Applied Physiology* 2002; 92(5): 2146-2152.

13 Ramsay R and Wolman R. Are synchronized swimmers at risk of amenorrhoea? *British Journal of Sports Medicine* 2001; 35(4): 242-244.

14 Hinton PS, Sanford TC, Davidson MM, Yakushko OF, and Beck NC. Nutrient intakes and dietary behaviors of male and female collegiate athletes. *International Journal of Sport Nutrition and Exercise Metabolism* 2004; 14(4): 389-405.

15 Sundgot-Borgen J. Eating disorders in athletes. In: *Nutrition in sport* (Ed. Maughan RJ). London: Blackwell Science. 2000: pp. 510-522.

16 Warren MP and Goodman LR. Exercise-induced endocrine pathologies. *Journal of Endocrinology Investigation* 2003; 26(9): 873-878.

17 Thompson RA and Trattner-Sherman R. *Helping athletes with eating disorders.* Champaign, IL: Human Kinetics. 1993.

18 Brownell KD and Rodin J. Prevalence of eating disorders in athletes. In: *Eating, body weight and performance in athletes: Disorders of modern society* (Ed. Brownell KD, Rodin J, and Wilmore JH). Philadelphia: Lea & Febiger. 1992: pp. 128-143.

19 Manore MM. Dietary recommendations and athletic menstrual dysfunction. *Sports Medicine* 2002; 32(14): 887-901.

20 Fogelholm GM, Koskinen R, and Lasko J. Gradual and rapid weight loss: Effects on nutrition and performance in male athletes. *Medicine and Science in Sports and Exercise* 1993; 25(3): 371-377.

21 Fogelholm M. Effects of bodyweight reduction on sports performance. *Sports Medicine* 1994; 18(4): 249-267.

22 Reading KJ, McCarger LI, and Harber VJ. Energy balance and luteal phase progesterone levels in elite adolescent aesthetic athletes. *International Journal of Sport Nutrition and Exercise Metabolism* 2002; 12(1): 93-104.

Chapter 13

1 Grivetti, L.E., and Applegate, E.A. 1997. From Olympia to Atlanta: A cultural-historical perspective on diet and athletic training. *J. Nutr.* 127 (5): 860S-868S.

2 Recht, L.D., Lew, R.A., and Schwartz, W.J. 1995. Baseball teams beaten by jet lag. *Nature* 377 (6550): 583.

3 Whitley, J.D., and Terrio, T. 1998. Changes in peak torque arm-shoulder strength of high school baseball pitchers during the season. *Percept. Motor Skills* 86: 1361-1362.

4 MacWilliams, B.A., Choi, T., Perezous, M.K., Chao, E.Y., and McFarland, E.G. 1998. Characteristic ground-reaction forces in baseball pitching. *Am. J. Sports Med.* 26: 66-71.

5 Palumbo CM and Clark N. Case problem: Nutrition concerns related to the performance of a baseball team. *Journal of the American Dietetic Association* 2000; 100(6): 704-707.

6 Yoshida, T., Nakai, S., Yorimoto, A., Kawabata, T., and Morimoto, T. 1995. Effect of aerobic capacity on sweat rate and fluid intake during outdoor exercise in the heat. *Eur. J. Appl. Physiol.* 71: 235-239.

7 Bast, S.C., Perry, J.R., Poppiti, R., Vangsness, C.T., and Weaver, F.A. 1996. Upper extremity blood flow in collegiate and high school baseball pitchers: A preliminary report. *Am. J. Sports Med.* 24 (6): 847-851.

8 Schulz, R., and Curnow, C. 1988. Peak performance and age among superathletes: Track and field, swimming, baseball, tennis, and golf. *J. Gerontology* 43 (5): 113-120.

9 van der Ploeg GE, Brooks AG, Withers RT, Dollman, J, Leaney F, Chatterton BE. Body composition changes in female bodybuilders during preparation for competition. *European Journal of Clinical Nutrition* 2001; 55(4): 268-277.

10 Morrison LJ, Gizis F, and Shorter B. Prevalent use of dietary supplements among people who exercise at a commercial gym. *International Journal of Sport Nutrition and Exercise Metabolism* 2004; 14(4): 481-492.

11 Hickson, J.F., Johnson, T.E., Lee, W., and Sidor, R.J. 1990. Nutrition and the precontent preparations of a male bodybuilder. *J. Am. Diet. Assoc.* 90 (2): 264-267.

12 Britschgi, F., and Zund, G. 1991. Bodybuilding: Hypokalemia and hypophosphatemia. *Schweiz Med. Wochenschr.* 121 (33): 1163-1165.

13 Hickson, J.F., Johnson, T.E., Lee, W., and Sidor, R.J. 1990. Nutrition and the precontent preparations of a male bodybuilder. *J. Am. Diet. Assoc.* 90 (2): 264-267.

14 Barron, R.L., and Vanscoy, G.J. 1993. Natural products and the athlete: Facts and folklore. *Ann. Pharmacother.* 27 (5): 607-615.

15 Kleiner, S.M., Bazzarre, T.L., and Litchford, M.D. 1990. Metabolic profiles, diet, and health practices of championship male and female bodybuilders. *J. Am. Diet. Assoc.* 90 (7): 962-967.

16 Bosselaers, I., Buemann, B., Victor, O.J., and Astrup, A. 1994. Twenty-four hour energy expenditure and substrate utilization in body builders. *Am. J. Clin. Nutr.* 59: 10-12.

17 Lambert CP, Frank LL, and Evans WJ. Macronutrient considerations for the sport of bodybuilding. *Sports Medicine* 2004; 34(5): 317-327.

18 Andersen, R.E., Barlett, S.J., Morgan, G.D., and Brownell, K.D. 1995. Weight loss, psychological, and nutritional patterns in competitive male body builders. *Int. J. Eat. Disord.* 181 (1): 49-57.

19 Jonnalagadda SS, Rosenbloom CA, and Skinner R. Dietary practices, attitudes, and physiological status of collegiate freshman football players. *Journal of Strength and Conditioning Research* 2001; 15(4): 507-513.

20 Kreider, R.B., Ferreira, M., Wilson, M., Grindstaff, P., Plisk, S., Reinardy, J., Cantler, E., and Almada, A.L. 1998. Effects of creatine supplementation on body composition, strength, and sprint performance. *Med. Sci. Sports Exerc.* 30 (1): 73-82.

21 Stone MH, Sanborn K, Smith LL, O'Bryant HS, Hoke T, Utter AC, Johnson RL, Boros R, Hruby J, Pierce KC, Stone ME, and Garner B. Effects of in-season (5 weeks) creatine and pyruvate supplementation on anaerobic performance and body composition in American Football Players. *International Journal of Sport Nutrition* 1999; 9(2): 146-165.

22 Mayhew DL, Mayhew JL, and Ware JS. Effects of long-term creatine supplementation on liver and kidney functions in American college football players. *International Journal of Sport Nutrition and Exercise Metabolism* 2002; 12(4): 453-460.

23 Clancy, S.P., Clarkson, P.M., DeCheke, M.E., Nosaka, K., Freedson, P.S., Cunningham, J.J., and Valentine, B. 1994. Effects of chromium picolinate supplementation on body composition, strength, and urinary chromium loss in football players. *Int. J. Sport Nutr.* 4 (2): 142-153.

24 Burke, L.M., and Hawley, J.A. 1997. Fluid balance in team sports: Guidelines for optimal practices. *Sports Med.* 24 (1): 38-54.

25 Criswell, D., Powers, D., Lawler, J., Tew, J., Dodd, S., Iryiboz, Y., Tulley, R., and Wheeler, K. 1991. Influence of a carbohydrate-electrolyte beverage on performance and blood homeostasis during recovery from football. *Int. J. Sport Nutr.* 1 (2): 178-191.

26 Parks, P.S., and Read, M.H. 1997. Adolescent male athletes: Body image, diet, and exercise. *Adolescence* 32 (127): 593-602.

27 Wang, M.Q., Downey, G.S., Perko, M.A., and Yesalis, C.E. 1993. Changes in body size of elite high school football players: 1963-1989. *Percept. Motor Skills* 76 (2): 379-383.

28 Gomez, J.E., Ross, S.K., Calmbach, W.L., Kimmel, R.B., Schmidt, D.R., and Dhanda, R. 1998. Body fatness and increased injury rates in high school football linemen. *Clin. J. Sport Med.* 8 (2): 115-120.

29 Kaplan, T.A., Digel, S.L., Scavo, V.A., and Arellana, S.B. 1995. Effect of obesity on injury risk in high school football players. *Clin. J. Sport Med.* 5 (1): 43-47.

30 Huddy, D.C., Nieman, D.C., and Johnson, R.L. 1993. Relationship between body image and percent body fat among college male varsity athletes and nonathletes. *Percept. Motor Skills* 77 (3): 851-857.

31 DePalma, M.T., Koszewski, W.M., Case, J.G., Barile, R.J., DePalma, B.F., and Oliaro, S.M. 1993. Weight control practices of lightweight football players. *Med. Sci. Sports Exerc.* 25 (6): 694-701.

32 Hickson, J.F., Jr., Duke, M.A., Risser, W.L., Johnson, C.W., Palmer, R., and Stockton, J.E. 1987. Nutritional intake from food sources of high school football athletes. *J. Am. Diet. Assoc.* 87 (12): 1656-1659.

33 Jehue, R., Street, D., and Huizenga, R. 1993. Effect of time zone and game time changes on team performance: National Football League. *Med. Sci. Sports Exerc.* 25 (1): 127-131.

34 Maddux, G.T. 1970. *Men's gymnastics.* Pacific Palisades, CA: Goodyear Publishing, 9.

35 Weimann E, Blum WF, Witzel C, Schwidergall S, and Bohles HJ. Hypoleptinemia in female and male elite gymnasts. *European Journal of Clinical Invesigation* 1999; 29(10): 853-860.

36 Weimann E, Witzel C, Schwidergall S, and Bohles HJ. Peripubertal perturbations in elite gymnasts caused by sport specific training regimes and inadequate nutritional intake. *International Journal of Sports Medicine* 2000; 21(3): 210-215.

37 Constantini NW, Eliakim A, Zigel L, Yaaron M, and Falk B. Iron status of highly active adolescents: Evidence of depleted iron stores in gymnasts. *International Journal of Sport Nutrition and Exercise Metabolism* 2000; 10(1): 62-70.

38 Houtkooper, L.B., and Going, S.B. 1994. Body composition: How should it be measured? Does it affect sport performance? *Gatorade Sports Sci. Inst.: Sports Sci. Exch.* 52: 7 (5s).

39 Bortz, S., Schoonen, J.C., Kanter, M., Kosharek, S., and Benardot, D. 1993. Physiology of anaerobic and aerobic exercise. In *Sports nutrition: A guide for the professional working with active people*, ed. Benardot, D., 2-10. Chicago, IL: American Dietetic Association.

40 Benardot, D., and Czerwinski, C. 1991. Selected body composition and growth measures of junior elite gymnasts. *J. Am. Diet. Assoc.* 91 (1): 29-33.

41 Benardot, D., Schwarz, M., and Heller, D.W. 1989. Nutrient intake in young, highly competitive gymnasts. *J. Am. Diet. Assoc.* 89: 401-403.

42 Benardot, D. 1996. Working with young athletes: Views of a nutritionist on the Sports Medicine team. *Int. J. Sport Nutr.* 6 (2): 110-120.

43 Loosli, A.R. 1993. Reversing sports-related iron and zinc deficiencies. *Phys. Sportsmed.* 21 (6): 70-78.

44 Burns, J., and Dugan, L. 1994. Working with professional athletes in the rink: The evolution of a nutrition program for an NHL team. *Int. J. Sport Nutr.* 4 (2): 132-134.

45 Akermark, C., Jacobs, I., Rasmussen, M., and Karlsson, J. 1996. Diet and muscle glycogen concentration in relation to physical performance in Swedish elite ice hockey players. *Int. J. Sport Nutr.* 6 (3): 272-284.

46 Davis JM, Welsh RS, and Alerson NA. Effects of carbohydrate and chromium ingestion during intermittent high-intensity exercise to fatigue. *International Journal of Sport Nutrition and Exercise Metabolism* 2000; 10(4): 476-485.

47 Houston, M.E. 1979. Nutrition and ice hockey performance. *Can. J. Appl. Sport Sci.* 4 (1): 98-99.

48 Tegelman, R., Aberg, T., Pousette, A., and Carlstrom, K. 1992. Effects of a diet regimen on pituitary and steroid hormones in male ice hockey players. *Int. J. Sports Med.* 13 (5): 424-430.

49 Glycogen synthetase is a hormone that is elevated as glycogen storage becomes depleted. Following a game or training session, the higher circulating glycogen synthetase enables an efficient replacement of glycogen if carbohydrates and fluids are consumed.

50 Horswill, C.A., Hickner, R.C., Scott, J.R., Costill, D.L., and Gould, D. 1990. Weight loss, dietary carbohydrate modifications, and high intensity, physical performance. *Med. Sci. Sports Exerc.* 22 (4): 470-476.

51 Sugiura K, Suzuki I, and Kobayashi K. Nutritional intake of elite Japanese track-and-field athletes. *International Journal of Sport Nutrition* 1999; 9(2): 202-212.

52 Nattiv A. Stress fractures and bone health in track and field athletes. *Journal of Science and Medicine in Sport* 2000; 3(3): 268-279.

53 Grediagin, M.A., Cody, M., Rupp, J., Benardot, D., and Shern, R. 1995. Exercise intensity does not effect body composition change in untrained, moderately overfat women. *J. Am. Diet. Assoc.* (95) 6: 661-665.

54 Kreider, R.B., Ferreira, M., Wilson, M., Grindstaff, P., Plisk, S., Reinardy, J., Cantler, E., and Almada, A.L. 1998. Effects of creatine supplementation on body composition, strength, and sprint performance. *Med. Sci. Sports Exerc.* 30 (1): 73-82.

55 Chwalbinska-Moneta J. Effect of creatine supplementation on aerobic performance and anaerobic capacity in elite rowers in the course of endurance training. *International Journal of Sport Nutrition and Exercise Metabolism* 2003; 13(2): 173-183.

56 Nevill, M.E., Williams, C., Roper, D., Slater, C., and Nevill, A.M. 1993. Effect of diet on performance during recovery from intermittent sprint exercise. *J. Sports Sci.* 11 (2): 119-126.

57 Sherman, W.M., Doyle, J.A., Lamb, D.R., and Strauss, R.H. 1993. Dietary carbohydrate, muscle glycogen, and exercise performance during seven days of training. *Am. J. Clin. Nutr.* 57 (1): 27-31.

58 Berning, J.R., Troup, J.P., VanHandel, P.J., Daniels, J., and Daniels, N. 1991. The nutritional habits of young adolescent swimmers. *Int. J. Sport Nutr.* 1(3): 240-248.

59 Braun WA, Flynn MG, Carl DL, Carroll KK, Brickman T, and Lambert CP. Iron status and resting immune function in female collegiate swimmers. *International Journal of Sport Nutrition and Exercise Metabolism* 2000; 10(4): 425-433.

60 Guinard, J.X., Seador, K., Beard, J.L., and Brown, P.L. 1995. Sensory acceptability of meat and dairy products and dietary fat in male collegiate swimmers. *Int. J. Sport Nutr.* 5(4): 315-328.

61 Lamb, D.R. *Basic principles for improving sport performance.* 1995. Gatorade Sports Science Exchange (#55) 8(2).

62 Microsoft. 1993-1996. "Wrestling." Encarta 97 Encyclopedia. CD-ROM: Microsoft Corporation.

63 Sossin, K., Gizis, F., Marquart, L.F., and Sobal, J. 1997. Nutrition beliefs, attitudes, and resource use of high school wrestling coaches. *Int. J. Sport Nutr.* 7 (3): 219-228.

64 Oppliger, R.A., Case, H.S., Horswill, C.A., Landry, G.L., and Shelter, A.C. 1996. American College of Sports Medicine position stand: Weight loss in wrestlers. *Med. Sci. Sports Exerc.* 28 (6): ix-xii.

65 Oppliger RA, Steen SA, and Scott JR. Weight loss practices of college wrestlers. *International Journal of Sport Nutrition and Exercise Metabolism* 2003; 13(1): 29-46.

66 Wroble, R.R., and Moxley, D.P. 1998. Weight loss patterns and success rates in high school wrestlers. *Med. Sci. Sports Exerc.* 30 (4): 625-628.

67 Wroble, R.R., and Moxley, D.P. 1998. Acute weight gain and its relationship to success in high school wrestlers. *Med. Sci. Sports Exerc.* 30 (6): 949-951.

68 Roemmich, J.N., and Sinning, W.E. 1997. Weight loss and wrestling training: Effects on growth-related hormones. *J. Appl. Physiol.* 82 (6): 1760-1764.

69 Roemmich, J.N., and Sinning, W.E. 1997. Weight loss and wrestling training: Effects on nutrition, growth, maturation, body composition, and strength. *J. Appl. Physiol.* 82 (6): 1751-1759.

70 Rankin, J.W., Ocel, J.V., and Craft, L.L. 1996. Effect of weight loss and refeeding diet composition on anaerobic performance in wrestlers. *Med. Sci. Sports Exerc.* 28 (10): 1292-1299.

71 Choma, C.W., Sforzo, G.A., and Keller, B.A. 1998. Impact of rapid weight loss on cognitive function in collegiate wrestlers. *Med. Sci. Sports Exerc.* 30 (5): 746-749.

72 Horswill, C.A. 1993. Weight loss and weight cycling in amateur wrestlers: Implications for performance and resting metabolic rate. *Int. J. Sport Nutr.* (3): 245-260.

73 Oppliger, R.A., Harms, R.D., Herrmann, D.E., Streich, C.M., and Clark, R.R. 1995. The Wisconsin wrestling minimum weight project: A model for weight control among high school wrestlers. *Med. Sci. Sports Exerc.* 27 (8): 1220-1224.

74 Burke DG, Silver S, Holt LE, Smith Palmer T, Culligan CJ, and Chilibeck PD. The effect of continuous low dose creatine supplementation on force, power, and total work. *International Journal of Sport Nutrition and Exercise Metabolism* 2000; 10(3): 235-244.

75 Ronsen O, Sundgot-Borgen J, and Maehlum S. Supplement use and nutritional habits in Norwegian elite athletes. *Scandinavian Journal of Medicine and Science in Sports* 1999; 9(1): 28-35.

76 Juzwiak CR and Ancona-Lopez F. Evaluation of nutrition knowledge and dietary recommendations by coaches of adolescent Brazilian athletes. *International Journal of Sport Nutrition and Exercise Metabolism* 2004; 14(2): 222-235.

77 Coyle EF. Fluid and fuel intake during exercise. *Journal of Sports Sciences* 2004; 22(1): 39-55.

Chapter 14

1 Sizer, F., and Whitney, E. 1997. *Nutrition: Concepts and controversies* (7th ed.). Albany, NY: West/Wadsworth: 383.

2 Pyruvate has been studied as an ergogenic aid to determine if supplemental doses improve performance. Since pyruvate infusion is a self-limiting pathway, it has not been found to be ergogenic. [Juhn MS. Ergogenic aids in aerobic activity. *Current Sports Medicine Reports* 2002; 1(4): 233-238.]

3 The tricarboxylic acid cycle is commonly referred to as the Krebs cycle, named for Hans Krebs, who first described the oxidative metabolic reactions. It is also referred to as the citric acid cycle because citric acid is required for one of the first reactions in the cycle. Therefore, the tricarboxylic acid cycle, Krebs cycle, and citric acid cycle are all referring to the same energy-yielding reactions.

4 Johnson NA, Stannard SR & Thompson MW. Muscle triglyceride and glycogen in endurance exercise: implications for performance. *Sports Medicine* 2004; 34(3): 151-64.

5 Uusitalo AL, Valkonen-Korhonen M, Helenius P, Vanninen E, Bergström KA, Kuikka JT. Abnormal serotonin reuptake in an overtrained, insomnic and depressed team athlete. *International Journal of Sports Medicine* 2004; 25(2): 150-53.

6 American College of Sports Medicine. 1999. Overtraining: Consensus statement. *Sports Medicine Bulletin* 31 (1): 29.

7 American College of Sports Medicine. 1999. Overtraining: Consensus statement. *Sports Medicine Bulletin* 31 (1): 29.

8 Asp, S., Rohde, T., and Richter, E.A. 1997. Impaired muscle glycogen resynthesis after a marathon is not caused by decreased muscle GLUT-4 content. *J. Appl. Physiol.* 83 (5): 1482-1485.

9 Naughton G, Farpour-Lambert NJ, Carlson J, Bradney M, and VanPraagh E. Physiological issues surrounding the performance of adolescent athletes. *Sports Medicine* 2000; 30(5): 309-325.

10 Farber, H.W., Schaefer, E.J., Franey, R., Grimaldi, R., and Hill, N.S. The endurance triathlon: Metabolic changes after

each event and during recovery. *Med. Sci. Sports Exerc.* 23 (8): 959-965.

11 Dressendorfer, R.H., and Wade, C.E. 1991. Effects of a 15-d race on plasma steroid levels and leg muscle fitness in runners. *Med. Sci. Sports Exerc.* 23 (8): 954-958.

12 Sherman, W.M., and Maglischo, E.W. 1991. Minimizing chronic athletic fatigue among swimmers: Special emphasis on nutrition. *Sports Sci. Exch.* 4(35).

13 Niekamp, R.A., and Baer, J.T. 1995. In-season dietary adequacy of trained male cross-country runners. *Int. J. Sport Nutr.* 5: 45-55.

14 Butterworth, D.E., Nieman, D.C., Butler, J.V., and Herring, J.L. 1994. Food intake patterns of marathon runners. *Int. J. Sport Nutr.* 4 (1): 1-7.

15 Houtkooper, L. 1992. Food selection for endurance sports. *Med. Sci. Sports Exerc.* 24 (9): S349-S359.

16 Hickner, R.C., Fisher, J.S., Hansen, P.A., Racette, S.B., Mier, C.M., Turner, M.J., and Holloszy, J.O. 1997. Muscle glycogen accumulation after endurance exercise in trained and untrained individuals. *J. Appl. Physiol.* 83 (3): 897-903.

17 Helmich, P., Christensen, S.W., Darre, E., Jahnsen, F., and Hartvig, T. 1989. Non-elite marathon runners: Health, training, and injuries. *Br. J. Sports Med.* 23 (3): 177-178.

18 Fogelholm, M., Tikkanen, H., Naveri, H., and Harkonen, M. 1989. High-carbohydrate diet for long distance runners: A practical view-point. *Br. J. Sports Med.* 23 (2): 94-96.

19 Nieman, D.C., Gates, J.R., Butler, J.V., Pollett, L.M., Dietrich, S.J., and Lutz, R.D. 1989. Supplementation patterns in marathon runners. *J. Am. Diet. Assoc.* 89 (11): 1615-1619.

20 Rokitzki, L., Hinkel, S., Klemp, C., Cufi, D., and Keul, J. 1994. Dietary, serum, and urine ascorbic acid status in male athletes. *Int. J. Sports Med.* 15 (7): 435-440.

21 Rokitzki, L., Sagredos, A.N., Reuss, F., Buchner, M., and Keul, J. 1994. Acute changes in vitamin B_6 status in endurance athletes before and after a marathon. *Int. J. Sport Nutr.* 4 (2): 154-165.

22 Terblanche, S., Noakes, T.D., Dennis, S.C., Marais, D., and Eckert, M. 1992. Failure of magnesium supplementation to influence marathon running performance or recovery in magnesium-replete subjects. *Int. J. Sport Nutr.* 2 (2): 154-164.

23 Barnett, D.W., and Conlee, R.K. 1984. The effects of a commercial dietary supplement on human performance. *Am. J. Clin. Nutr.* 40 (3): 586-590.

24 Sloniger, M.A., Cureton, K.J., and O'Bannon, P.J. 1997. One-mile run-walk performance in young men and women: Role of anaerobic metabolism. *Can. J. Appl. Physiol.* 22 (4): 337-350.

25 Penn, I.W., Wang, Z.M., Buhl, K.M., Allison, D.B., Burastero, S.E., Heymsfield, S.B. 1994. Body composition and two-compartment model assumptions in male long-distance runners. *Med. Sci. Sports Exerc.* 26: 392-397.

26 Reeder, M.T., Dick, B.H., Atkins, J.K., Pribis, A.B., and Martinez, J.M. 1996. Stress fractures: Current concepts of diagnosis and treatment. *Sports Med.* 22 (3): 198-212.

27 Deuster, P.A., Kyle, S.B., Moser, P.B., Vigersky, R.A., Singh, A., and Schoomaker, E.B. 1986. Nutritional intakes and status of highly trained amenorrheic and eumenorrheic women runners. *Fertil. Steril.* 46 (4): 636-643.

28 Beidleman, B.A., Puhl, J.L., and DeSouza, M.J. 1995. Energy balance in female distance runners. *Am. J. Clin. Nutr.* 61: 303-311.

29 Rontoyannis, G.P., Skoulis, T., and Pavlou, K.N. 1989. Energy balance in ultramarathon running. *Am. J. Clin. Nutr.* 49: 976-979.

30 Eden, B.D., and Abernethy, P.J. 1994. Nutritional intake during an ultraendurance running race. *Int. J. Sport Nutr.* 4: 166-174.

31 Millard-Stafford, M.L., Sparling, P.B., Rosskopf, L.B., and DiCarlo, L.J. 1992. Carbohydrate-electrolyte replacement improves distance running performance in the heat. *Med. Sci. Sports Exerc.* 24 (8): 934-940.

32 Hedley AM, Climstein M, and Hansen R. The effects of acute heat exposure on muscular strength, muscular endurance, and

muscular power in the euhydrated athlete. *Journal of Strength and Conditioning Research* 2002; 16(3): 353-358.

33 Noakes, T.D., Adams, B.A., Myburgh, K.H., Greeff, C., Lotz, T., and Nathan, M. 1988. The danger of an inadequate water intake during prolonged exercise: A novel concept re-visited. *Eur. J. Appl. Physiol.* 57 (2): 210-219.

34 Dennis, S.C., and Noakes, T.D. 1999. Advantages of a smaller body mass in humans when distance-running in warm, humid conditions. *Eur. J. Appl. Physiol.* 79 (3): 280-284.

35 Schumacher YO, Schmid A, Grathwohl D, Bultermann D, and Berg A. Hematological indices and iron status in athletes of various sports and performances. *Medicine and Science in Sports and Exercise* 2002; 34(5): 869-875.

36 Erythropoietin is associated with multiple deaths because it may cause a dangerously high increase in blood viscosity.

37 Tokish JM, Kocher MS, and Hawkins RJ. Ergogenic aids: A review of basic science, performance, side effects, and status in sports. *American Journal of Sports Medicine* 2004; 32(6): 1543-1553.

38 Lamanca JJ, Haymes EM, Daly JA, Moffatt RJ, and Waller MF. Sweat iron loss of male and female runners during exercise. *International Journal of Sports Medicine* 1988; 9(1): 52-55.

39 Selby GB and Eichner ER. Endurance swimming, intravascular hemolysis, anemia, and iron depletion: New perspective on athlete's anemia. *American Journal of Medicine* 1986; 81(5): 791-794.

40 Ehn L, Carlmark B, and Hoglund S. Iron status in athletes involved in intense physical activity. *Medicine and Science in Sports and Exercise* 1980; 12(1): 61-64.

41 Noakes T. *Lore of running.* Champaign, IL: Human Kinetics. 1991: p. 695.

42 Bentley, D.J., Wilson, G.J., Davie, A.J., and Zhou, S. 1998. Correlations between peak power output, muscular strength, and cycle time trial performance in triathletes. *J. Sports Med. Phys. Fitness* 38 (3): 201-207.

43 Laurenson, N.M., Fulcher, K.Y., and Korkia, P. 1993. Physiological characteristics of elite and club level female triathletes during running. *Int. J. Sports Med.* 14 (8): 455-459.

44 Gulbin, J.P., and Gaffney, P.T. 1999. Ultraendurance triathlon participation: Typical race preparation of lower-level triathletes. *J. Sports Med. Phys. Fitness* 39 (1): 12-15.

45 Banister, E.W., Carter, J.B., and Zarkadas, P.C. 1999. Training theory and taper: Validation in triathlon athletes. *Eur. J. Appl. Physiol.* 79 (2)182-191.

46 Guezennec, C.Y., Chalabi, H., Bernard, J., Fardellone, P., Krentowski, R., Zerath, E., and Meunier, P.J. 1998. Is there a relationship between physical activity and dietary calcium intake? A survey in 10,373 young French subjects. *Med. Sci. Sports Exerc.* 30 (5): 732-739.

47 Kerr, C.G., Trappe, T.A., Starling, R.D., and Trappe, S.W. 1998. Hyperthermia during Olympic triathlon: Influence of body heat storage during the swimming stage. *Med. Sci. Sports Exerc.* 30 (1): 99-104.

48 Rogers, G., Goodman, C., and Rosen, C. 1997. Water budget during ultra-endurance exercise. *Med. Sci. Sports Exerc.* 29 (11): 1477-1481.

49 O'Toole, M.L., Douglas, P.S., Laird, R.H., and Hiller, D.B. 1995. Fluid and electrolyte status in athletes receiving medical care at an ultradistance triathlon. *Clin. J. Sport Med.* 5 (2): 116-122

50 Speedy, D.B., Faris, J.G., Hamlin, M., Gallagher, P.G., and Campbell, R.G. 1997. Hyponatremia and weight changes in an ultradistance triathlon. *Clin. J. Sport Med.* 7 (3): 180-184.

51 Speedy DB, Noakes TD, Kimber NE, Rogers IR, Thompson JM, Boswell DR, Ross JJ, Campbell RG, Gallagher PG, and Kuttner JA. Fluid Balance During and After an Ironman Triathlon. *Clinical Journal of Sport Medicine* 2001; 11(1): 44-50.

52 Rehrer, N.J., van Kemenade, M., Meester, W., Brouns, F., and Saris, W.H. 1992. Gastrointestinal complaints in relation to dietary intake in triathletes. *Int. J. Sport Nutr.* 2 (1): 48-59.

53 Clark, N., Tobin, J., Jr., and Ellis, C. 1992. Feeding the ultraendurance athlete: Practical tips and a case study. *J. Am. Diet. Assoc.* 92 (10): 1258-1262.

54 Frentsos, J.A., and Baer, J.T. 1997. Increased energy and nutrient intake during training and competition improves elite triathletes' endurance performance. *Int. J. Sport Nutr.* 7 (1): 61-71.

55 Ribeiro, J.P., Cadavid, E., Baena, J., Monsalvete, E., Barna, A., and DeRose, E.H. 1990. Metabolic predictors of middle-distance swimming performance. *Br. J. Sports Med.* 24 (3): 196-200.

56 Lee, E.J., Long, K.A., Risser, W.L., Poindexter, H.B., Gibbons, W.E., and Goldzieher, J. 1995. Variations in bone status of contralateral and regional sites in young athletic women. *Med. Sci. Sports Exerc.* 27 (10): 1354-1361.

57 Berning, J.R., Troup, J.P., VanHandel, P.J., Daniels, J., and Daniels, N. 1991. The nutritional habits of young adolescent swimmers. *Int. J. Sport Nutr.* 1 (3): 240-248.

58 Saris, W.H., Schrijver, J., van Erp Baart, M.A., and Brouns, F. 1989. Adequacy of vitamin supply under maximal sustained workloads: The Tour de France. *Int. J. Vitam. Nutr. Res. Suppl.* 30: 205-212.

59 Brouns, F., Saris, W.H., Stroecken, J., Beckers, E., Thijssen, R., Rehrer, J.N., and ten Hoor, F. 1989. Eating, drinking, and cycling: A controlled Tour de France simulation study, Part II. Effect of diet manipulation. *Int. J. Sports Med.* 10 (S1): S41-S48.

60 Weiler, J.M., Layton, T., and Hunt, M. 1998. Asthma in United States Olympic athletes who participated in the 1996 Summer Games. *J. Allergy Clin. Immunol.* 102 (5): 722-726.

61 Brown RC. Nutrition for optimal performance during exercise: Carbohydrate and fat. *Current Sports Medicine Reports* 2002; 1(4): 222-229.

62 Miller SL and Wolfe RR. Physical exercise as a modulator of adaptation to low and high carbohydrate and low and high fat intakes. *European Journal of Clinical Nutrition* 1999; 53(suppl. 1): S112-S119.

63 Graham TE. Caffeine and exercise: Metabolism, endurance and performance. *Sports Medicine* 2001; 31(11): 785-807.

64 Hunter AM, St. Clair Gibson A, Collins M, Lambert M, and Noakes TD. Caffeine ingestion does not alter performance during a 100-km cycling time-trial performance. *International Journal of Sport Nutrition and Exercise Metabolism* 2002; 12(4): 438-452.

Chapter 15

1 Bangsbo J. Team sports. In: *Nutrition in sport* (Ed. Maughan R). London: Blackwell Science. 2000: pp. 574-587.

2 Davis, M. 1995. Repeated sprint work is enhanced with consumption of a carbohydrate-electrolyte beverage. *Med. Sci. Sports Exerc.* 27: S223.

3 Nicholas, C.W., Williams, C., Phillips, G., and Nowitz, A. 1995. Influence of ingesting a carbohydrate-electrolyte solution on endurance capacity during intermittent, high intensity shuttle running. *J. Appl. Sports Sci. Res.* 13: 282-290.

4 Below, P.R., Mora-Rodrigues, R., Gonzalez-Alonso, J., and Coyle, E.F. 1995. Fluid and carbohydrate ingestion independently improve performance during one hour of intense exercise. *Med. Sci. Sports Exerc.* 27 (2): 200-210.

5 Murray, R., Paul, G.L., Seifert, J.G., and Eddy, D.E. 1991. Responses to varying rates of carbohydrate ingestion during exercise. *Med. Sci. Sports Exerc.* 23 (6): 713-718.

6 Gisolfi, C.V., Summers, R.W., Schedl, H.P., and Bleiler, T.L. 1992. Intestinal water absorption from select carbohydrate solutions in humans. *J. Appl. Physiol.* 73: 2142-2150.

7 Lambert, C.P. 1991. Effects of carbohydrate feeding on multiple-bout resistance exercise. *J. Appl. Sports Sci. Res.* 5: 129-197.

8 Ryan, A.J., Lambert, G.P., Shi, X., Chang, R.T., Summers, R.W., and Gisolfi, C.V. 1998. Effect of hypohydration on gastric emptying and intestinal absorption during exercise. *J. Appl. Physiol.* 84 (5): 1581-1588.

9 Horswill, C.A. 1998. Effective fluid replacement. *Int. J. Sport Nutr.* 8: 175-195.

10 American College of Sports Medicine. 1996. Position stand on exercise and fluid replacement. *Med. Sci. Sports Exerc.* 28: i-vii.

11 Corley, G., Demarest-Litchford, M., and Bazzarre, T.L. 1990. Nutrition knowledge and dietary practices of college coaches. *J. Am. Diet. Assoc.* 90 (5): 705-709.

12 Dubnov G and Constantini NW. Prevalence of iron depletion and anemia in top-level basketball players. *International Journal of Sport Nutrition and Exercise Metabolism* 2004; 14(1): 30-37.

13 Nowak, R.K., Knudsen, K.S., and Schulz, L.O. 1988. Body composition and nutrient intakes of college men and women basketball players. *J. Am. Diet. Assoc.* 88 (5): 575-578.

14 Schroder H, Navarro E, Mora J, Galiano D, and Tramullas A. Effects of alpha-tocopherol, beta-carotene and ascorbic acid on oxidative, hormonal and enzymatic exercise stress markers in habitual training activity of professional basketball players. *European Journal of Nutrition* 2001; 40(4): 178-184.

15 Schroder H, Navarro E, Tramullas A, Mora J, and Galiano D. Nutrition antioxidant status and oxidative stress in professional basketball players: Effects of a three compound antioxidative supplement. *International Journal of Sports Medicine* 2000; 21(2): 146-150.

16 Maughan R. Contamination of supplements: An interview with professor Ron Maughan by Louise M. Burke. *International Journal of Sport Nutrition and Exercise Metabolism* 2004; 14(4): 493.

17 Mannix, E.T., Healy, A., and Farber, M.O. 1996. Aerobic power and supramaximal endurance of competitive figure skaters. *J. Sports Med. Phys. Fitness* 36 (3): 161-168.

18 Delistray, D.A., Reisman, E.J., and Snipes, M. 1992. A physiological and nutritional profile of young female figure skaters. *J. Sports Med. Phys. Fitness* 32 (2): 149-155.

19 Ziegler PJ, Nelson JA, and Jonnalagadda SS. Use of dietary supplements by elite figure skaters. *International Journal of Sport Nutrition and Exercise Metabolism* 2003; 13(3): 266-276.

20 Ziegler, P., Hensley, S., Roepke, J.B., Whitaker, S.H., Craig, B.W., and Drewnowski, A. 1998. Eating attitudes and energy intakes of female skaters. *Med. Sci. Sports Exerc.* 30 (4): 583-586.

21 Ziegler PJ, Jonnalagadda SS, Nelson JA, Lawrence C, and Baciak B. Contribution of meals and snacks to nutrient intake of male and female elite figure skaters during peak competitive season. *Journal of American Collegiate Nutrition* 2002; 21(2): 114-119.

22 Smith, A.D., and Ludington, R. 1989. Injuries in elite pair skaters and ice dancers. *Am. J. Sports Med.* 17 (4): 482-488.

23 Kjaer, M., and Larsson, B. 1992. Physiological profile and incidence of injuries among elite figure skaters. *J. Sports Sci.* 10 (1): 29-36.

24 Ziegler PJ, Nelson JA, and Jonnalagadda SS. Nutritional and physiological status of U.S. national figure skaters. *International Journal of Sport Nutrition* 1999; 9(4): 345-360.

25 Tumilty, D. 1993. Physiological characteristics of elite soccer players. *Sports Med.* 16 (2): 80-96.

26 Wittich, A., Mautalen, C.A., Oliveri, M.B., Bagur, A., Somoza, F., and Rotemberg, E. 1998. Professional football (soccer) players have a markedly greater skeletal mineral content, density, and size than age- and BMI-matched controls. *Calcif. Tissue Int.* 63 (2): 112-117.

27 Duppe, H., Gardsell, P., Johnell, O., and Ornstein, E. 1996. Bone mineral density in female junior, senior, and former football players. *Osteoporos. Int.* 6 (6): 437-441.

28 Tumilty, D. 1993. Physiological characteristics of elite soccer players. *Sports Med.* 16 (2): 80-96.

29 Rico-Sanz, J. 1998. Body composition and nutritional assessments in soccer. *Int. J. Sport Nutr.* 8 (2): 113-123.

30 Maughan, R.J. 1997. Energy and macronutrient intakes of professional football (soccer) players. *Br. J. Sports Med.* 31 (1): 45-47.

31 Clark, K. 1994. Nutritional guidance to soccer players for training and competition. *J. Sports Sci.* 12: S43-S50.

32 Kirkendall, D.T. 1993. Effects of nutrition on performance in soccer. *Med. Sci. Sports Exerc.* 25 (12): 1370-1374.

33 Clark M, Reed DB, Crouse SF, and Armstrong RB. Pre- and post-season dietary intake, body composition, and performance indices of NCAA division I female soccer players. *International Journal of Sport Nutrition and Exercise Metabolism* 2003; 13(3): 303-319.

34 Hargreaves, M. 1994. Carbohydrate and lipid requirements of soccer. *J. Sports Sci.* 12: S13-S16.

35 Davis JM, Welsh RS, and Alerson NA. Effects of carbohydrate and chromium ingestion during intermittent high-intensity exercise to fatigue. *International Journal of Sport Nutrition and Exercise Metabolism* 2000; 10(4): 476-485.

36 Ostojic SM. Creatine supplementation in young soccer players. *International Journal of Sport Nutrition and Exercise Metabolism* 2004; 14(1): 95-103.

37 Maughan RJ, Merson SJ, Broad NP, and Shirreffs SM. Fluid and electrolyte intake and loss in elite soccer players during training. *International Journal of Sport Nutrition and Exercise Metabolism* 2004; 14(3): 333-346.

38 Groppel, J.L., and Roetert, E.P. 1992. Applied physiology of tennis. *Sports Med.* 14 (4): 260-268.

39 Bergeron, M.F., Maresh, C.M., Kraemer, W.J., Abraham, A., Conroy, B., and Gabaree, C. 1991. Tennis: A physiological profile during match play. *Int. J. Sports Med.* 12 (5): 474-479.

40 Vergauwen, L., Brouns, F., and Hespel, P. 1998. Carbohydrate supplementation improves stroke performance in tennis. *Med. Sci. Sports Exerc.* 30 (8): 1289-1295.

41 Bergeron, M.F., Maresh, C.M., Armstrong, L.E., Signorile, J.F., Castellani, J.W., Kenefick, R.W., LaGasse, K.E., and Riebe, D.A. 1995. Fluid-electrolyte balance associated with tennis match play in a hot environment. *Int. J. Sport Nutr.* 5 (3): 180-193.

42 Baxter-Jones, A.D., Helms, P., Baines-Preece, J., and Preece, M. 1994. Menarche in intensively trained gymnasts, swimmers, and tennis players. *Ann. Hum. Biol.* 21 (5): 407-415.

43 Harris MB. Weight concern, body image, and abnormal eating in college women tennis players and their coaches. *International Journal of Sport Nutrition and Exercise Metabolism* 2000; 10(1): 1-15.

Index

Note: Page numbers followed by an italicized *f* or *t* represent the figure or table on that page, respectively.

About the Author

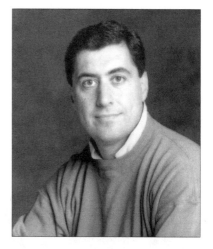

Dan Benardot, PhD, DHC, RD, LD, FACSM, is an associate professor in the nutrition division of the School of Health Professions at Georgia State University and an associate professor in the department of kinesiology and health, also at Georgia State University. He serves as codirector of the Laboratory for Elite Athlete Performance, where athletes receive training and nutrition plans that assist them in their pursuit of athletic excellence.

As the national team nutritionist and a founding member of the Athlete Wellness Program for USA Gymnastics, Benardot worked with the gold-medal-winning women's gymnastics team at the 1996 Olympic Games in Atlanta and also worked with the medal-winning USA marathoners at the 2004 Olympic Games in Athens. He has served as an officer of the US Figure Skating Sports Medicine Society and has had his research funded by several organizations, including the United States Olympic Committee. In addition to working with top athletes from a variety of professional individual and team sports, Benardot serves as the head scientific advisor for Calorie & Pulse Technologies, LLC, which has developed a Web site (www.SportsNutrition Clinic.com) that assists athletes in achieving top performance.

Benardot received his PhD in human nutrition and health planning from Cornell University and a doctor of humane letters, honoris causa, from Marywood University. He is a registered and licensed (Georgia) dietitian of the American Dietetic Association (ADA) and is a fellow of the American College of Sports Medicine (ACSM). In addition to authoring numerous journal publications, he served as editor in chief of ADA's *Sports Nutrition: A Guide for Professionals Working With Active People* (2nd edition), is the author of *Nutrition for Serious Athletes*, and is a coauthor of the *ACSM Fitness Book* (3rd edition). Born in Salonika, Greece, Benardot gained his love for sport while growing up in the Lake Placid region of northern New York. He now lives in Atlanta, Georgia, where he enjoys tennis and photography.

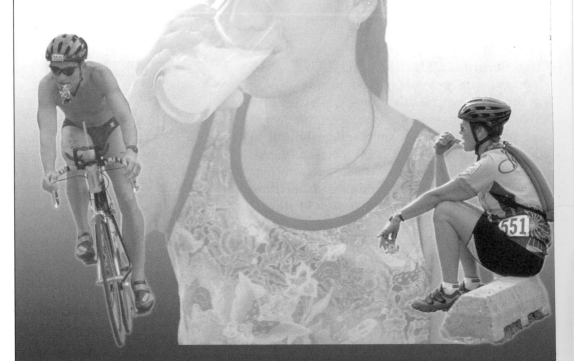

You'll find other outstanding sports nutrition resources at

http://sportsnutrition.humankinetics.com

In the U.S. call 1-800-747-4457

Australia 08 8372 0999 • Canada 1-800-465-7301
Europe +44 (0) 113 255 5665 • New Zealand 0064 9 448 1207

HUMAN KINETICS
The Premier Publisher for Sports & Fitness
P.O. Box 5076 • Champaign, IL 61825-5076 USA